Atlas of Clinical Positron Emission Tomography

Second edition

Sally F Barrington MSc MD FRCP
Consultant Physician in Nuclear Medicine at the PET Imaging Centre at
St Thomas', Guy's, King's and St Thomas' School of Medicine, London, UK

Michael N Maisey BSc MD FRCP FRCR
Emeritus Professor of Radiological Sciences, Guy's, King's and St Thomas' School of Medicine, London, UK

Richard L Wahl MD FANCP
Professor of Radiology and Oncology, Director, Division of Nuclear
Medicine/PET, Henry N. Wagner Professor of Nuclear Medicine, Johns Hopkins
Medical Institutions, Baltimore, Maryland, USA

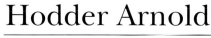

Hodder Arnold

A MEMBER OF THE HODDER HEADLINE GROUP

First published in Great Britain in 2006 by
Hodder Arnold, an imprint of Hodder Education and a member of the
Hodder Headline Group
338 Euston Road, London NW1 3BH

http://www.hoddereducation.com

Distributed in the United States of America by
Oxford University Press Inc.,
198 Madison Avenue, New York, NY10016
Oxford is a registered trademark of Oxford University Press

Whilst the advice and information in this book are believed to be true and
accurate at the date of going to press, neither the author[s] nor the publisher
can accept any legal responsibility or liability for any errors or omissions
that may be made. In particular, (but without limiting the generality of the
preceding disclaimer) every effort has been made to check drug dosages;
however it is still possible that errors have been missed. Furthermore,
dosage schedules are constantly being revised and new side-effects
recognized. For these reasons the reader is strongly urged to consult the
drug companies' printed instructions before administering any of the drugs
recommended in this book.

Disclaimer: The discussion in the text and on the DVD is not a comprehensive
interpretation of all aspects of the PET/CT images but emphasizes the key
teaching points for educational purposes only.

British Library Cataloguing in Publication Data
A catalogue record for this book is available from the British Library

Library of Congress Cataloging-in-Publication Data
A catalog record for this book is available from the Library of Congress

ISBN-10:   0-340-81693 7
ISBN-13:   978-0-340-816936

1 2 3 4 5 6 7 8 9 10

Commissioning Editor: Joanna Koster
Development Editor: Sarah Burrows
Project Manager: Gavin Smith
Production Controller: Joanna Walker
Cover Design: Georgina Hewitt

Typeset in 11 on 13 pt Minion by Phoenix Photosetting
Printed and bound in Italy by Printer Trento

What do you think about this book? Or any other Hodder Arnold
title? Please visit our website at www.hoddereducation.com

For Lewis, Irene, and Sandy

CONTENTS

CONTRIBUTORS

Nicholas R Maisey MBBS MRCP MD
Consultant Physician in Medical Oncology at Guy's and St Thomas' NHS
Foundation Trust, London, UK

Paul K Marsden PhD
Senior Lecturer, The PET Imaging Centre at St Thomas' Hospital, Guy's, King's and
St Thomas' School of Medicine, London, UK

Eva A Wegner BMed, FRACP
Consultant Physician, Department of Nuclear Medicine, The Prince of Wales and
Sydney Children's Hospitals, Randwick, New South Wales, Australia;
Formerly The PET Imaging Centre at St Thomas', Guy's, King's and St Thomas'
School of Medicine, London, UK

Making the diagnosis

In the diagnostic process, the nuclear physician or radiologist converts the evidence in the images before him or her into the name of a particular disease. This is a matter of judgment, which, in turn, depends on the care, dedication, education, and experience of the interpreting physician. The process is not an arcane 'natural art' or 'process based on pure intuition' that would make it no more than hand waving. 'Making the diagnosis' is a rational process involving both inductive and deductive reasoning that (when successful) culminates in the interpreting physician's commitment to a particular diagnosis or diagnoses, presented to the referring physician together with a probability statement of his or her degree of certainty.

The diagnostic process is a matter of expert judgment, honed by a wealth of observation and experience. It is the product of the process of reasoning, informed by a history of relevant experience. This is not to deny that, at times, upon confronting all the available data, including 'molecular images', a good radiologist or nuclear medicine physician, rather like a good car mechanic, may make a correct diagnostic judgment almost instantly; but then the initial 'impression' must be subject to analysis of all the available data. The authors have great personal experience, and illustrate how expert diagnostic thinking is applied in the interpretation of the images, with emphasis on PET and PET/CT. They present what could become the basis for designing successful expert PET and PET/CT systems of the future. Students and practitioners of nuclear imaging would do well to start their journey by studying this book.

Henry N. Wagner Jr. MD
Professor Emeritus of Medicine and Radiology and Radiological Science;
Professor of Environmental Health Sciences; and
Director, Division of Radiation Health Sciences
Johns Hopkins Bloomberg School of Public Health, Baltimore, MD, USA

PREFACE

The first edition of this book was written in the early days of clinical PET. Its purpose was to share experience from the first 5 years of our institutions and hopefully to shorten the learning curve of others entering the field. Since the first edition, the number of PET centers in the world has increased markedly and PET has become an integral part of the diagnostic work-up and management of patients in oncology while continuing to be applied in neurology and cardiology. PET is no longer regarded as a 'niche' imaging tool but has become part of mainstream diagnostics alongside CT, MR, and ultrasound. Improvements in camera technology have contributed to better PET image quality and the emergence of PET/CT has been the most significant recent advance. PET/CT has provided us with new challenges and this second edition is timely as it attempts once more to share our combined experience in this rapidly changing field. The development of PET/CT requires new skills to be learnt and the sharing of established skills with greater cooperation and integration between nuclear medicine and radiology.

The same format has been used as the first edition. Each chapter gives clinical background information, including the relevant epidemiology, pathology, and staging (for the oncology chapters) and lists the key management issues followed by clinical cases. Each case represents a real patient seen in one of our departments with PET, CT, and fused images shown and the key points highlighted. We think it is a major advance that a DVD is included with this edition enabling the reader to view selected cases chosen to illustrate key management issues as though he/she were reporting 'in the clinic'. Each chapter concludes with a summary of the clinical indications for PET/CT imaging and a set of references for further reading about the topic.

This second edition has been expanded because the use of PET for imaging certain cancers, which were featured in the first edition as 'emerging applications' have now become established applications. We have also extended the book to cover pediatric PET applications, and infection and inflammation imaging to reflect the increasing breadth of PET and PET/CT imaging. The main emphasis, however, remains on oncology, mostly with FDG, which continues to represent 90% of the workload in our two centers.

PET and PET/CT continues to be a fascinating and fast-moving imaging specialty. We hope we have conveyed our enthusiasm for PET and PET/CT in these pages and that you the reader will come to share in that enthusiasm. We further hope that our state-of-the-art images and clinical case material illustrating key teaching points will prove useful in educating both the novice and experienced practitioners regarding PET and PET/CT.

SFB, MNM, RLW
London and Baltimore, 2005

ACKNOWLEDGMENTS

PET/CT is a multidisciplinary modality. It requires a dedicated team of scientists, doctors, radiographers, and administration staff to offer a high-quality clinical service. It is crucial to have a good relationship with referring clinicians to make the best use of the knowledge provided by PET and to incorporate that knowledge into improved patient management. We wish to acknowledge the support, hard work, and dedication of our colleagues, which is so important in maintaining the service we offer to our patients. This book would not have been possible without them.

St Thomas' PET Imaging Centre

Clinical Manager: M Dakin
Cyclotron: P Halsted, M Kelly, A Page
Radiochemistry: G D'Costa, K Kahlon, N Ossoulyan
Physicists and Computer Scientists: Dr PK Marsden, E Somer, J MacKewn, P Schleyer, P Liepins
Clinicians: Dr MJ O'Doherty, Professor I Fogelman, Dr TO Nunan, Dr SF Barrington, Dr SC Rankin, Dr S Vijayanathan
Radiographers/Nuclear Medicine Technologists : N Benatar (superintendent) R Dobbin, S Bray, M Cunneen, K Hau
Imaging Assistant: Dr K Curran
Secretary: M Maureso

Johns Hopkins PET Centre

Clinical Manager: J Nieve
Cyclotron: Professor R Dannals
Radiochemistry: H Ravert, W Mathews, R Smoot, A Horti
Physicists and Computer Scientists: Mr JP Leal and Professor J Links
Clinicians: Dr K Friedman, Professor Z Szabo, Professor RL Wahl, Professor H Ziessman, Dr H Jacene, Dr C Cohade, Dr R Rosen, Dr P Patel, Dr J Frost
Radiographers/Nuclear Medicine Technologists: L King, L Kerin, D Franz
Secretary/Service Coordinators: M Willett, A Herbert, N Cooper

Specifically we would like to acknowledge the contributions of Paul Marsden who has again provided an excellent introductory chapter covering the basic science and outlining the elements involved in PET. We would like to thank Eva Wegner for sharing with us with the expertise in pediatric PET that she developed during the 3 years she spent at St Thomas'. We are especially grateful to Nick Maisey for his oncological expertise and for advising us on the epidemiology, pathology, and staging in the chapters that focus on cancer. We would also like to thank Jeff Grenier and Susan Ellan from Nuclear Diagnostics for working with us to develop the interactive DVD that comes with this edition.

It was because of the pivotal role of our colleagues in our working lives that the first edition of this book was dedicated to those who helped us to establish and run our joint Centres. We continue to be extremely grateful to them. We also wish to acknowledge the unwavering support and love of our families, which is the foundation for our working and home lives. It is for this reason that the second edition of this book is dedicated to our spouses, Lewis, Irene, and Sandy.

LIST OF ABBREVIATIONS

CEA	carcinoembryonic antigen
CLL	chronic lymphatic leukemia
CNS	central nervous system
CT	computed tomography
CTAC	CT attenuation correction
DTC	differentiated thyroid cancer
EBV	Epstein–Barr virus
ED	effective dose
EEG	electroencephalography
EUS	endoscopic ultrasound
FDG	$[^{18}F]$2-fluoro-2-deoxy-D-glucose
FUO	fever of unknown origin
HD	Hodgkin disease
HIV	human immunodeficiency virus
HPV	human papilloma virus
IVC	inferior vena cava
MALT	mucosa-associated lymphoid tissue
MEN	multiple endocrine neoplasia
MRI	magnetic resonance imaging
NEC	noise equivalent count
NHL	non-Hodgkin disease
NSCLC	nonsmall-cell lung cancer
NSGCT	nonseminomatous germ cell tumors
OSEM	ordered subsets expectation maximization
PET	positron emission tomography
PGL	persistent generalized lymphadenopathy
RCA	right coronary artery
rh TSH	recombinant human thyrotropin
SCLC	small-cell lung cancer
SPECT	single photon emission computed tomography
SPN	solitary pulmonary nodule
SUV	standardized uptake value
TLE	temporal lobe epilepsy
TSH	thyroid stimulating hormone

About the *Atlas of Clinical Positron Emission Tomography* DVD
Powered by HERMES RAPID™

The Atlas DVD with HERMES RAPID™ (Run Anywhere Patient Image Display) software is designed to be a dynamic, interactive, educational complement to the *Atlas of Clinical Positron Emission Tomography*. The Atlas DVD contains 30 specially selected PET/CT patient cases with clinical histories, PET/CT findings and key points included. These 30 featured cases correspond by chapter and case number to cases in the Atlas itself. The complete patient PET/CT datasets are also included for every case with HERMES RAPID™ software. The DVD also includes video interviews with the authors, allowing you to quickly learn more about their experience and expertise in the field of Nuclear Medicine/PET.

The Atlas DVD with HERMES RAPID™ is intended for use on personal computers with DVD Rom capability and Windows NT, 2000 or XP operating system. Once the DVD is loaded into your computer the interactive session will launch automatically, and begins with a guided video and voice tour of HERMES RAPID™ software, which will show you how to utilize the software in the most optimal way to view the selected cases. The Atlas DVD with HERMES RAPID™ is very straightforward and easy to use. In addition to the software tour, there is also a complete HERMES RAPID™ handbook on the main menu for your reference.

Once you are in the main menu of the Atlas DVD, you can easily select the case of interest, and by clicking you will see the clinical history, PET/CT findings and key points for that particular case. From here, you are also able to launch the case in the viewing software by clicking on 'LAUNCH CASE' which will start the diagnostic program called HERMES RAPID™.

About HERMES RAPID™ Software

HERMES RAPID™ software, provided by the company Hermes Medical Solutions, is an application for the display and analysis of PET, SPECT, CT, MRI & ultrasound studies and Maximum Intensity Projection (MIP) movie data. It is packaged as a standalone PC application.

RAPID provides a MIP movie and splash display, and can also show three orthogonal views simultaneously, with cross-modality image fusion capability, image reorientation, volume of interest (VOI) generation and standard uptake value (SUV) calculation.

Key RAPID features:

- RAPID has a powerful yet simple user interface, with all common functions easily accessible for daily clinical use.
- Manual manipulation, thresholding, triangulation, and full standard uptake value (SUV) capabilities for PET studies, including 3D automatic region growing.
- Fusion of two studies with variable overlay, triangulation of two studies in synchrony and MIP movie generation.
- No network is required and HERMES RAPID™ auto-runs when inserted into a Windows PC.

Hermes Medical Solutions, www.hermesmedical.com, is proud to support the second edition of the *Atlas of Clinical Positron Emission Tomography* with HERMES RAPID™ software and this Atlas DVD.

PART I
Introduction

CHAPTER 1

PRINCIPLES AND METHODS

PAUL K MARSDEN

INTRODUCTION

The introduction of combined PET/CT scanners which have the ability to acquire accurately registered functional and anatomic images in under 30 minutes has been one of the major contributing factors to positron emission tomography (PET) at last being adopted as a routine clinical imaging modality.

Unlike computed tomography (CT) and magnetic resonance imaging (MRI), PET has taken several decades since its initial development to become widely adopted. One of the reasons for this has certainly been the large amount of infrastructure that it requires, in particular the cyclotron and radiochemistry facilities necessary to provide a reliable supply of tracer. Another reason has been the long scan times (~1 hour) required for whole-body (^{18}F)2-fluoro-2-deoxy-D-glucose (FDG) PET studies. FDG is now readily available, and with PET/CT the scan time approaches half that of PET-only systems.

In the current generation of PET/CT scanners, a CT and PET are mounted in-line in a single gantry, and the two scans are carried out in quick succession while the patient remains in the same position on the couch. This results in the second major advantage of PET/CT, the acquisition of accurately registered functional and anatomic images in a single scanning session. Great advances have been made in the development of algorithms that can accurately register images acquired on different scanners and at different times. However PET/CT has, at a stroke, provided simple and accurate image registration with no complex logistics.

Despite the great excitement about PET/CT, there have to date been few serious trials to evaluate the additional clinical value over independently acquired PET and CT scans, and most of the evidence remains anecdotal. Certainly the ability to locate disease accurately increases the confidence of reporting clinicians, and there will be obvious advantages when more specific tracers, without the anatomic detail demonstrated by FDG, begin to be used clinically. As detailed trials of the efficacy of PET/CT start to emerge, it will be surprising if they do not demonstrate significant advantages of this exciting new technology.

PET AND PET/CT SCANNING TECHNOLOGY

The PET component

POSITRON ANNIHILATION AND COINCIDENCE DETECTION

The radionuclides used in PET decay by the emission of a positron which behaves in a similar way to an electron but has a positive charge. At the end of its range, which is about 0.6 mm in tissue for the most common PET radionuclide ^{18}F, the positron undergoes mutual annihilation with an electron, resulting in the production of two 511 keV gamma (γ) rays which are emitted at 180 degrees to each other as shown in Figure 1.1. A PET scanner consists of thin rings of scintillation detectors around the patient. If both γ rays are detected by the scanner within a certain time of one another (i.e. within a 'coincidence time window'), then it is assumed that both originated from the same annihilation, and that the original disintegration occurred along a line joining the two detection positions.

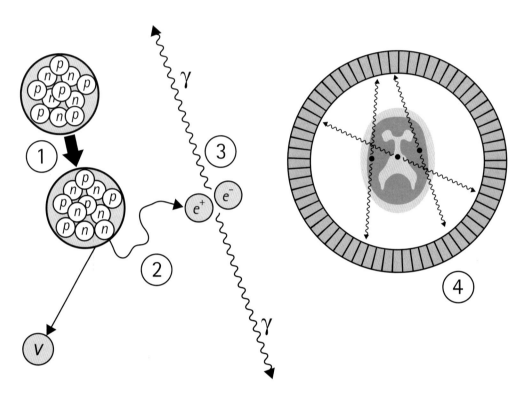

Figure 1.1   *Annihilation coincidence detection. A positron and a neutrino are emitted by a proton-rich nucleus (1). The positron follows a convoluted path (2) of a millimeter or so. At the end of its path the positron interacts with an electron to produce two antiparallel 511 keV photons (3), which are detected in coincidence (4) by the PET scanner*

Data acquired in this manner can be reconstructed into an image of the original radionuclide distribution. The combination of high sensitivity (tracers are usually present in picomolar concentrations or less) that results from the absence of collimators, and the ability to perform an accurate correction for attenuation of the photons as they pass through tissue, results in images of higher quality and quantitative accuracy than those that can be obtained using single photon emitters. The finite range of positrons in tissue and the non-colinearity of the annihilation γ rays (~0.25 degrees) impose a limit on the spatial resolution obtainable with PET, but this limit has not been reached by PET scanners in operation today. The spatial resolution is usually approximately equal to the width of the scanner detector elements (currently typically ~5 mm), however in practice the need to smooth images to reduce noise usually degrades the resolution beyond this.

ATTENUATION CORRECTION

The half-value layer for 511 keV γ rays in tissue is 7 cm. γ Rays originating in the center of the body are therefore attenuated to a much greater extent than are those originating at the edge. Central regions will appear relatively less bright and there appears to be activity in the skin unless an attenuation correction is performed as shown in Figure 1.2. Correction factors are obtained by taking an additional 'transmission' scan with the patient in position on the couch. In a PET-only system the transmission scan is performed using positron-emitting sources housed in the gantry and takes 15–20 minutes. In a PET/CT the CT scan itself is used to correct for attenuation, reducing this time to less than a minute.

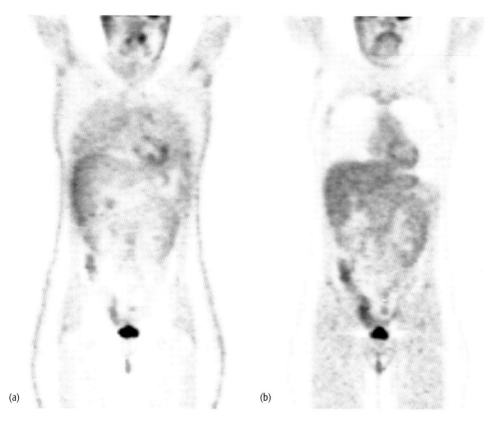

(a)   (b)

Figure 1.2   *Whole-body PET image (a) without attenuation correction and (b) with attenuation correction*

SCATTER, RANDOM COINCIDENCES, AND NOISE EQUIVALENT COUNT RATE

Ideally all the coincidence pairs detected by the PET scanner would be 'true' coincidences that contribute to forming the image. Unfortunately a large fraction (often more than 50 percent) of the data collected consists of scatter and random coincidences that significantly degrade the image quality. Scatter coincidences arise when one or both of the two annihilation γ rays are scattered in the body before they are detected, and random coincidences arise when unconnected single γ rays from different disintegrations are detected within the coincidence time window (Fig. 1.3). Both scatter and random coincidences add background noise to the image which results in poorer detection of small and low-contrast objects. The signal-to-noise ratio of the scanner is one of the key performance parameters and is often characterized by the 'noise equivalent count rate' or NEC (Strother *et al.*, 1990). The NEC accounts for the relative amounts of true, scatter, and random coincidences that the scanner detects in a given imaging situation and provides a crude indicator of image quality – it is usually expressed on a graph as a function of activity concentration in the field of view, as shown in Figure 1.4.

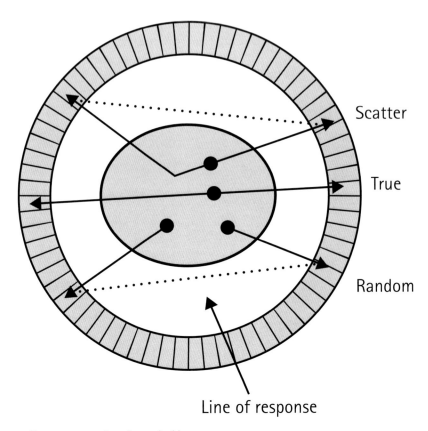

Figure 1.3   *True, scatter, and random coincidences*

TWO-DIMENSIONAL (2D) AND THREE-DIMENSIONAL (3D) ACQUISITION MODE

A multislice PET scanner consists of a stack of ~25 independent detector rings. Each ring is ~5 mm thick and the images acquired from the individual rings are arranged into a contiguous three-dimensional (3D) dataset for display – this is referred to as two-dimensional (2D) acquisition mode. The sensitivity (i.e. the fraction of radioactive decays in the field of view that are detected) of PET scanners can be increased by a large factor by removing the interslice septa from the field of view and acquiring coincidence pairs between detectors in different planes of the scanner, as shown in Figure 1.5. This is referred to as 3D acquisition mode. While 3D mode increases the sensitivity to true coincidences it also increases the sensitivity to scatter and randoms, particularly those arising from activity outside the field. This means that the NEC does not always increase as dramatically as might be expected. 3D mode is gradually becoming standard as new scintillation materials that minimize scatter and randoms are introduced, and it is the only option on many systems. However 2D mode is still widely used, particularly for large patients. 3D acquisition benefits greatly from positioning the patient's arms above their head and not at their side. This is facilitated by the faster overall scan times possible with PET/CT.

DETECTOR DESIGN

The most common detector design is the 'block detector' consisting of block of scintillator (typically 5 cm × 5 cm × 3 cm) which is divided up into an 8 × 8 or 12 × 12 matrix of detector elements. Four photomultiplier tubes attached to the back of the block detect the scintillation light emitted from the scintillator and identify the

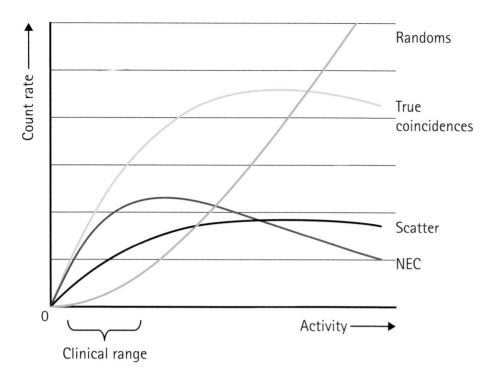

Figure 1.4 *PET scanner count rates as a function of activity administered to the patient. Noise equivalent count (NEC) rate can give an indication of overall performance. Adapted with kind permission of Elsevier from Marsden PK (2003) Detector technology challenges for nuclear medicine and PET Nucl Inst Meth Phys Res A* **513**, *1–7 (Fig. 4).*

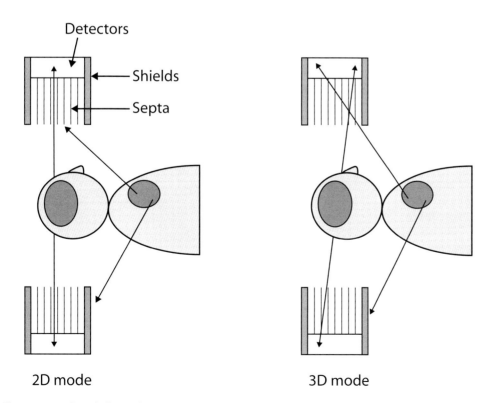

Figure 1.5 *2D and 3D acquisition. In 3D mode, the larger solid angle results in not only a higher sensitivity to true coincidences but also a higher sensitivity to scattered and random coincidences, particularly to those originating from outside the field of view*

element in which an interaction occurred (Fig. 1.6). The block detector is a cost-effective solution for the construction of high-resolution scanners with large numbers of contiguous rings. Detectors for PET must stop high-energy 511 keV γ rays with high efficiency and at high rates. Sodium iodide (NaI) is not effective at this energy and the scintillator materials used in current scanners are bismuth germanate (BGO), lutetium oxyorthosilicate (LSO), and gadolinium oxyorthosilicate (GSO). The properties of these scintillators are shown in Table 1.1. The overall imaging performance of a PET scanner is the result of careful trade-offs between the overall geometry of the scanner, the scintillator material and detector design, shielding, electronics, and many other factors. The choice of scintillator is probably the most important of these, however, and in general scanners using BGO have a slightly higher sensitivity whereas LSO has better timing properties and energy resolution.

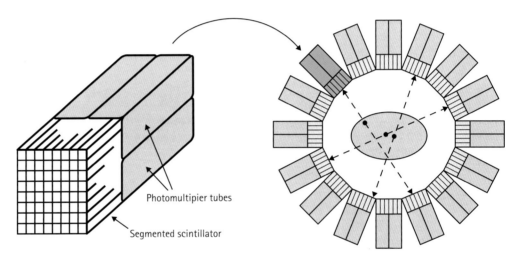

Photomultipier tubes

Segmented scintillator

Figure 1.6 *Block detector. A 511 keV γ ray interacts in one of the segments of the crystal block. The interaction position is determined by comparing the amount of scintillation light that reaches each of the four photomultiplier tubes. The total amount of light collected reflects the energy deposited in the crystal*

Table 1.1 Physical properties of scintillators used in PET cameras				
	NaI (Tl)	**BGO**	**LSO**	**GSO**
Density (g/cc)	3.67	7.13	7.4	6.7
Effective atomic number	51	75	66	59
Attenuation length* (mm)	25.6	11.2	11.4	15
Relative light yield	100	15	75	22
Decay time (ns)	230	300	~40	43

*Distance in which a 511keV photon beam is attenuated by a factor of 2.72.

The CT component

The CT components of current PET/CT models are all state-of-the-art multislice helical scanners (Flohr *et al.*, 2005) that are also available as stand-alone systems and have the same imaging and radiation dose characteristics. Most have full diagnostic capabilities (and indeed can operate independently of the PET) and options to increase the number of slices, currently to around 64. For PET/CT cardiac applications, the ability to perform rapid dynamic scanning with many slices is likely to become important, however for general oncology use no major advantages of using more than ~8 slices have yet been demonstrated. Increasing the number of slices permits faster scanning and reduces artefacts in the CT image. However, this does not in itself address the issues of mismatch between the CT and PET images in the presence of motion (see below).

The ability to incorporate respiratory gated CT data into the PET/CT procedure is currently work-in-progress, however this is likely to become important as respiratory gating techniques begin to be used in radiotherapy (Nehmeh *et al.*, 2002). It is important that there is a lot of flexibility in the CT operation, for instance the ability to reduce the beam current to very low values (~10 mA or below) to reduce radiation dose for some studies (e.g. pediatrics), and that dose reduction/optimization methods are implemented. In most respects though the features required for the CT are the same as those for stand-alone CT. The CT protocols used in PET/CT are usually much simpler than used in diagnostic CT, because the standard breath-hold is not used, to aid registration with PET, and to minimize radiation dose, given that the patient will often already have had a diagnostic CT. A typical protocol currently would be to acquire 3–5 mm slices with a beam current of 80 mA and 0.8 s rotation time (64 mAs – resulting in doses several times lower than for diagnostic CT), to obtain images adequate for 'localization'. As it becomes established how PET/CT is integrated into the patient management for different diseases, a range of different CT protocols will evolve.

PET/CT scanners

COMMERCIAL PET/CT SYSTEMS

The configuration of most PET/CT scanners available commercially is to have the PET and CT components mounted in-line in a single gantry as in Figure 1.7. The first models were assembled from existing CT and PET components which operated essentially independently (Beyer *et al.*, 2000), however more recent systems (Bettinardi *et al.*, 2004; Erdi *et al.*, 2004) have a much greater degree of hardware and software integration, leading to greater ease of use and a more compact gantry. The CT components are fully specified multislice helical systems with the same capabilities (in particular number of slices) as the equivalent stand-alone models. The development of stand-alone PET systems has ceased for the time being and all new PET systems are being designed as an integral part of a PET/CT, nevertheless there are some differences between these and the previous generation of PET scanners. In particular most PET/CTs no longer include transmission rod sources for attenuation correction as an alternative to CT attenuation correction, and most have a patient aperture of at least 70 cm, which facilitates radiotherapy planning applications but offers less shielding to out of field of view activity. In general, whereas the motivation for stand-alone PET was quantitative accuracy, the emphasis with PET/CT has been firmly placed on high throughput FDG whole-body studies and this is reflected in the available features, for example most PET/CTs can perform the PET scan in about 20 minutes *c.f.* 30–40 minutes previously, and a complete PET/CT in under 25 minutes. The 15 cm PET field of view is typically about 75 cm apart from the CT, with the CT at the front so that the patient's head remains outside the scanner bore for the majority of the scan. Another key component is a purpose-designed patient couch which must be extremely rigid and not sag between the PET and CT acquisitions, in order to maintain exact registration. The main features of some commercial PET/CT systems are given in Table 1.2.

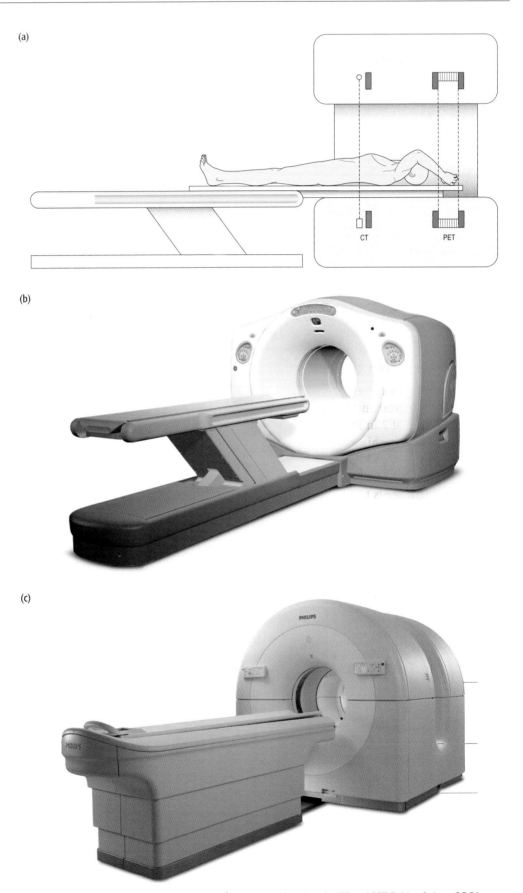

Figure 1.7 *(a) Schematic diagram of a PET/CT scanner showing the CT and PET fields of view. GE Discovery ST (b) and Philips Gemini (c) PET/CT scanners. (Photographs courtesy of GE Healthcare and Philips Medical Systems)*

Table 1.2 Features of some commercial PET/CT scanners

	Scintillator material	Detector element dimensions (mm)	PET axial field of view (cm)	Transmission rod sources	Patient aperture diameter	PET acquisition modes
GE Discovery ST	BGO	6.3 × 6.3	15.7	No	70 cm	2D/3D
Philips Gemini	GSO	4.0 × 6.0	18.0	Yes	62 cm (PET) 70 cm (CT)	3D
Siemens	LSO	4.0 × 4.0	16.2	No	70 cm	3D

With large investment from the major manufacturers, PET/CT technology is advancing rapidly. Future developments will include larger CT axial fields of view particularly for enhanced cardiac studies, time of flight acquisition and new scintillation materials to improve PET image quality, and closer integration with the radiotherapy planning process. Also in the pipeline is the integration of the PET and CT detectors themselves, allowing very compact gantries, near simultaneous PET and CT acquisition, and better image registration.

CT ATTENUATION CORRECTION

A CT scan is used to correct the PET emission data for attenuation. Combined with incremental improvements to the PET scanner design, this has resulted a reduction in almost a factor of 2 in scan time for PET/CT relative to stand alone PET systems. Using the CT scan in this way does not actually enhance the PET image quality in any way, in fact it introduces several complications. As the CT data are acquired at a much lower energy than is the PET, a procedure to convert the measured attenuation coefficients to 511 keV is necessary. The CT attenuation correction (CTAC) is usually accomplished by assuming a simple bilinear relationship between the CT number in Hounsfield Units (linearly related to the CT attenuation coefficient), and the 511 keV attenuation coefficients required for PET, as shown in Figure 1.8 (Kinahan et al., 1998). The relation is actually more complex than this and the current methods do not account correctly for, in particular, contrast agents and other high-Z materials. At best this can lead to inaccurate quantification, and at worst to artefacts in the PET image. More sophisticated algorithms are under development but in the meantime the consequences of using CTAC have to be addressed empirically (e.g. by modifying the contrast agents and protocols) as described below. CTAC also of course leads to an additional radiation dose to the patient.

ARTEFACTS AND OTHER ISSUES ARISING FROM CTAC

- **Breathing artefacts**

CTAC can result in artefacts related to respiratory motion (Goerres et al., 2002). One of these is the so-called 'mushroom' artefact sometimes seen at the base of the lung on the CT image. This occurs when the lung is at different phases of the respiratory cycle for different parts of the acquisition, e.g. as may happen when a breath-hold or shallow breathing protocol is not adhered to. This CT artefact can lead to severe artefacts in the PET image via the CTAC as shown in Case 2.21 (Chapter 2). The artefact is common for 1- and 2-slice CTs but is less likely to occur with multislice systems capable of faster imaging times.

A second effect, that is not addressed by faster scanning times, is that whereas the PET emission part of a PET/CT scan is acquired over several minutes for each bed position, the CT scan is acquired in just a few seconds. A perfect anatomic match

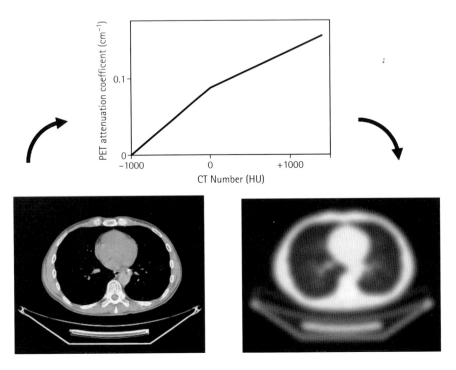

Figure 1.8 *CT attenuation correction. The CT numbers in the original CT image (left) are scaled using a bilinear relationship to obtain the 511 keV PET attenuation coefficients necessary to attenuation correct the PET image. The scaled CT image (right) is also smoothed to match the spatial resolution of the PET data*

between the two is therefore not possible. The standard diagnostic CT protocol is to scan the whole chest within one breath-hold at maximum inspiration. However, this position is very poorly matched to the 'time averaged' PET image. Mismatches between the reconstructed PET and CT images make interpretation difficult, but equally importantly create artefacts in the PET image via the CTAC. Various empirical breathing protocols are therefore employed to address this problem (Goerres, 2003a). A well-validated protocol is for the patient to hold their breath at the end of a normal expiration for the section of the scan covering the lower lung and a short region beyond (the region that can be covered will depend on the speed of the CT). This protocol nevertheless requires careful coaching and some centers have reported that simple shallow breathing produces equally acceptable results without the risk of serious artefacts that can occur if the breath-hold protocol is performed incorrectly. Artefacts due to PET/CT mismatch commonly occur above the diaphragm in the corrected PET images, as shown in Figure 1.9b, and can in some cases lead to lesions at the base of the lung disappearing altogether. The uncorrected PET images are not subject to these artefacts (or the mushroom artefact) and so should always be reviewed if a mismatch is suspected.

None of the protocol-based solutions to motion artefacts are ideal and, in the medium term, solutions will probably emerge that employ some form of motion tracking with associated correction algorithms (Nehmeh *et al.*, 2002).

- **Contrast agents**
CT in general makes extensive use of oral and intravenous contrast agents, however, with the CTAC algorithms currently available, iodine- and barium-based contrast agents can cause artefacts, appearing as areas of apparently elevated tracer uptake, in PET images (Figs 1.10 and 1.11) (Antoch *et al.*, 2004). Artefacts can also arise when movement of contrast between or during scans occurs. One solution to this problem

(a)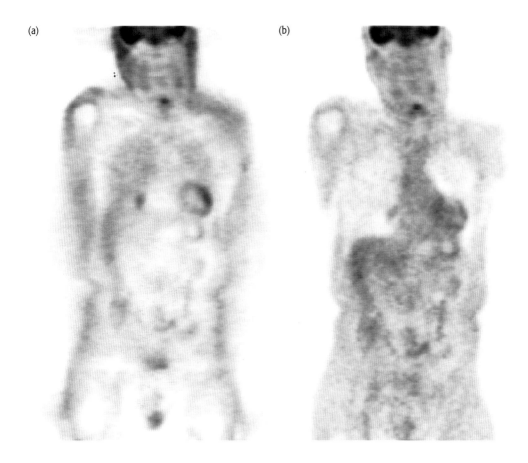

(b)

(c)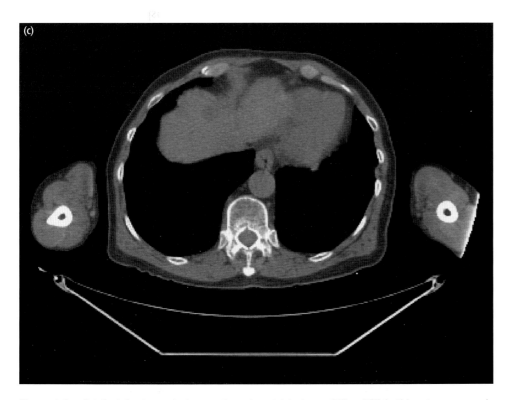

Figure 1.9   *Artefact due to respiratory motion mismatch between PET and CT. In this extreme example a region of abnormal uptake in the liver is clearly seen on the non attenuation-corrected PET (a), but is not seen on the attenuation-corrected PET (b). The region of abnormal uptake is confirmed by the CT (c)*

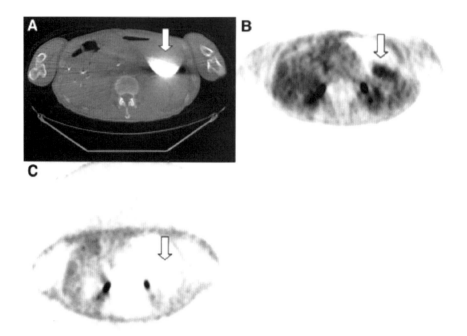

Figure 1.10   *Example of an artefact due to oral contrast. This man with a history of pancreatic cancer and rising tumor markers was evaluated by PET/CT. The patient had ingested barium for an upper gastrointestinal study 1 week before the PET/CT without additional contrast being administered. CT showed residual, dense barium in a distended stomach (a). CT attenuation-corrected PET emission images showed an area of increased activity in stomach corresponding to the area of barium retention on CT (b). However, no increased uptake was seen in the stomach in non attenuation-corrected images (c). Reprinted with kind permission of the Society of Nuclear Medicine from Cohade C, Osman M, Nakamoto Y et al. (2003) Initial experience with oral contrast in PET/CT: Phantom and clinical studies.* J Nucl Med **44**, *412 (Fig. 1)*

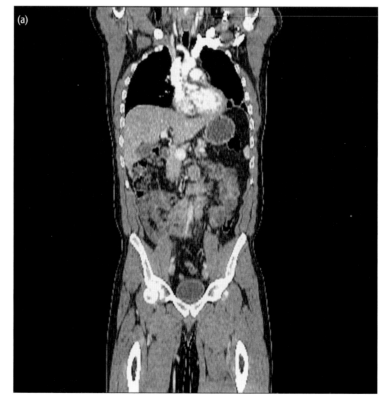

Figure 1.11   *Example of artefacts due to intravenous contrast: (a) CT, (continued over)*

(b)

(c)

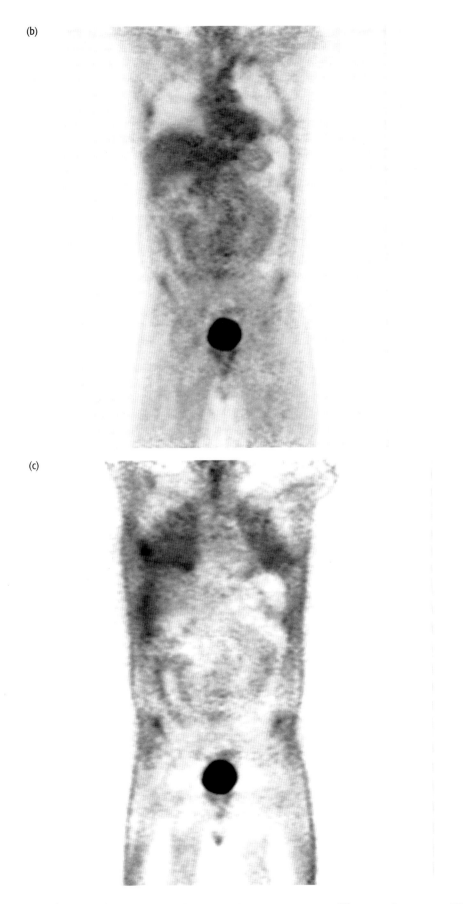

Figure 1.11   *(continued) Example of artefacts due to intravenous contrast: (b) attenuation-corrected PET, (c) non attenuation-corrected PET. (Images courtesy of T Beyer)*

is to perform a 'standard' PET/CT protocol and then administer contrast prior to an additional CT. The second CT may be performed (half an hour later for oral contrast) with a breath-hold and a full diagnostic protocol, but in general will not be well registered to the PET/CT. This solution also makes inefficient use of scanner time. A second approach is to modify the contrast protocol so that it can be integrated into the standard PET/CT procedure without creating artefacts on the PET image. This is an evolving area and, once again, the emphasis tends to be on developing protocols that produce 'clinically acceptable' images rather than highly accurate quantification.

Iodine- or barium-based oral contrast agents can be used with caution in most circumstances, though they will result in small changes to standard uptake values (SUVs) (Dizendorf et al., 2002). An alternative solution is to use water-equivalent contrast agents, which are treated correctly by the CTAC algorithm. Several studies indicate that the clinical significance of artefacts and quantitative changes arising from the use of intravenous contrast is small in most cases, however artefacts mimicking focal tracer uptake can occur (Antoch et al., 2002) and specific contrast administration protocols have been described in order to minimize any such artefacts. For example, in the protocol described by Beyer et al. (2005) contrast is administered in two phases over ~60 s, the CT scan is delayed until 50 s after the start of administration, and the CT is performed in the reverse (i.e. craniocaudal) direction, resulting in reproducible, high-quality CT and artefact-free PET images.

- Metal implants and prostheses

Dental fillings, prostheses, artificial joints, and other metallic items create artefacts on CT and additionally are not correctly dealt with by the CTAC algorithm, and so create artefacts in the PET images (Goerres et al., 2003; Kamel et al., 2003). Unlike the case for contrast agents, there are no protocol-based solutions and the artefacts can sometimes be severe, as shown in Figure 1.12. As for all the CTAC-related artefacts, inspection of the non attenuation-corrected PET image is helpful but large, highly attenuating items (i.e. artificial hip joints) can also create artefacts directly on the PET scan. Conversely, small items such as fillings may cause streaking on the CT but still have no discernable effect on the PET. Some CT scanners have algorithms to reduce artefacts arising from high CT numbers but these are not implemented as standard. Artefacts are generally more severe when there is PET/CT misregistration, and are generally less so when iterative reconstruction algorithms are employed.

- Truncation artefact

The field of view of the PET component of PET/CT systems is wide enough that the arms are always included, even when they are at the patient's side. However, the CT field of view is usually limited to 50 cm and activity outside this limit will not be reconstructed correctly, as shown in Figure 1.13. If tracer is present outside the CT field of view, there is also a small effect on the quantitative accuracy of the PET image within the CT field of view. There are several straightforward technical solutions to this problem (Schaller et al., 2002), though currently none is implemented and the only solution is to ensure that, whenever possible, the patient remains within the CT field of view.

- Photon starvation

Photon starvation occurs when too few x-rays pass through the patient along certain directions, resulting in noisy projection data and streaking artefacts in the

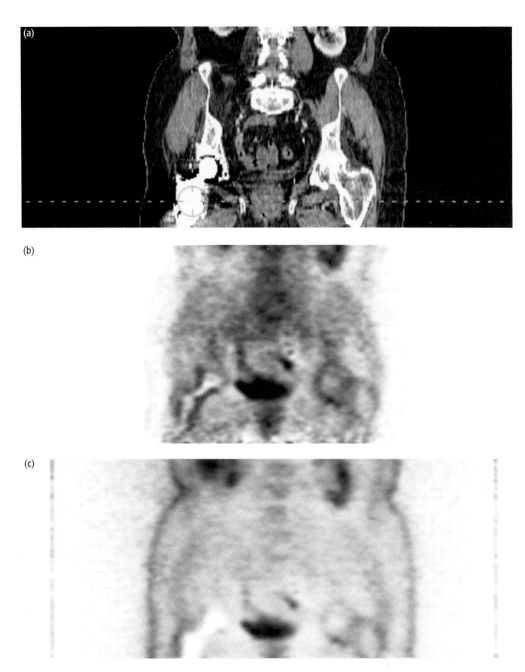

Figure 1.12 *Artefacts in the region of an artificial hip joint: (a) CT, (b) attenuation-corrected PET, (c) non attenuation corrected PET. (Images courtesy of T Beyer)*

reconstructed CT images. This may occur, for example, when imaging with the arms at the patient's side, and in very-low-dose protocols. Solutions therefore can be found in increasing the dose and in imaging with the arms above the patient's head. If this is not possible, placing the arms over the abdomen will remove the longest beam paths. Photon starvation is often confused with beam hardening, which is a consequence of the multispectral nature of the x-ray beam. Beam hardening refers to the increase in average x-ray energy as the beam proceeds through the body, and results in the CT 'cupping artefact'. This appears as an apparent decrease in CT number in the center of the body and is corrected for in the CT reconstruction software.

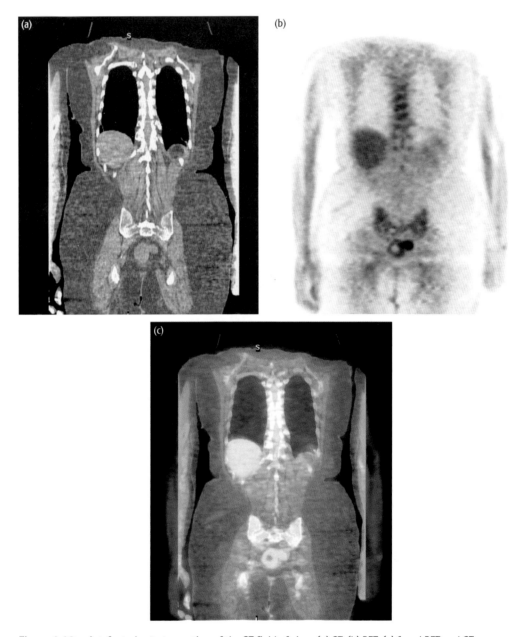

Figure 1.13 *Artefacts due to truncation of the CT field of view: (a) CT, (b) PET, (c) fused PET and CT*

- CT scan parameters

For the reasons given above, the CT part of a PET/CT scan is not usually suitable as a substitute for a diagnostic CT. The scan is required for attenuation correction of the PET data and to provide anatomic localization only, and the acquisition parameters are chosen to achieve both of these while minimizing the radiation dose. The main relevant variable is the beam current (combined with the rotation speed of typically 0.5–0.8 s) and, for attenuation correction only, this can be reduced to extremely low values. For most patients scanned with their arms raised, there is no loss of PET image quality or quantitative accuracy by reducing the beam current to around 10 mA at 0.5 s rotation time (Kamel *et al.*, 2002). The visual quality of these images is poor; however, when smoothed to the PET spatial resolution, they are still superior to the transmission images previously obtained with PET transmission rod sources. Defining the necessary CT image quality for clinical interpretation in conjunction with the PET is difficult and may vary for different applications. However, there is a general consensus that a current of ~80 mA (0.5–0.8 s rotation time) is most appropriate. Images are usually acquired with a 5 mm slice thickness, CT pitch of 1.5, and at 140 kVp. Depending on the details of the CT scanner, this protocol results in a radiation dose (ED) to the patient of ~8 mSv, which is 2–3 times less than that for an equivalent diagnostic study and adds to the ~10 mSv from the tracer. Even for this 'low-dose' protocol the radiation dose is seen to be significant (Brix *et al.*, 2005) and the availability of CT dose reduction/optimization techniques is likely to become important. There are few data available yet as to what protocol will provide acceptable 'low-dose' images for pediatric PET/CT, although reducing the kVp is likely to be effective in this situation.

Image reconstruction and software

PET AND CT IMAGE RECONSTRUCTION

All PET images are reconstructed using iterative algorithms, which explicitly model the statistical properties of the data, resulting in improved image quality over filtered back-projection-type algorithms (Meikle *et al.*, 1994). More advanced algorithms also model other aspects of the data acquisition process (attenuation, scatter, and the scanner itself), resulting in a more accurate reconstruction. For 2D data the ordered subsets expectation maximization (OSEM) algorithm is standard. For 3D data there are several options, the most common being a sophisticated rebinning algorithm ('Fourier rebinning' or FORE) that rearranges the 3D dataset into a set of 2D slices which are then reconstructed by OSEM. Most manufacturers now also provide a fully 3D iterative algorithm that provides improved image quality but requires (substantially) more computing power. The helical CT data are reconstructed using one of the many algorithms now established (Flohr *et al.*, 2005). At present, iterative techniques are not used for CT reconstruction. The CT image must be reconstructed first so that the CTAC attenuation map can be created and used in the PET reconstruction. The CT images are available immediately at the end of the CT acquisition, whereas the PET will may take a minute or so after the last bed position has been acquired.

IMAGE DISPLAY AND ANALYSIS

PET/CT requires sophisticated display tools. Not only must all the standard CT and PET tools be available, but also methods that enable the reporting physician to navigate rapidly through several linked images. It is often necessary (e.g. when evaluating response to therapy) to display more than one study at a time, each linked to its own CT, and the number of images on the screen at any time can multiply rapidly. PET and CT datasets can be displayed side by side or as a fused image. Tools for display and evaluation of SUVs are usually incorporated, and many PET/CT workstations include sophisticated registration software that can be used, for example, to register the PET scan with MR using the CT to obtain a more accurate transformation. All commercial systems are able to export PET/CT images in DICOM format, including to hospital PACS systems. However, it should be noted that at present the tools available for display and analysis of PET data on PACS systems are extremely crude and not adequate for clinical reporting, similarly for tools for viewing registered PET/CT datasets. DICOM formats for PET/CT images and region of interest information attached to them (e.g. tumor margins) are also available for exporting data to radiotherapy planning systems.

PET TRACERS

Radionuclides for PET

The positron-emitting radionuclides relevant to clinical imaging are listed in Table 1.3. Positrons from a given radionuclide are emitted over a continuous range of energies, but are characterized by a maximum energy E_{max}. Higher-energy positrons have a longer range in tissue, however in practice the effect of positron range on spatial resolution is very small. The low-Z cyclotron-produced radionuclides – ^{15}O, ^{13}N, ^{11}C, and ^{18}F – all have high branching ratios for positron emission, however some of the higher-Z nuclides have other emissions resulting in less favorable radiation dosimetry.

Table 1.3 Properties and production routes for PET radionuclides

Radionuclide	Half-life	E_{max} (MeV)	Production reaction	Target	Product
^{11}C	20.4 min	0.96	$^{14}_{7}N(p,\alpha)^{11}_{6}C$	$^{nat}N_2$ gas	$^{11}CO_2$ gas
^{13}N	9.96 min	1.19	$^{16}_{8}O(p,\alpha)^{13}_{7}N$	^{nat}O water	$^{13}NH_4^+$ ion
^{15}O	2.07 min	1.72	$^{15}_{7}N(p,n)^{15}_{8}O$	$^{15}N_2$ gas	$^{15}O_2$ gas
			$^{14}_{7}N(d,n)^{15}_{8}O$	$^{nat}N_2$ gas	$^{15}O_2$ gas
^{18}F	109.8 min	0.635	$^{18}_{8}O(p,n)^{18}_{9}F$	^{18}O water	$^{18}F^-$ ion
			$^{20}_{10}Ne(d,\alpha)^{18}_{9}F$	^{nat}Ne gas	$^{18}F\text{-}F_2$ gas
^{68}Ga	68 min	1.9	$^{68}Ge \rightarrow {}^{68}Ga$	(Generator)	Ga metal
^{82}Rb	75 s	3.36	$^{82}Sr \rightarrow {}^{82}Rb$	(Generator)	RbCl

PET tracer production

THE CYCLOTRON

The standard low-Z PET radionuclides are all produced in a cyclotron in which a high-energy proton (usually) beam is fired into an appropriate target. To produce ^{18}F an [^{18}O]water target undergoes the nuclear reaction $^{18}O(p,n)^{18}_{9}F$, indicating that a proton (p) is absorbed and a neutron (n) lost. The most common cyclotron configuration for PET is the negative ion design, shown in Figure 1.14, which consists of two 'dee' electrodes, which are about 1 m in diameter. Negative ions (usually H$^-$, i.e. a proton and two electrons) are produced from an ion source at the center of the dees, and an alternating voltage is applied so that the ions move back and forth between the dees. A strong magnetic field constrains the path of the ions to a circular orbit, which increases in diameter as the ions pick up energy from the electric field. On passing through a thin carbon stripping foil, inserted into the beam at the edge of the dees, two electrons are stripped from each H$^-$ ion. The resulting H$^+$ ions move out of the beam under the influence of the magnetic field and are directed onto the target. Cyclotrons designed for PET are usually limited to relatively low energies, and hence in the range of nuclear reactions they can induce. A maximum energy of 11 MeV is sufficient to obtain adequate yields of ^{11}C, ^{13}N, ^{15}O, and ^{18}F. For example, bombardment of a small volume (~1 mL) of [^{18}O]water for ~2 hours will produce ~100 GBq of ^{18}F – enough to supply FDG to several scanners for a half day's operation. Most cyclotrons for routine FDG production are self-shielded, and can be opened for maintenance within several hours of bombardment.

(a)

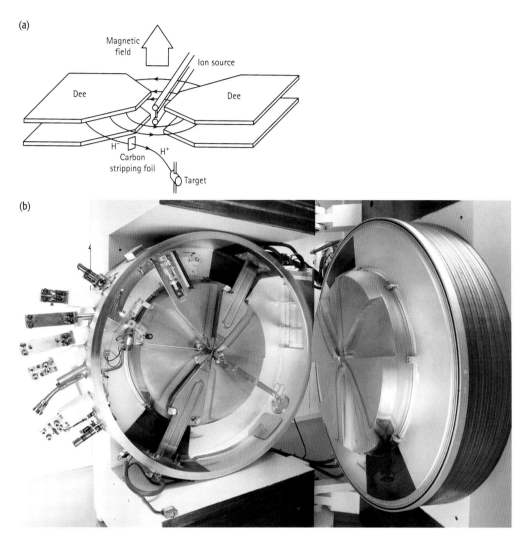

(b)

Figure 1.14 *Schematic diagram of cyclotron operation (a) and commercial PET cyclotron (b). (Photograph courtesy of GE Healthcare)*

TARGET CHEMISTRY AND TRACER SYNTHESIS

The yield of the required radionuclide from the cyclotron target depends on many factors relating both to the bombardment process and to the target chemistry, both of which also determine the initial chemical form of the radionuclide. Target materials and the chemical form of the products are given in Table 1.3. The chemical form of the radionuclide will determine what radiopharmaceuticals can be labeled with it. For example, $^{18}F^-$ produced from an $[^{18}O]$ water target can be used to produce ^{18}FDG via nucleophilic substitution; however, it is very difficult to label fluorodopa with ^{18}F in this form. Fluorodopa is more readily labeled with $^{18}F\text{-}F_2$ obtained from the $^{20}_{10}Ne(d,\alpha)^{18}_{9}F$ reaction. In many cases the target product is converted into a reactive intermediate, which is subsequently reacted with a stable precursor to obtain the final radiopharmaceutical. For example, $[^{11}C]$methyl-iodide can be used to incorporate ^{11}C-labeled methyl groups into many complex organic molecules, and this route is used routinely for the production of ^{11}C-labeled methionine. The final stage of production usually involves the separation of the radioactive product from nonradioactive byproducts using high performance liquid chromatography (HPLC) or other standard separation techniques.

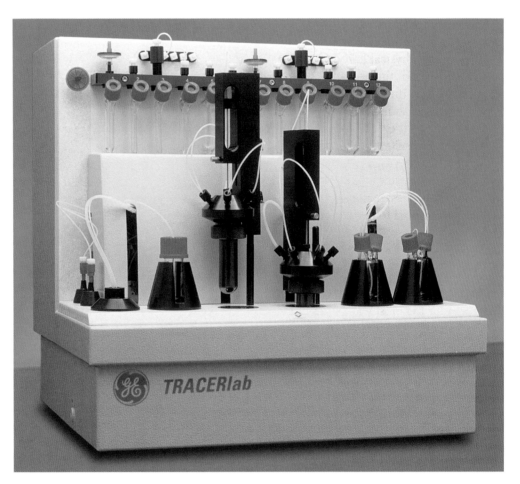

Figure 1.15 *Automated FDG synthesis unit. (Courtesy of GE Healthcare)*

All processes must be performed under the constraints imposed by the short half-life of the radionuclide, the large amounts of radioactivity and the small (picomolar) quantities of material involved. Consequently, a great deal of effort has gone into automating the syntheses, and commercial systems are available (Fig. 1.15) that can complete synthesis of FDG from packaged reagents in about 40 minutes.

RADIOPHARMACEUTICAL QUALITY CONTROL AND QUALITY ASSURANCE

Quality control and quality assurance procedures are an integral part of the routine production of PET radiopharmaceuticals. All aspects of production and quality control must conform to good manufacturing practice (GMP) standards, and the tracer must pass the tests below before administration to a patient. Most of the tests are performed using HPLC techniques, and for FDG they can be completed in ~30 minutes.

- Chemical purity is defined as the fraction of tracer in the formulated radiopharmaceutical that is in the desired molecular form. A test is performed to ensure that no compounds are present in sufficient quantities to cause toxicity or to be pharmacologically active. Such compounds should of course normally all be removed as part of the tracer preparation procedure.
- Radiochemical purity is defined as the fraction of the PET radionuclide in the desired chemical form and molecular position. Radiochemical impurities usually originate from radionuclide production, side reactions and incomplete removal of protecting groups.

- Radionuclidic purity is defined as the fraction of total radioactivity present as the specified radionuclide, and is determined either by measurements of energy spectra and physical half-life, or indirectly using HPLC or gas chromotography. If the half-lives of the impurities are much shorter than that of the desired radionuclide, the purity can be improved by simply letting the impurities decay. For example, short-lived ^{13}N and ^{15}O impurities are often present when ^{18}F is produced via the $^{18}_{8}O(p,n)^{18}_{9}F$ reaction.
- Microbiological testing is performed to ensure that the radiopharmaceutical is sterile and free from pyrogens. Tests for sterility and pyrogens are too time consuming to be performed prior to patient administration; however, the *Limulus* amebocyte lysate (LAL) test is a less general test for pyrogenicity which can be performed in about an hour and is used to test multidose vial preparations of ^{18}FDG.

FDG

KINETICS AND DISTRIBUTION OF FDG

FDG is by far the most widely used PET tracer. Following administration to the patient, FDG is rapidly taken up into tissue and over a period of 1–2 hours is trapped in proportion to the rate of glucose utilization. Much of clinical PET is based on the fact that diseased tissues, and in particular tumors, exhibit a high rate of glucose utilization. The straightforward kinetics of FDG, its ease of production and distribution, and demonstrated utility in very many different clinical conditions have resulted in FDG becoming almost synonymous with clinical PET as currently practiced.

FDG is taken up into all normal tissue except fat, with a large fraction of the administered activity accumulating in the brain (~ 6 percent) and myocardium (~ 4 percent). Unlike glucose, FDG is excreted via the kidneys and accumulates rapidly in the bladder (~ 20 percent in the first 2 hours). The kinetics of FDG can be described by a simple three-compartment model (Phelps *et al.*, 1979) as shown in Figure 1.16. This atlas describes the wide and expanding range of clinical applications of FDG. Although FDG is a nonspecific tracer, its proven utility means that it is likely to remain the cornerstone of clinical PET imaging for the forseeable future.

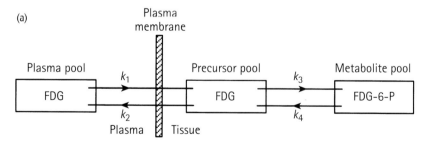

Figure 1.16   (a) Three-compartment model of FDG kinetics. The compartments represent (1) free FDG in plasma, (2) free FDG in tissue, and (3) FDG 6-phosphate (FDG 6-P). Free FDG is phosphorylated by the action of hexokinase to FDG 6-phosphate but is not metabolized further. It may be dephosphorylated on a timescale of several hours. The rate constants k_1, k_2, k_3, k_4 (in units of min^{-1}) represent the extraction of tracer from plasma into tissue, the return of free FDG to plasma, the rate of phosphorylation, and the rate of dephosphorylation, respectively. In many tissues k_4 is very low, in which case the metabolic rate for glucose is given by the expression $\dfrac{[glc]}{LC} \times \dfrac{k_1 \times k_3}{k_2 + k_3}$ where [glc] is the plasma glucose concentration and LC (~0.5) is the lumped constant which accounts for differences in the kinetics of glucose and FDG (continued over)

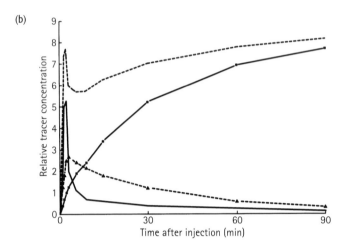

Figure 1.16 (continued) *(b) Time-activity curves for FDG in tissue and in plasma (corrected for radioactive decay). Extraction into tissue is rapid over the first 10 minutes until equilibrium with the plasma concentration is achieved, when it start to fall. FDG 6-P accumulates rapidly at first and continues to rise over the next hour or so. At 30 minutes the ratio between trapped and free FDG is about 4:1. The total labeled FDG, as registered by a PET scanner, includes contributions from FDG in tissue and in plasma as well as FDG 6-P. The 2-hour half-life of ^{18}F is well suited to the rate of uptake for FDG and permits acquisition of images at reasonable count rates. Most clinical protocols consist of a 30–60-minute uptake period after tracer administration followed by a static scan over a period of ~1–10 minutes, which results in an image where the grayscale level is roughly proportional to the rate of glucose utilization*

QUANTIFICATION OF FDG UPTAKE

In clinical PET and PET/CT studies quantification of tracer uptake is becoming increasingly important, in measuring changes in tracer uptake to assess response to therapy, in differentiating benign and malignant tumors, identifying the stage of disease, and in indicating prognosis (Hoekstra *et al.*, 2000; Hallett 2004; Lucignani *et al.*, 2004; Visvikis *et al.*, 2004). Absolute quantification with the aim of measuring glucose utilization in mol/min/g requires complex acquisition protocols and is rarely performed. In practice quantification usually refers to the much simpler standardized uptake value (SUV), which provides an index of tracer uptake that can be compared between patients and between scans. While SUVs are usually used to quantify uptake of FDG in oncology studies, the basic principle can readily be applied to other tracers and disease. The SUV is defined as follows:

$$SUV = \frac{Tracer\ uptake\ (MBq/mL)}{Administered\ activity\ (MBq)/(Patient\ weight\ (kg) \times 1000)}$$

Tracer uptake is determined from a small region of interest placed over the tumor in an attenuation-corrected image, and a scanner calibration factor is required to convert the value measured from the image into MBq/mL. SUVs are based on the approximation that the tracer is distributed uniformly throughout the body, so in normal tissue SUVs are very roughly equal to one. However, since little FDG accumulates in normal fat in fasting patients, many vascular tissues have an SUV greater than this. For malignant tumors, where the metabolic rate is higher, SUVs may range from 2 to as high as 15 or more.

Limitations of SUVs

Despite their widespread use, SUVs are subject to several limitations, and when SUV values are quoted, or compared with threshold values taken from the literature, care must be taken to see which of the various corrections have been applied:

- *Correlation with body weight.* ^{18}FDG is not taken up into adipose tissue and some studies have shown that SUVs are more reproducible when the lean body mass or body surface area (derived from measurements of both height and weight) is substituted for patient weight in the expression above; however, there is still no general consensus on which variation should be used (Zasadny *et al.*, 1993; Erselcan *et al.*, 2002).

- *Blood glucose concentration.* Likewise a blood glucose correction can be made which accounts for competition between ^{18}FDG and glucose, but again there is no general consensus if or when this correction should be used (Hallett *et al.*, 2001).

- *Measurement time.* FDG uptake may continue to increase for several hours after administration, and that the shape of the uptake curve is variable. To minimize errors due to these effects, SUVs should always be acquired at the same time post-injection (Hustinx *et al.*, 1999; Lodge *et al.*, 1999).

- *Partial volume effect.* All quantification performed in PET is subject to the limitations imposed by poor spatial resolution, which manifests itself as the 'partial volume effect'. For objects of dimensions less than twice the spatial resolution (FWHM) in the image, the apparent activity in the object is decreased as seen in Figure 1.17. For objects of diameter equal to the spatial resolution the maximum apparent activity concentration will be less than 50 percent of the true value, and quantification of uptake for small objects must be treated with great caution.

- *ROI placement.* Since tumors often have heterogeneous distributions of tracer uptake, SUVs are generally evaluated for the hottest part of the tumor, which is assumed to be the most malignant. Either SUV_{max} or SUV_{av} may be quoted.

- *Respiratory motion.* SUVs are reduced for small lesions in the lower lobes of the lung due to the blurring effect of respiratory motion (Nehmeh *et al.*, 2002).

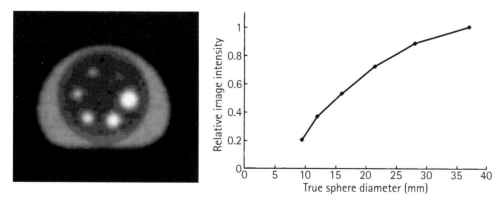

Figure 1.17 *Partial volume effect. Each sphere in the phantom contains the same activity concentration. The apparent activity is dramatically reduced for the smaller spheres*

Other tracers

[^{13}N]AMMONIA

^{13}N-labeled ammonia is rapidly extracted into the myocardium with a 70 percent extraction fraction (falling to ~35 percent at high coronary flows), and is trapped by the glutamic acid–glutamate reaction. It has been suggested that the degree to which ammonia is trapped depends to some extent on the metabolic state of the myocardium; however, due to its ease of use, and the high-quality images that can be obtained, [^{13}N]ammonia is the standard tracer for PET myocardial perfusion studies. Clinical protocols consist of a static scan beginning a few minutes after tracer injection to allow for clearance of the blood pool activity. Parametric images of myocardial perfusion can be obtained, however these are complicated by the appearance of labeled metabolites in the blood which become significant a few minutes after injection. Ammonia scans are usually performed in a rest/stress protocol with a pharmacologic cardiac stressing agent (e.g. adenosine) and/or combined with an FDG metabolic study, in which case successive tracer injections must be arranged such that an emission scan does not begin until the count rate from the previous administration has fallen to a sufficiently low level. Cardiac studies are usually performed as simple static emission scans. Higher resolution and more accurate quantitative values can be obtained by performing gated emission scans. The cardiac cycle is divided into ~8 separate images, each of which can be processed in the same way as a static cardiac scan. Estimates of wall motion and wall thickening can be made from gated cardiac studies if the acquisition time is extended to account for the smaller number of counts in each image.

[^{11}C]METHIONINE

Accumulation of [^{11}C]L-methionine into tumor tissue is believed to be due to increased transport of amino acids and incorporation of amino acids into protein fractions, although it is not clear which of these mechanisms is predominant in PET tumor imaging. Further metabolism also results in the label being incorporated into lipids and nucleic acids. [^{11}C]L-methionine can be used to delineate tumor extent, and to some extent tumor proliferation rate.

FLUORINE-18

Uptake of ^{18}F$^-$ provides an index of bone metabolism, and has a long history of use in skeletal imaging to investigate focal bone disease such as tumors or infection. ^{18}F$^-$ is rapidly cleared from the blood by renal excretion, and by incorporation into bone by exchanging with the hydroxyl ion in hydroxyapatite crystal in bone to form fluoroapatite. Imaging is performed ~60 minutes after tracer injection.

RUBIDIUM-82

^{82}Rb is used to measure myocardial perfusion. It is an analogue of potassium, and its kinetics are similar to those of the single-photon emitter ^{201}Tl. Rb is extracted rapidly into the myocardium with a 50–60 percent extraction fraction which falls to 25–30 percent at high flows. The short half-life (75 s) of ^{82}Rb means that repeat studies can be performed in rapid succession. ^{82}Rb is generated by the decay of ^{82}Sr ($t_{1/2} = 25$ days) in a generator, and an automated system for rapid elution of the generator directly into an intravenous catheter is used.

CLINICAL PROTOCOLS AND PRACTICAL ISSUES

Standard whole-body acquisition protocol

A conventional whole-body PET/CT protocol is described below and shown schematically in Figure 1.18. It is necessary for the patient to fast for 6 hours prior to FDG scanning in order to maximize FDG uptake. Insulin-dependent diabetic

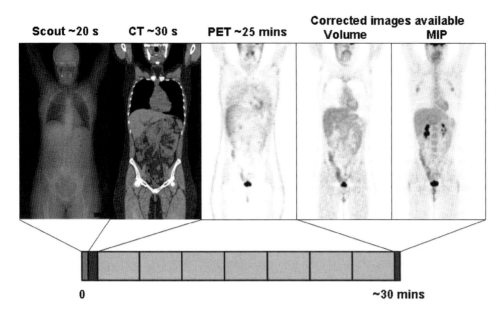

| Scout ~20 s | CT ~30 s | PET ~25 mins | Corrected images available Volume | MIP |

Figure 1.18 *PET/CT whole-body imaging protocol. A scout scan is performed followed by the CT and PET scans. The CT is used to attenuation correct the PET data, and corrected images are available at the end of study. The PET takes up the vast majority of the scanning time*

patients are not required to fast. Intravenous administration of the tracer is performed in a separate room to the scanning suite and the patient is left quietly, preferably lying down, for the tracer uptake period of 60–90 minutes. Injected doses tend to be lower (400 MBq, 10 mCi) in Europe and higher (400–800 MBq, 10–20 mCi) in the USA. Some sites use the same dose for all patients whereas many scale the dose with patient's weight – there are few definitive data on this and the optimum protocol will depend on the scanner used. As scan times have decreased, there will always be at least two or three highly radioactive patients waiting to be scanned, and purpose designed waiting rooms are therefore required that incorporate a significant amount of radiation shielding. The increased patient throughput can also potentially lead to high radiation doses to radiographers who should avoid close proximity with active patients.

Prior to starting the acquisition the patient should be coached in the breathing protocol if one is to be used. Acquisition with the arms above the head is preferred as this results in improved image quality for both CT and PET (particularly for 3D mode). This can usually be tolerated for up to a maximum of about 30 minutes, and total scanning times are now usually well below this. Head and neck scans should be performed with arms at the patient's side.

The region to be scanned is specified using a CT scout scan (or topogram) which provides a single projection view of the whole patient. This is immediately followed by the CT (see above for typical scan parameters) starting with the head. As the lung region is scanned instructions are given to the patient as to the breathing protocol if one is used.

The PET scan immediately follows the CT. Opinion varies as to how much time should be spent at each bed position, and this will vary for different scanner models (Halpern *et al.*, 2004). Most studies are performed with between 1 and 5 minutes per bed position. Images are available rapidly after the acquisition and may be examined for artefacts or relevant clinical information prior to releasing the patient.

In some cases additional local views of suspicious regions may be requested.

There is great interest in using PET to aid target volume definition in radiotherapy planning (Ciernik *et al.*, 2003), however until much more extensive evaluation is completed this cannot be considered a routine procedure. The proposed treatment position must be exactly reproduced for the PET/CT scan using the various radiotherapy immobilization devices and standard radiotherapy positioning lasers installed in the scanning suite. Usually only a scan of a limited area is required, nevertheless experience so far indicates that great attention must be paid to setting up the patient for the PET/CT scan, making the whole process very time consuming.

Brain and heart imaging protocols

Brain imaging protocols are straightforward. An uptake period of 30 minutes is standard with an emission acquisition time of 5–10 minutes. The brain is always imaged in 3D mode. The radiation dose from the CT will be low compared to that from the radiotracer due to the small region being scanned and the CT image can be used to facilitate registration of the PET image with MR. A reliable method of preventing head movement is essential.

There is relatively little experience in cardiac PET/CT imaging, and protocols for FDG and ammonia are essentially the same as for imaging with stand-alone PET. Although the use of CTAC might be expected to cause problems, it appears that for both static and gated studies a standard CTAC procedure is effective (Souvatzoglou *et al.*, 2004).

Radiation dose

Table 1.4 shows the whole-body effective dose (ED) values for common PET radiopharmaceuticals. Values are on the whole less than for single-photon emitters, primarily due to the short half-lives of the PET radionuclides. For children, administration of activities reduced in proportion to body weight results in images which are of at least as good quality as those obtained in adults. EDs from the CT scan are typically about 8 mSv.

Table 1.4 Effective dose (ED) values for common PET radiopharmaceuticals		
Tracer	**Typical activity in MBq (mCi)**	**EDE in mSv (mR)**
^{18}FDG	250 (7)	6.8 (705)
^{18}F$^-$	250 (7)	6.7 (693)
[^{11}C]Methionine	370 (10)	4.6 (460)
[^{15}O]Water	2000 (55)	2.3 (234)
[^{13}N]Ammonia	550 (15)	1.5 (150)
^{82}Rb	2000 (55)	2.4 (244)

REFERENCES AND FURTHER READING

Antoch G, Freudenberg LS, Egelhof T *et al.* (2002) Focal tracer uptake: A potential artefact in contrast-enhanced dual-modality PET/CT scans. *J Nucl Med* **43**, 1339–42.

Antoch G, Freudenberg LS, Beyer T, Bockisch A, Debatin JF (2004) To enhance or not to enhance? F-18-FDG and CT contrast agents in dual-modality F-18-FDG PET/CT. *J Nucl Med* **45**, 56S–65S.

Bettinardi V, Danna M, Savi A *et al.* (2004) Performance evaluation of the new whole-body PET/CT scanner: Discovery ST. *Eur J Nucl Med Mol Imaging* **31**, 867–81.

Beyer T, Townsend DW, Brun T *et al.* (2000) A combined PET/CT scanner for clinical oncology. *J Nucl Med* **41**, 1369–79.

Beyer T, Antoch G, Bockisch A, Stattaus J (2005) Optimized intravenous contrast administration for diagnostic whole-body F-18-FDG PET/CT. *J Nucl Med* **46**, 429–35.

Brix G, Lechel U, Glatting G *et al.* (2005) Radiation exposure of patients undergoing whole-body dual-modality F-18-FDG PET/CT examinations. *J Nucl Med* **46**, 608–13.

Ciernik IF, Dizendorf E, Baumert BG *et al.* (2003) Radiation treatment planning with an integrated positron emission and computer tomography (PET/CT): A feasibility study. *Int J Radiat Oncol Biol Phys* **57**, 853–63.

Dizendorf EV, Treyer V, von Schulthess GK, Hany TF (2002) Application of oral contrast media in coregistered positron emission tomography-CT. *AJR Am J Roentgenol* **179**, 477–81.

Erdi YE, Nehmeh SA, Mulnix T, Humm JL, Watson CC (2004) PET performance measurements for an LSO-based combined PET/CT scanner using the National Electrical Manufacturers Association NU 2–2001 standard. *J Nucl Med* **45**, 813–21.

Erselcan T, Turgut B, Dogan D, Ozdemir S (2002) Lean body mass-based standardized uptake value, derived from a predictive equation, might be misleading in PET studies. *Eur J Nucl Med* **29**, 1630–38.

Flohr TG, Schaller S, Stierstorfer K *et al.* (2005) Multi-detector row CT systems and image-reconstruction techniques. *Radiology* **235**, 756–73.

Goerres GW, Kamel E, Heidelberg TNH, Schwitter MR, Burger C, von Schulthess GK (2002) PET/CT image co-registration in the thorax: influence of respiration. *Eur J Nucl Med Mol Imaging* **29**, 351–60.

Goerres GW, Burger C, Schwitter MR *et al.* (2003a) PET/CT of the abdomen: optimizing the patient breathing pattern. *Eur Radiol* **13**, 734–9.

Goerres GW, Ziegler SI, Burger C *et al.* (2003b) Artefacts at PET and PET/CT caused by metallic hip prosthetic material. *Radiology* **226**, 577–84.

Hallett WA (2004) Quantification in clinical fluorodeoxyglucose positron emission tomography. *Nucl Med Commun* **25**, 647–50.

Hallett WA, Marsden PK, Cronin BF, O'Doherty MJ (2001) Effect of corrections for blood glucose and body size on (^{18}F)FDG standardized uptake values in lung cancer. *Eur J Nucl Med* **28**, 919–22.

Halpern BS, Dahlbom M, Quon A *et al.* (2004) Impact of patient weight and emission scan duration on PET/CT image quality and lesion detectability. *J Nucl Med* **45**, 797–801.

Hoekstra CJ, Paglianiti I, Hoekstra OS *et al.* (2000) Monitoring response to therapy in cancer using (^{18}F)-2-fluorodeoxy-D-glucose and positron emission tomography: an overview of different analytical methods. *Eur J Nucl Med* **27**, 731–43.

Hustinx R, Smith RJ, Benard F *et al.* (1999) Dual time point fluorine-18 fluorodeoxyglucose positron emission tomography: a potential method to differentiate malignancy from inflammation and normal tissue in the head and neck. *Eur J Nucl Med* **26**, 1345–8.

Kamel E, Hany TF, Burger C *et al.* (2002) CT vs Ge-68 attenuation correction in a combined PET/CT system: evaluation of the effect of lowering the CT tube current. *Eur J Nucl Med Mol Imaging* **29**, 346–50.

Kamel EM, Burger C, Buck A, von Schulthess GK, Goerres GW (2003) Impact of metallic dental implants on CT-based attenuation correction in a combined PET/CT scanner. *Eur Radiol* **13**, 724–8.

Kinahan PE, Townsend DW, Beyer T, Sashin D (1998) Attenuation correction for a combined 3D PET/CT scanner. *Med Phys* **25**, 2046–53.

Lodge MA, Lucas JD, Marsden PK, Cronin BF, O'Doherty MJ (1999) A PET study of ^{18}FDG uptake in soft tissue masses. *Eur J Nucl Med* **26**, 22–30.

Lucignani G, Paganelli G, Bombardieri E (2004) The use of standardized uptake values for assessing FDG uptake with PET in oncology: a clinical perspective. *Nucl Med Commun* **25**, 651–6.

Meikle SR, Hutton BF, Bailey DL, Hooper PK, Fulham MJ (1994) Accelerated EM reconstruction in total-body PET – potential for improving tumor detectability. *Phys Med Biol* **39**, 1689–704.

Nehmeh SA, Erdi YE, Ling CC *et al.* (2002) Effect of respiratory gating on reducing lung motion artifacts in PET imaging of lung cancer. *Med Phys* **29**, 366–71.

Phelps ME, Huang SC, Hoffman EJ *et al.* (1979) Tomographic measurement of local cerebral glucose metabolic rate in humans with (F-18)2-fluoro-2-deoxy-D-glucose: validation of method. *Ann Neurol* **6**, 371–88.

Schaller S, Sembritzki O, Beyer T *et al.* (2002) An algorithm for virtual extension of the CT field of measurement for application in combined PET/CT scanners. *Radiology* **225**, 497.

Souvatzoglou M, Bengel F, Fernolendt H, Schwaiger M, Nekolla S (2004) Different CT protocols for attenuation correction in cardiac FDG imaging with PET/CT: a comparison with conventional PET. *Eur J Nucl Med Mol Imaging* **31**, S317–S318.

Strother SC, Casey ME, Hoffman EJ (1990) Measuring PET scanner sensitivity – relating countrates to image signal-to-noise ratios using noise equivalent counts. *IEEE Trans Nucl Sci* **37**, 783–8.

Visvikis D, Turzo A, Bizais Y, Rest CCL (2004) Technology related parameters affecting quantification in positron emission tomography imaging. *Nucl Med Commun* **25**, 637–41.

Zasadny KR, Wahl RL (1993) Standardized uptake values of normal tissues at PET with 2-(fluorine-18)-fluoro-2-deoxy-D-glucose: variations with body weight and a method for correction. *Radiology* **189**, 847–50.

CHAPTER 2
NORMAL VARIANTS AND POTENTIAL PROBLEMS/PITFALLS

INTRODUCTION AND BACKGROUND

Glucose acts as the basic energy substrate for many tissues so variations in distribution of [^{18}F]2-fluoro-2-deoxy-D-glucose (FDG) can cause considerable difficulties in interpretation of clinical positron emission tomography (PET) scans. The most difficult thing to learn when first starting to report whole-body FDG scans is appreciating the normal variation which can occur. High uptake of FDG is seen in the brain, approximately 6 percent of administered activity is taken up in brain. Hence some brain metastases such as those from lung cancer may be difficult to distinguish from normal cortical uptake and the sensitivity for detection of metastatic disease in the brain can be low. The myocardium also accumulates FDG, although uptake is lower in the fasted than the fed state and this is one of the reasons why patients are fasted for 4–6 hours prior to scanning to minimize uptake in normal tissues. In the fed state there is secretion of endogenous insulin which further increases uptake in skeletal and cardiac muscle, which is desirable for cardiac imaging but highly undesirable for whole-body oncology imaging. It is tempting, but not advisable, to give additional insulin to diabetic patients who arrive for their whole-body scans with high blood sugar concentrations (see Case 2.19). This can result in a nondiagnostic scan with extensive uptake in muscle and little elsewhere. Although glucose and FDG compete for uptake into tumors, in our experience it is rare for uptake into tumor to be completely saturated even with high glucose concentration and to miss tumor altogether. It is, however, important to know that the blood sugar is high as this may affect scan quality and interpretation, and we routinely measure blood sugar prior to FDG injection. Caffeine increases levels of free fatty acids and either black coffee or a diet cola can be used to suppress myocardial uptake.

FDG is excreted in the urine and approximately 20 percent of the administered activity accumulates in the bladder in the first two hours. Administration of furosemide and good hydration can help minimize urinary uptake in patients with abdominopelvic disease. Some centers advocate catheterizing patients and bladder washouts, although this is not performed at our institutions.

Variable uptake also occurs in other body tissues including the gastrointestinal system. Physiologic uptake is often seen in bowel, especially in the colon and cecum. It is not clear whether uptake is extraluminal – perhaps occurring in smooth muscle or lymphoid tissue which could explain why the cecum tends to have high uptake in some individuals – or if FDG is secreted into the bowel lumen or taken up by bowel organisms. Glucagon, antimicrobials, and laxatives have all been used to try to reduce bowel uptake, with limited success. PET/computed tomography (CT) is making it easier to avoid some of these pitfalls by localizing uptake to normal structures. PET/CT helps to differentiate physiologic uptake in bowel from disease and to identify physiologic uptake in brown fat and muscle, which can often be asymmetric.

PHYSIOLOGICAL UPTAKE

High uptake occurs in:
  Brain
  Urinary system
Variable uptake occurs in:
  Salivary glands
  Tonsils
  Larynx
  Myocardium
  Thymus (children and young adults)
  Breast (lactating, premenopausal and HRT treatment)
  Stomach
  Bowel, especially colon and cecum
  Bone marrow
  Ovary (mid-cycle)
  Uterus (ovulatory phase and menstruation)
  Brown fat and muscle

The uptake of FDG in brown fat has a distinct pattern with marked uptake in the neck, upper chest, and thoracic paraspinal regions. When it was first reported by us, we postulated that this uptake might reside in muscle and that diazepam could reduce or abolish the uptake. However, with the introduction of PET/CT it has become clear that at least some of the uptake localizes to fat. The uptake occurs more frequently in patients with low body mass index and in cold weather. In the cold the sympathetic nervous system stimulates brown fat to generate heat by fatty acid oxidation. This 'nonshivering' response to cold is more likely to occur in thin people who are more prone to feel the cold. Anaerobic glycolysis then becomes the main source of ATP production instead of lipid metabolism, and glucose turnover within brown fat is increased. This may be the mechanism for FDG uptake in brown fat. Diazepam may work by an indirect effect on the sympathetic nervous system rather than as a muscle relaxant, to reduce uptake in patients with suspected cervical or mediastinal disease.

METHODS TO REDUCE PHYSIOLOGIC UPTAKE

1 Urinary uptake : good hydration ± furosemide
2 Larynx: patients with head and neck cancer remain silent during uptake period
3 Myocardial uptake: fasting ± caffeine
4 Brown fat: keep warm ± diazepam
5 Muscle : inject lying down, relaxing in a comfortable position for uptake period
6 Brain scans: inject in silence in quiet darkened room; avoid stimulation during uptake period; avoid any sedation for uptake period; no glucose-containing sedation prior to visit to PET centre

However, PET/CT is introducing a few new problems and potential pitfalls of its own. The CT acquisition typically takes 20–30 seconds whereas PET takes 20–30 minutes. This means it is possible to image the base of the lungs and the liver during a single breath-hold on CT whereas on PET the position of the diaphragm is 'averaged' over many respiratory cycles. Hence there is potential for significant misregistration of lesions situated close to the diaphragm. The best way to approximate the position of the diaphragm on the two studies appears to be to acquire the CT scan at the end of a normal expiration. The patient is 'coached' in the technique prior to scanning, but ability to comply can vary considerably, especially in elderly patients or patients with breathing difficulties. For this reason some centers prefer to adopt quiet shallow breathing for the CT scan. Whatever approach is used, it is important to recognize that misregistration may occur in the craniocaudal direction of up to 2–3 cm but careful evaluation of the two scans usually enables the PET uptake to be correctly ascribed to the correct CT lesion. A further potential problem is the use of intravenous or bowel contrast. High-density contrast results in overattenuation of the PET image and artifactual 'hot spots' can be introduced. The same occurs around metallic implants and prostheses. This can be circumvented by viewing the nonattenuation-corrected PET images, which do not display the artifact. The decision whether to use contrast is an issue of debate, with some advocating the use of intravenous contrast but perhaps slowing the rate of injection to avoid high density in the arterial contrast phase, and others advocating the use of low-density or negative oral contrast.

TECHNICAL PROBLEMS AND SOME SOLUTIONS

1 Injection artefacts: scan injection site when axillary uptake seen
2 Breathing artifacts, 'banana sign', 'mushrooms on the diaphragm': quiet breathing or end expiration during CT
3 Misregistration: scroll up and down or forwards and backwards on adjacent slices to 'match' lesions on PET + CT
4 Movement artifacts (especially brain scanning): always check scan prior to leaving department, consider acquiring brain scans as series of static frames and reject those with movement
5 Attenuation artefacts with contrast media, implants, pacemakers, and prostheses: view nonattenuation-corrected scan data

Apart from problems caused by confusion with physiologic uptake, 'technical' problems can also give rise to artifacts, which may be misinterpreted. Careful inspection of images before the patient leaves the department can often help to avoid misinterpretation, e.g. the injection site must be scanned in the case of axillary uptake to avoid misinterpreting axillary uptake as disease when it is the result of a tissued injection.

Recent surgery or radiotherapy may give rise to inflammatory uptake and a good history can help to spot potential sources of false-positive uptake such as these. Surgery and radiotherapy may also influence the distribution of 'normal' uptake. For example, physiologic uptake in salivary glands may be abolished with radiotherapy on the side of treatment with unilateral but 'normal' uptake occurring on the opposite side.

'FALSE-POSITIVE' UPTAKE

1 Inflammation associated with recent surgery
2 Inflammatory response to radiotherapy
3 Uptake associated with intravenous lines: take a note of all lines (current and recent); avoid using these lines for injection of tracer
4 Uptake associated with bowel stoma or urinary diversion/ileal conduit

Taking a good history from the patient can help to reduce misinterpretation of scan findings.

In this chapter we have attempted to document as many of the important variations that can cause problems in interpretation. It is not intended to be a totally comprehensive account, but should provide a helpful guide to those new to the field and prevent unnecessary false-positive interpretations with their potential for inappropriate management. Perhaps the best advice that can be offered is: take a good history from the patient, which can help you to spot many potential problems and pitfalls, and check every scan before the patient leaves the department.

EXAMPLES TO ILLUSTRATE KEY ISSUES

CASE 2.1	Normal female scan

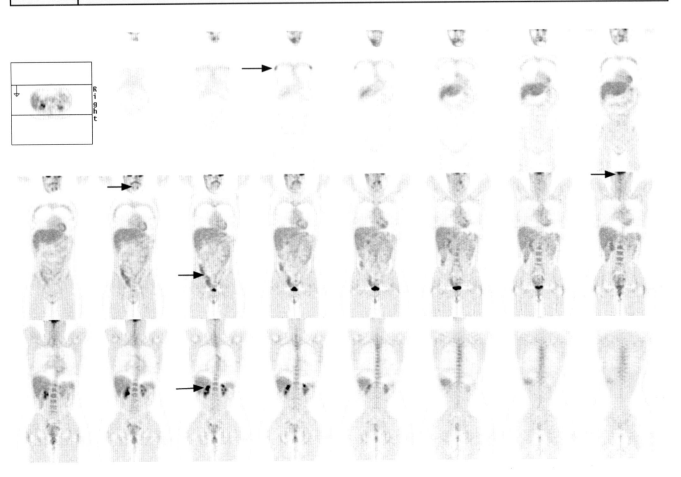

PET/CT findings:

Coronal slices are shown of a normal FDG PET half-body scan of a female. Note there is high uptake in the brain at the edge of the field of view. FDG has been excreted into the renal calyces and bladder. There is also physiologic uptake associated with the bowel, seen best in the cecum/ascending colon. Nipple uptake is a common finding in women. In the head and neck, normal uptake can be seen in the palate and sublingual salivary glands.

CASE 2.2	Normal male scan

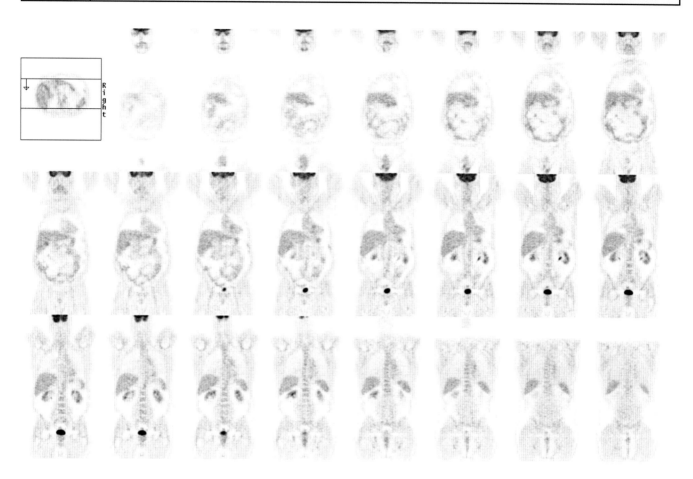

PET/CT findings:

Coronal slices are shown of a normal FDG PET half-body scan of a male. Note again there is significant physiologic uptake associated with large bowel.

CASE 2.3	Normal urinary uptake

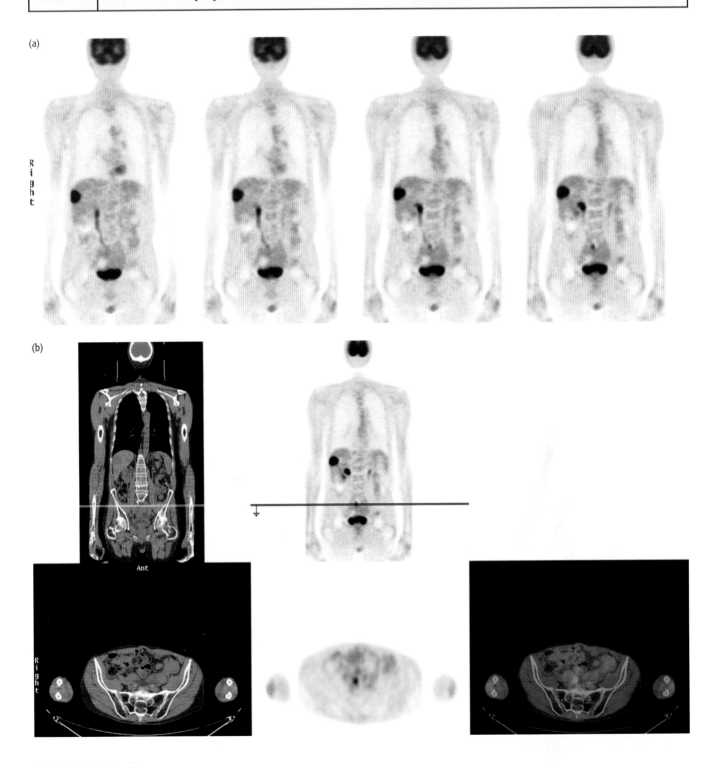

PET/CT findings:

Note there is hold up of tracer in the right ureter in this patient with a solitary liver metastasis from rectal cancer (a). The uptake can be clearly localized to the ureter on the fused image (b).

| CASE 2.4 | Iliac lymphadenopathy mimicking urinary uptake |

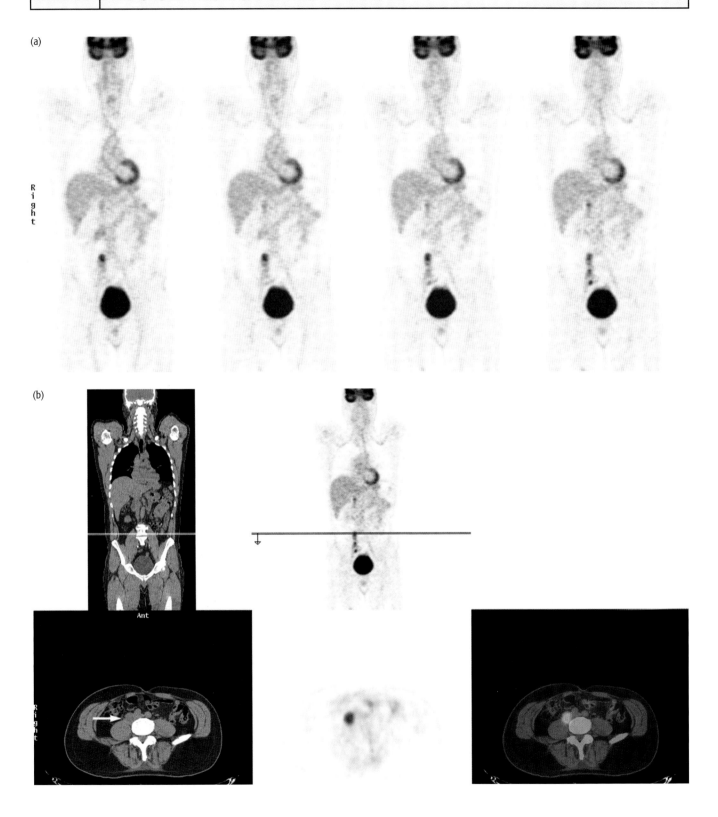

(c)

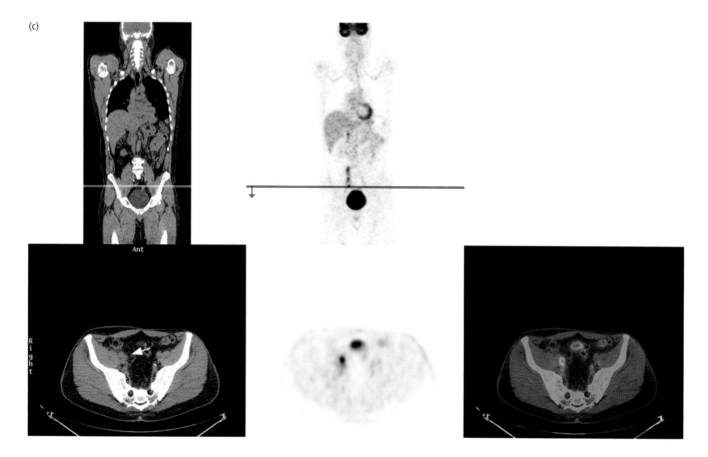

PET/CT findings:

Contrast these images with those of the former case. This patient with a history of melanoma and colon cancer has uptake which looks as though it could be within the right ureter (a) but is clearly located within right common iliac lymph nodes (b) and right external iliac lymph nodes (c) representing metastatic disease.

| CASE 2.5 | Myocardial uptake |

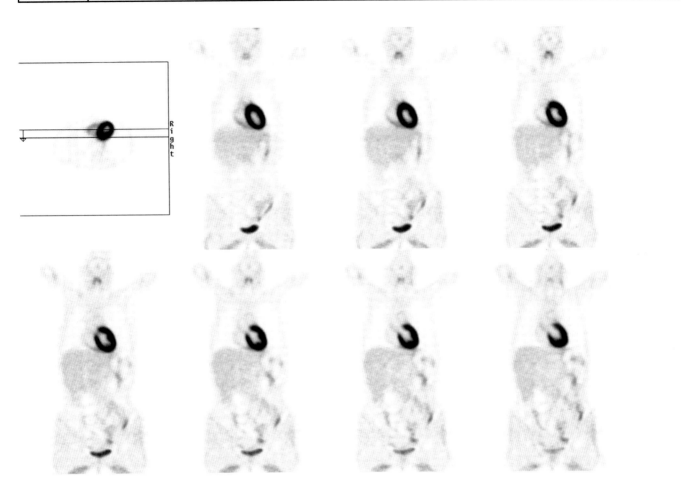

PET/CT findings:

Marked physiologic uptake is seen in the myocardium in this patient.

CASE 2.6	Thymus uptake

(a)

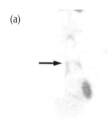

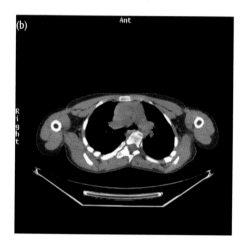

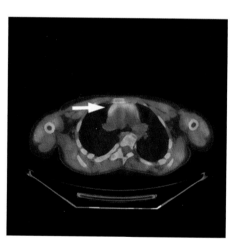

PET/CT findings:

This shows normal thymic uptake in a young patient (aged 12) being scanned for assessment of neurofibroma. Note the typical appearance on coronal PET images (a) and PET/CT axial images (b).

| CASE 2.7 | Stomach uptake |

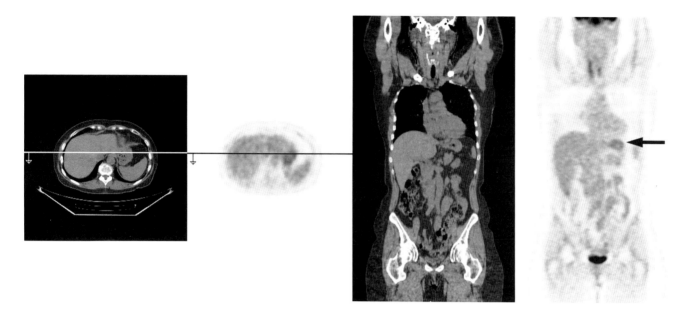

PET/CT findings:

Typical appearances of normal gastric uptake are shown (arrowed).

CASE 2.8	Bowel uptake

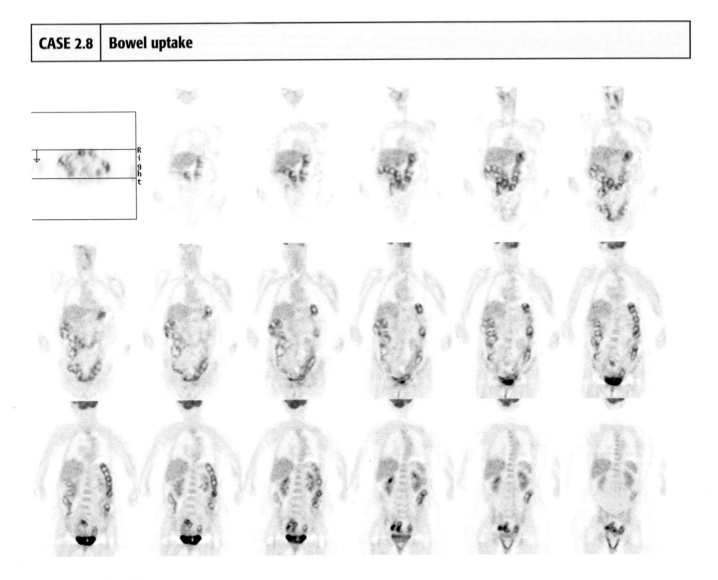

PET/CT findings:

Physiologic uptake within bowel can be marked in some patients.

CASE 2.9 | Bowel uptake and diverticular disease

(a)

(b)

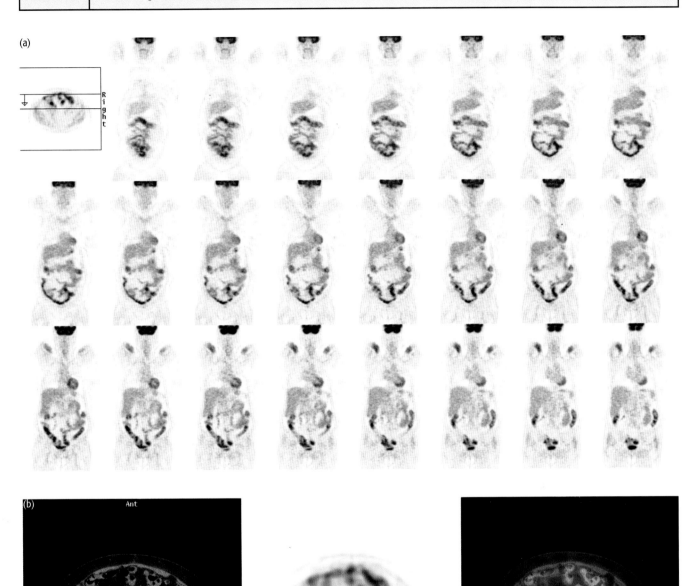

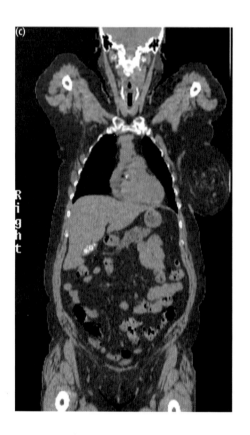 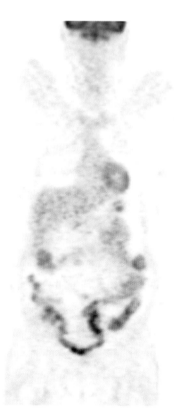 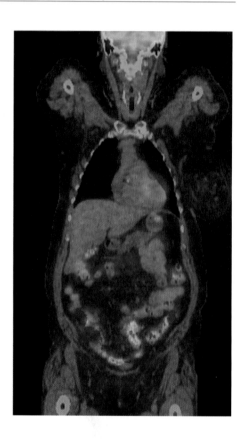

PET/CT findings:

This patient has marked uptake in the bowel associated with diverticular disease. Note the patient has had a right mastectomy.

CASE 2.10	Abdominal hernia

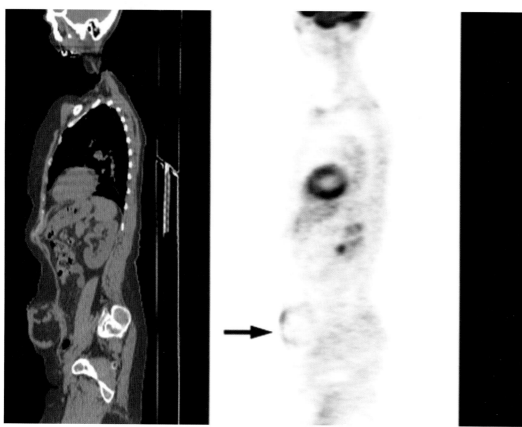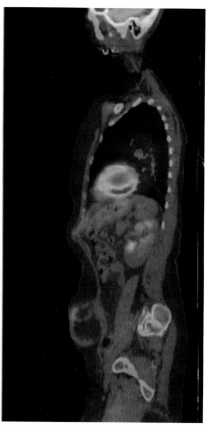

PET/CT findings:

Note uptake in a large abdominal hernia in this patient.

| CASE 2.11 | Bowel stoma |

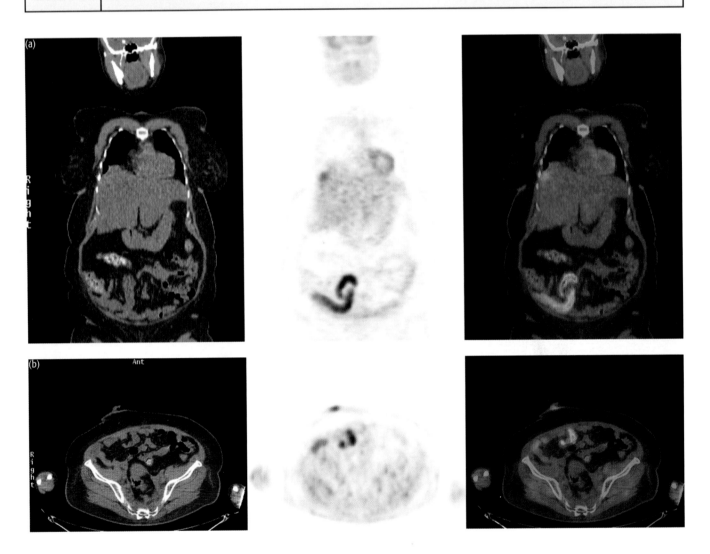

PET/CT findings:

Uptake is commonly seen in bowel stoma, in this case the patient had a defunctioning ileostomy (a, b) while undergoing chemoradiotherapy for rectal cancer. A liver metastasis is seen on the coronal image (a).

CASE 2.12	Ovarian uptake

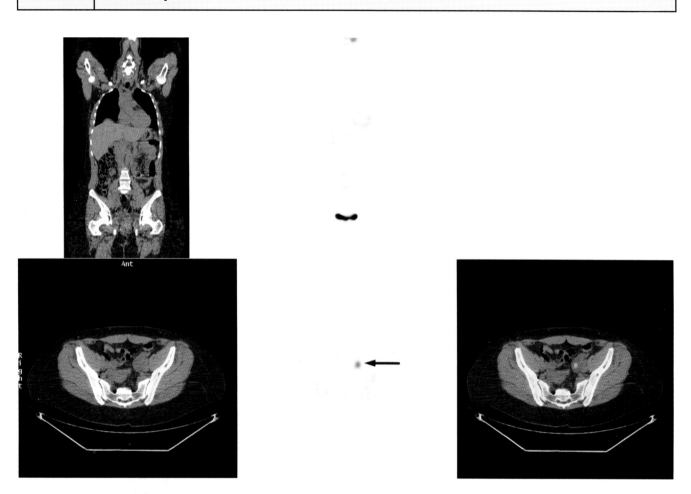

PET/CT findings:

There is uptake in the left ovary. Increased uptake may be seen in premenopausal women without ovarian malignancy, usually at mid-cycle. Increased uptake in postmenopausal women, however, may be associated with malignancy (contrast this case with Case 10.4 in Chapter 10). Normal endometrial uptake in premenopausal women also changes cyclically, increasing during the ovulatory and menstrual phases.

CASE 2.13 | Brown fat

(a)

(b)

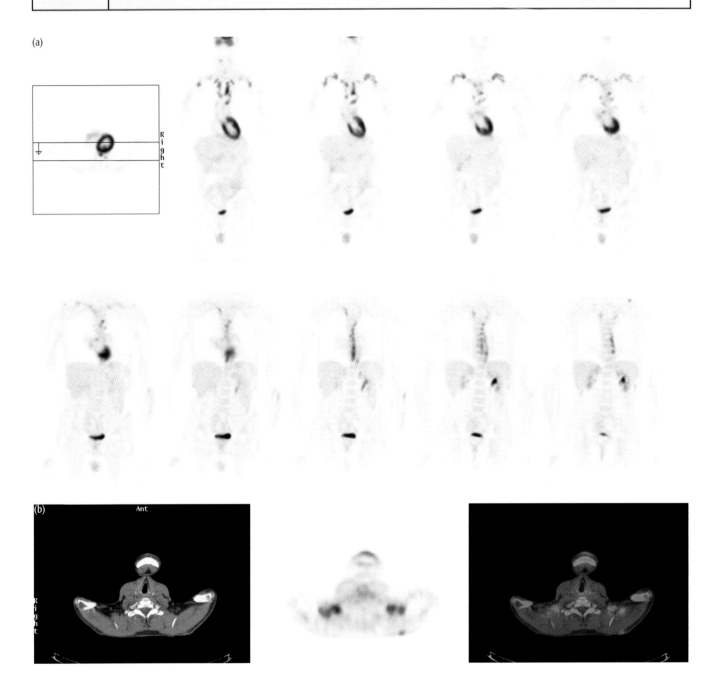

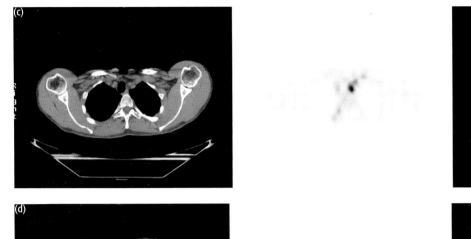

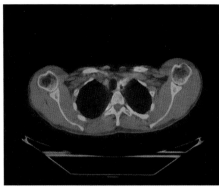

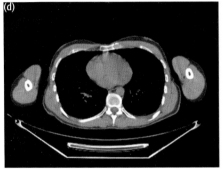

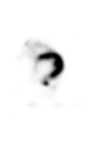

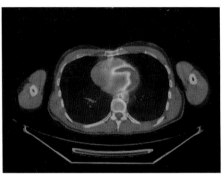

PET/CT findings:

Extensive uptake is associated with brown fat in the neck, upper chest, and paravertebral regions (a). The CT component makes interpretation easier especially where there is asymmetric uptake. The uptake localizes to brown fat in the neck (b), in the fat adjacent to the vessels in the superior mediastinum (c), and in the aortocaval region in the thorax (d). There is also low-grade uptake in a subcutaneous nodule which represents a neurofibroma (b).

CASE 2.14	Brown fat

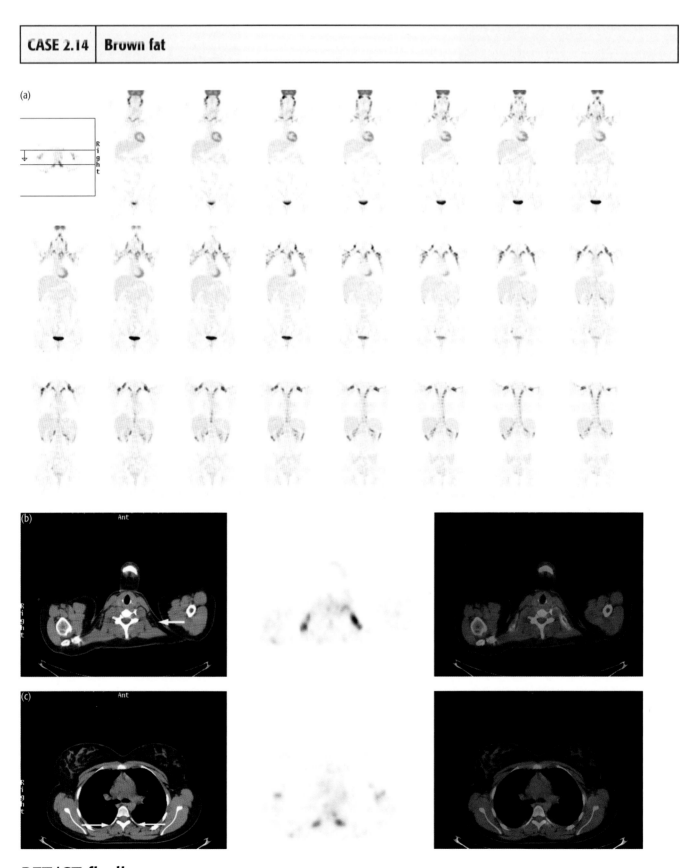

PET/CT findings:

Here is a further example of uptake within brown fat and muscle. Note marked uptake in the neck, upper chest, and paraspinal regions.

CASE 2.15	Muscle uptake – pterygoid muscles

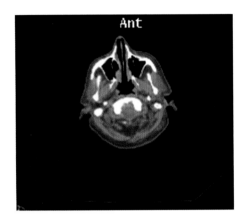
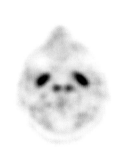
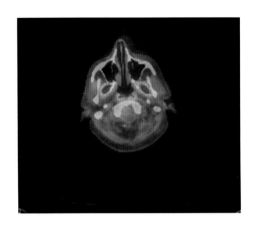

PET/CT findings:

Note in this patient there is symmetric uptake in the pterygoid muscles (and in the adenoids which is physiologic).

CASE 2.16	Muscle uptake – diaphragm uptake with rib fracture

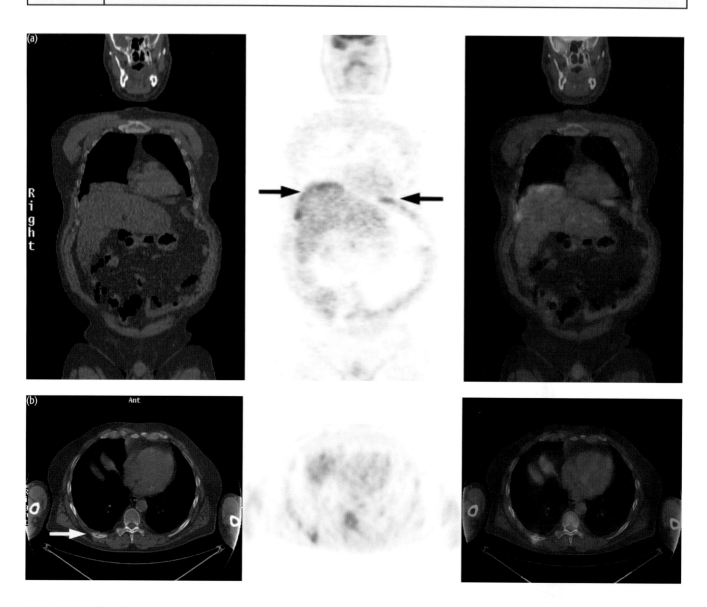

PET/CT findings:

This patient had a recent fracture of the right ninth rib and was experiencing pain in the right posterior chest associated with breathing. There was extensive physiologic uptake seen in the diaphragm bilaterally (a), presumably due to 'splinting' of the diaphragm due to pleuritic pain. Note also the low-grade uptake in the recent fracture (b). Physiologic uptake has also been reported in association with hyperventilation in patients with marked intercostal muscle activity.

CASE 2.17	Bone marrow uptake post chemotherapy

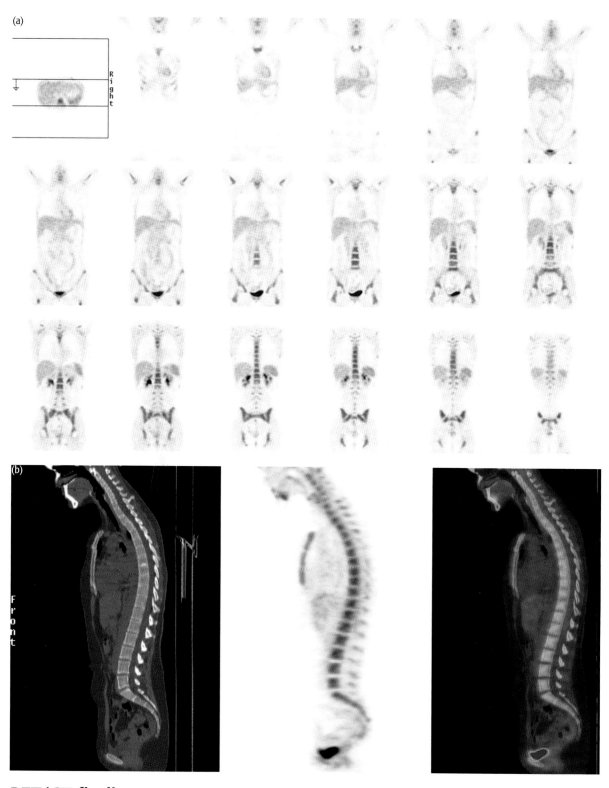

(a)

(b)

PET/CT findings:

Marked physiologic uptake is seen in this patient following chemotherapy reflecting marrow activation. This level of uptake can also be seen following administration of granulocyte colony-stimulating factor.

CASE 2.18	Skin contamination

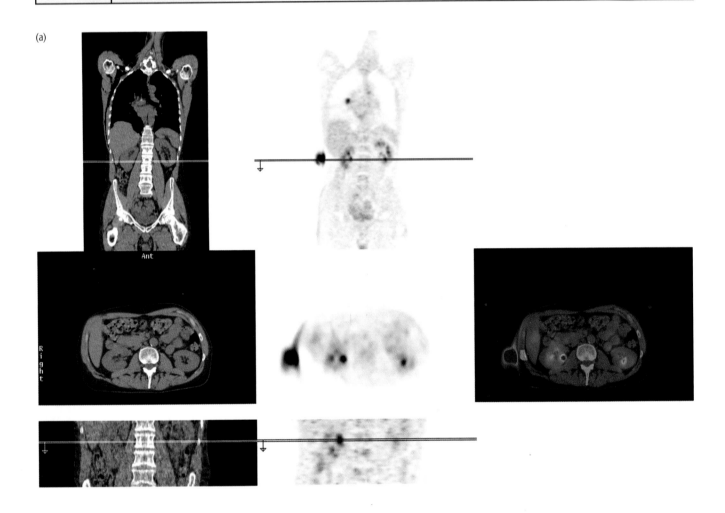

(a)

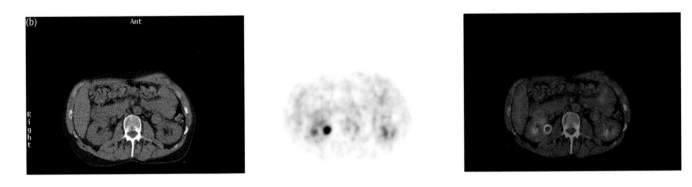

(b)

PET/CT findings:

Skin contamination was present in this patient (a). After checking the images, the area of skin was washed and a local view over the area repeated (b).

CASE 2.19	Insulin administration

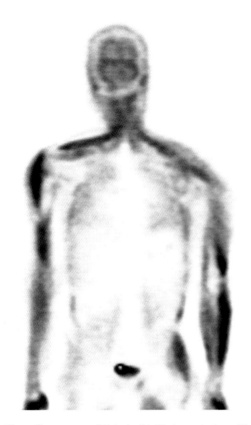 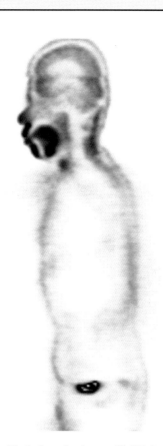

These figures are published with kind permission of Springer Science and Business Media from Barrington SF, O'Doherty MJ (2003) Imaging Limitations of PET for imaging lymphoma. Eur J Nucl Med Mol Imaging 30(Suppl 1), *S117–S127*

PET/CT findings:

This diabetic patient was given insulin in an attempt to lower the blood glucose. Insulin caused marked FDG uptake in skeletal muscle, resulting in a nondiagnostic scan.

| CASE 2.20 | Tissued injection with axillary uptake |

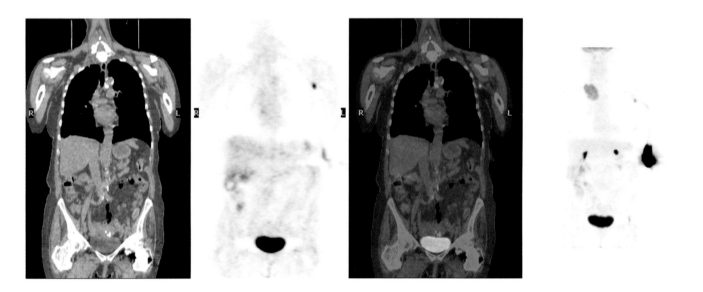

PET/CT findings:

This patient with right upper lobe adenocarcinoma had a tissued injection in the left antecubital fossa. Note uptake in the left axillary lymph node due to subcutaneous tracer tracking along lymphatic channels in the arm. Unless the injection site is scanned, the axillary uptake might be misinterpreted as pathologic. Note also the importance of injecting on the opposite side to known pathology.

CASE 2.21 | **Respiratory motion**

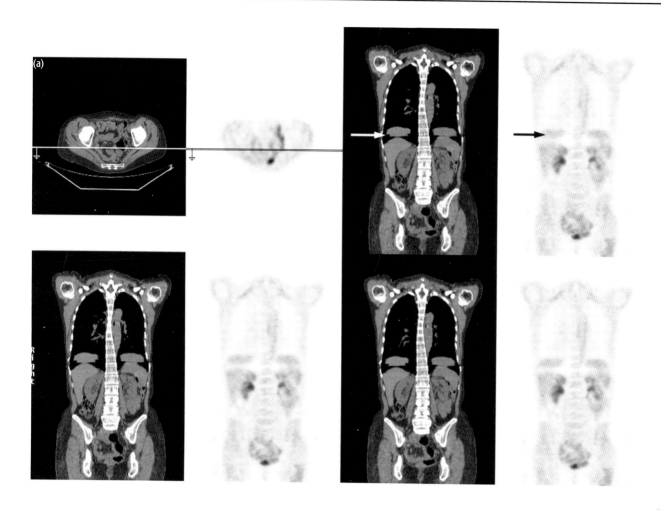

(b)

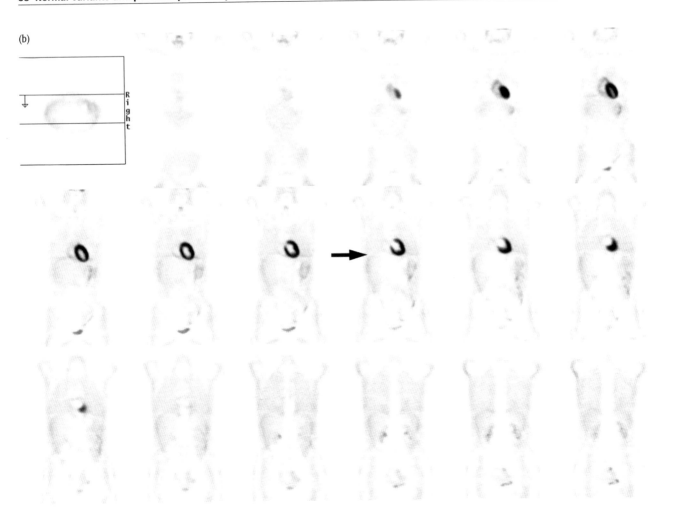

PET/CT findings:

There is a 'double' diaphragm in this patient, sometimes also referred to as 'mushroom' artifact (a). This is due to respiratory motion on the CT component of the scan. Overcorrection of the PET image using the CT data leads to the artifact being seen in the attenuation-corrected PET image (a). It is not present in the nonattenuation-corrected PET image (b).

CASE 2.22 | Misregistration

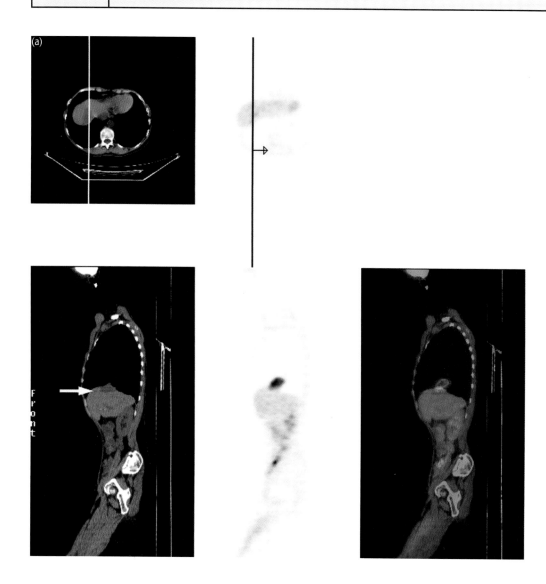

(b)

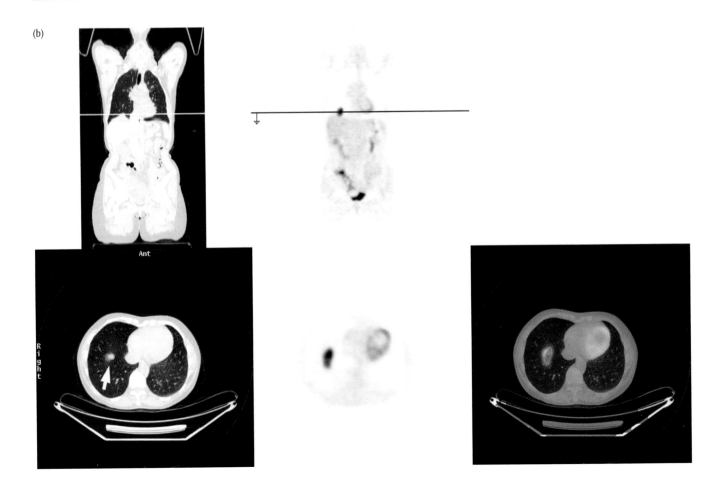

PET/CT findings:

This scan demonstrates focal uptake on the PET scan with a low-attenuation lesion in the dome of the liver on the CT scan (a) consistent with liver metastasis. Note that there is significant misregistration between the PET and the CT because of respiratory motion. The 'mushroom' effect seen at the junction of the liver/lungs is indicative of this (b). Without careful review of the CT scan, the focus of increased uptake on the PET could be mistakenly thought to be located in the base of the right lung (b).

| CASE 2.23 | Truncation of PET data using CT attenuation correction |

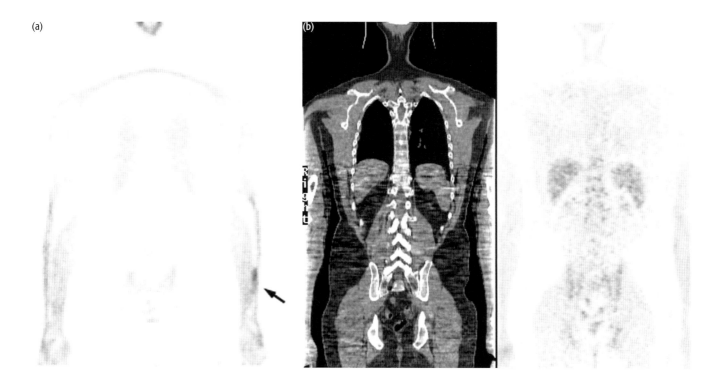

(a)　　(b)

PET/CT findings:

This patient had a metastatic lesion on the left forearm. Uptake is clearly seen on the nonattenuation PET image in the left forearm (a). The CT axial field of view is smaller than the PET and the lesion is not within the field of view. If the CT data are used for attenuation correction of the PET then the lesion is not seen (b).

| CASE 2.24 | Intramuscular injection |

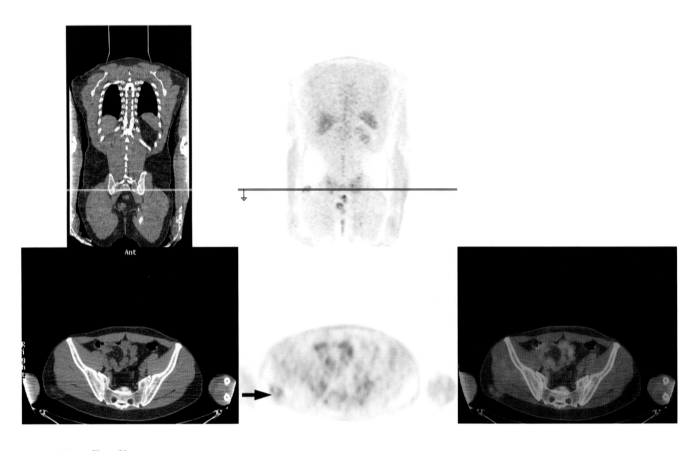

PET/CT findings:

Uptake in the buttocks can be seen as in this patient following intramuscular injection. Subcutaneous deposits can occur in up to 10 percent of patients with cancer, most commonly melanoma breast and lung. A history of recent injections helps to exclude disease.

CASE 2.25	Esophagitis

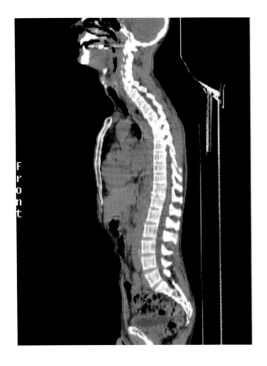 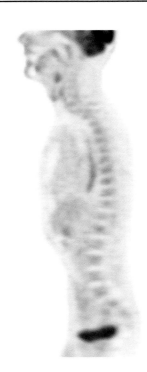 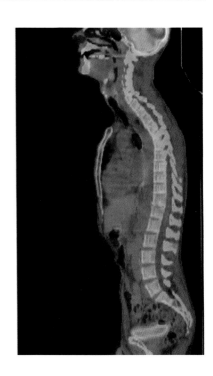

PET/CT findings:

Increased uptake is seen in association with esophagitis.

CASE 2.26	Femoral prosthesis

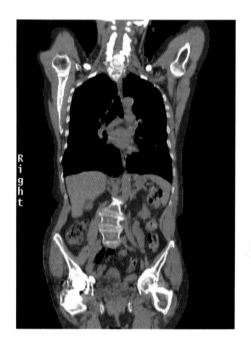  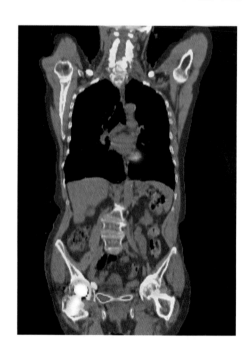

PET/CT findings:

There is inflammatory uptake around the femoral prosthesis.

CASE 2.27	Following mediastinotomy

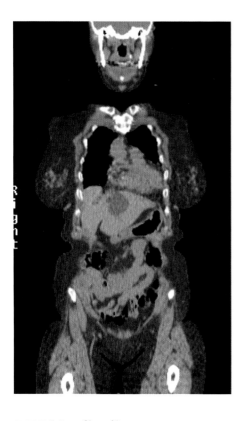 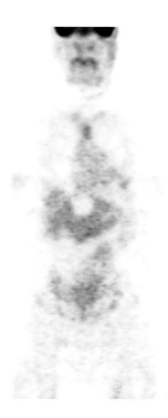 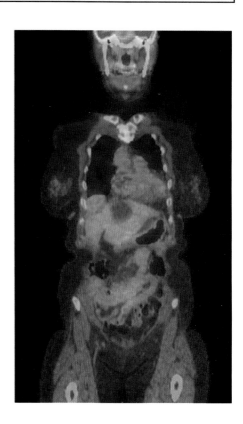

PET/CT findings:

This patient had uptake in the sternum and substernal area following recent mediastinotomy for aortic valve surgery. A liver cyst which is not FDG avid is also seen.

CASE 2.28	Hickman line

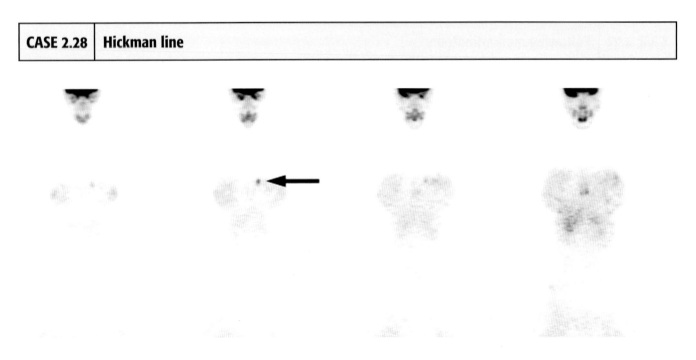

PET/CT findings:

This patient had uptake around the site of a recent Hickman line removed because of infection.

CASE 2.29	Thyroiditis

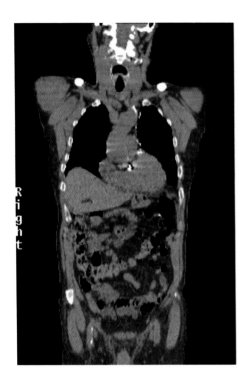 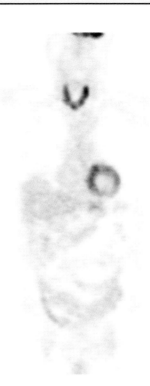 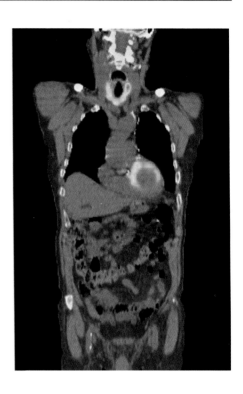

PET/CT findings:

There was marked uptake in the thyroid gland in this patient with known thyroiditis. Increased diffuse uptake can be seen as a normal variant particularly in young women. Focal increased uptake, however, warrants further investigation to exclude a thyroid neoplasm.

FURTHER READING

Bakheet S, Powe J (1998) Benign causes of 18-FDG uptake on whole body imaging. *Semin Nucl Med* 1998, 352–8.

Barrington SF, Maisey MN (1996) Skeletal muscle uptake of fluorine-18-FDG: effect of oral diazepam. *J Nucl Med* 37, 1127–9.

Brink I, Reinhardt M, Hoegerle S *et al.* (2001) Increased metabolic activity in the thymus gland studied with 18F-FDG PET: age dependency and frequency after chemotherapy. *J Nucl Med* 42, 591–5.

Cook GJ, Maisey MN, Fogelman I (1999) Normal variants, artefacts and interpretative pitfalls in PET imaging with 18-fluoro-2-deoxyglucose and carbon-11 methionine. *Eur J Nucl Med* 26, 1363–78.

Cook GJR, Wegner EA, Fogelman I (2004) Pitfalls and artifacts in [18]FDG PET and PET/CT oncologic imaging. *Semin Nucl Med* 34, 122–33.

Gordon BA, Flanagan FL, Dehdashti F. (1997) Whole body positron emission tomography: normal variations, pitfalls and technical considerations. *Am J Roentgenol* 169, 1675–80.

Hany TF, Gharehpapagh E, Kamel E *et al.* (2002) Brown adipose tissue: a factor to consider in symmetrical tracer uptake in the neck and upper chest region. *Eur J Nucl Med* 29, 1393–8.

Lerman H, Metser U, Grisaru D *et al.* (2004) Normal and abnormal 18F-FDG endometrial and ovarian uptake in pre and post menopausal patients: assessment by PET-CT. *J Nucl Med* 45, 266–71.

Miraldi FDG, Vesselle H, Faulhaber PF, Adler LP, Leisure GP (1998) Elimination of artifactual accumulation of FDG in PET imaging of colorectal cancer. *Clin Nucl Med* 23, 3–7.

Nakahara T, Fujii H, Ide M *et al.* (2001) FDG uptake in the morphologically normal thymus: comparison of FDG positron emission tomography and CT. *Br J Radiol* 74, 821–4.

Stokkel MP, Bongers V, Hordijk GJ, van Rijk PP (1999) FDG positron emission tomography in head and neck cancer: pitfall or pathology? *Clin Nucl Med* **24**, 950–4.

Sugawara Y, Fisher SJ, Zasadny KR *et al.* (1998) Preclinical and clinical studies of bone marrow uptake of fluorine-1-flourodeoxyglucose with or without granulocyte colony-stimulating factor during chemotherapy. *J Clin Oncol* **16**, 173–80.

Sugawara Y, Zasadny KR, Kison PV, Baker LH, Wahl RL (1999) Splenic fluorodeoxyglucose uptake increased by granulocyte colony-stimulating factor therapy: PET imaging results. *J Nucl Med* **40**, 1456–62.

PART II
Applications of PET in oncology

CHAPTER 3
OVERVIEW OF ONCOLOGIC APPLICATIONS OF PET AND PET/CT

INTRODUCTION

At present, in nearly all clinical positron emission tomography (PET) imaging centers, imaging of cancer with [^{18}F]2-fluoro-2-deoxy-D-glucose (FDG) represents the vast majority of the clinical PET volume, usually representing over 90 percent of total clinical workload. Of interest is that PET/computed tomography (CT) scanners now account for nearly all of the new PET scanner sales in the world, and currently, it would appear that PET/CT will replace PET imaging of cancer. Indeed, this transformation has already occurred at our PET centers. This extensive use of PET (and PET/CT) in cancer imaging is not surprising given that cancer recently became the most common cause of death in the USA, surpassing cardiovascular disease in frequency. These demographic trends are also seen in other Western industrialized countries. The incidence of cancer is increasing in most age groups. The reasons for this continuing rise in cancer frequency include increasing levels of environmental carcinogens, increasing age of the population, and other factors. Tobacco use and dietary fat play major etiological roles in several types of cancer, notably lung and colorectal. There is now over a one in three chance of an individual contracting cancer at some time during his or her lifetime. Although many of these cancers are now curable, many others remain incurable; though most are 'treatable' and the most appropriate selection of therapy for the individual patient is highly desirable.

Complete surgical excision remains the best means for treating and curing cancers diagnosed when the primary cancers are small and localized, but far too many patients are found to be inoperable at surgery, or experience relapse soon after, because undetected spread of cancer has already occurred. The problem of operations being performed on inoperable cancers has a significant cost to the patient as well as creating an enormous inefficiency in the use of healthcare resources. For example, the 5-year survival of patients with mediastinal spread of lung cancer is approximately 5–10 percent, whereas those patients without mediastinal spread have a 5-year survival of approximately 45–50 percent. PET is now commonly used to reduce the frequency of unnecessary surgery by selecting patients with resectable disease. A randomized trial of PET versus no PET use in lung cancer staging showed a 50 percent reduction in the frequency of unnecessary thoracotomy in the PET group.

Radiation therapy and chemotherapy are both alternative and additional methods of treatment. Rational delivery of radiation therapy requires accurate delineation of target tumor volume. This can be achieved well with PET and treatment plans can differ markedly from those plans without PET, and PET/CT can improve the accuracy of planning still further. Chemotherapy in particular is increasingly used both as primary treatment and adjuvant or neoadjuvant therapy in an effort to render inoperable cancer operable or to cure some tumors such as lymphomas. PET scanning is increasingly being applied to the problem of rapidly assessing and predicting the response to treatment. Efforts are also being made to provide early prediction of the effectiveness of a chemotherapy regimen, which if successful will significantly improve patient management outcome and cost-effectiveness of treatment regimens. In many instances PET scanning is providing more accurate information than anatomic imaging methods; in other cases it provides unique additional information. One of the most important challenges is to define the most accurate and cost-effective diagnostic pathway for any individual clinical situation.

PET and PET/CT are used in several clinical situations. In some instances, the characterization of a lesion, which has been identified in screening programs using anatomic methods or has been found incidentally as part of evaluation of an unrelated condition, as benign or malignant may be needed. This is quite commonly done in cases of solitary pulmonary nodules, where PET has an accuracy in excess of 90 percent in characterization of lesions above 1 cm in size. When cancer is present at initial diagnosis, an important question is whether the tumor is localized or disseminated. This often determines whether the tumor is resectable for cure by surgical techniques, or whether it has disseminated to such an extent that it cannot be successfully removed by surgery and needs additional treatment with radiation therapy or chemotherapy. Basic approaches to tumor staging are quite similar from disease to disease. They generally consider:

• the size of the primary lesion and whether it has invaded local structures (**T stage**)
• whether the primary tumor has spread to regional lymph nodes (**N stage**)
• whether the tumor has spread beyond the regional lymph nodes to the rest of the body (**M stage**).

Resecting a primary tumor when disease has disseminated systemically will not be curative. Indeed, such an endeavor can be counterproductive as there are major risks of morbidity and mortality and costs associated with surgical procedures, which are not curative. As an example, for elderly patients with impaired pulmonary function, thoracotomy can result in a mortality of 5–10 percent. Such a risk, along with a cost of over $30 000, cannot be justified if the disease has spread beyond the surgical field and satisfactory local tumor control can be achieved by nonsurgical methods. This scenario occurs in several common cancers, and accurate diagnostic tests are needed to ensure that aggressive or radical surgical procedures are not undertaken in patients who are unlikely to benefit from them, and are indeed more likely to be harmed. Using accurate staging information, a rational choice of therapy can be made. One of the first rules in medicine is 'do no harm'. An accurate understanding of the location(s) of tumors is one of the pieces of information needed for this to be achieved, and PET has been shown to be an excellent method for staging many cancers. Where directly compared, PET/CT has generally performed better than PET in diagnostic accuracy. It is important to realize that PET and PET/CT, although powerful methods, have limitations as regards the size of the lesion detected. The reconstructed resolution of modern PET systems is typically about 1 cm. Although lesions smaller than the resolution can be detected, the efficiency of lesion detection falls in lesions under 5 mm in size. PET and PET/CT are not equivalent to a microscope and proper direct histologic inspection of regional lymph nodes, such as following sentinel node surgery, is a more sensitive method than PET or PET/CT in low tumor burden nodal disease.

Once cancer is diagnosed, determining how to treat it or whether the treatment has been effective can be challenging. Since many chemotherapeutic agents work in less than half the patients receiving them, a rapid identification of which tumors are responding and which are resistant at an early time point will be extremely valuable as a means of individualizing therapy. Most responding tumors will eventually shrink in size with effective treatments, but the shrinkage can be slow and sometimes incomplete even though the tumor is 'dead' and has been replaced with scar. PET with FDG can often detect the early metabolic changes that occur soon after effective treatment is initiated. For instance in lymphoma, interim assessment of treatment after two cycles of chemotherapy may be a better predictor of disease-free survival than CT assessment at the end of six cycles. In other situations, the area of the tumor may be hard to assess after surgery or radiation therapy because of treatment-induced changes in anatomy. One of the more empirical aspects of cancer management is the choice of which chemotherapeutic agent to use, how to determine if the treatment is working, and to determine how much treatment is sufficient … or too much. Since chemotherapy causes major toxicity and has substantial costs, excessive treatment is undesirable. Treating a scar with chemotherapy is not particularly useful. However, it is very important to treat residual living cancer aggressively. These determinations are not made optimally with current imaging methods but are increasingly made earlier and with greater accuracy using PET and PET/CT.

CT and magnetic resonance imaging (MRI), while cornerstones of cancer imaging, have major limitations for staging. FDG PET is consistently more sensitive and specific than CT in staging mediastinal lymph nodes for metastases of nonsmall cell lung cancer – and FDG PET/CT is more accurate than PET alone. CT and MRI have difficulty in assessing the entire body for cancer and extreme difficulty in separating benign postoperative/postradiation changes from viable tumor. PET/CT currently appears to be the best single modality for assessing the presence/absence of active cancer in the whole body.

LIMITATIONS OF ANATOMIC IMAGING METHODS

1 Inability to determine if a mass is benign or malignant based on size/shape
2 Inability to determine if enlarged lymph nodes contain cancer
3 Inability to detect small tumor foci in lymph nodes or elsewhere
4 Inability to predict or to rapidly assess the response of a cancer to treatment
5 Inability to determine whether a residual abnormality present after treatment represents scar or tumor
6 Difficulty in assessing the entire body for cancer
7 Most contrast-enhancing agents are not specific for cancer

ADVANTAGES OF PET MOLECULAR IMAGING

1 Ability to distinguish viable metabolically active tissue from scar
2 Potential to use a variety of metabolic tracers to assess spectrum of tissue function
3 Ability to provide quantitative measurements of metabolic activity of cancer cells
4 Ability to rapidly detect treatment-induced change before there is any change in size of a mass
5 Detection is highly dependent on the intensity of the signal and less so on the tumor size
6 Postsurgical or postradiation distortion of anatomy is less important for accurate interpretation than with MRI or CT. CT and PET can be combined as PET/CT

PET offers the proved ability to improve on CT and MRI in these difficult clinical settings. Metabolic imaging complements anatomic imaging and addresses the shortfalls. PET/CT combines both anatomic and functional imaging using strengths from both methods.

PET AND THE CANCER CELL

In the late 1980s and early 1990s the use of PET for imaging cancer was considered a research endeavor, requiring a team of various kinds of researcher. PET cameras remain expensive, but in most current clinical PET centers, FDG (the most commonly used PET cancer imaging radiopharmaceutical) can be purchased from a regional cyclotron facility, and it is not necessary for a cyclotron to be owned by a clinical PET imaging center to perform clinical PET or PET/CT imaging. Similarly, powerful image processing computers are routinely available with modern PET and PET/CT systems. Thus, PET and PET/CT imaging can be initiated for the cost of purchasing and installing a PET or PET/CT scanning system, which can be less than US$2 million. While still expensive, this cost is not vastly beyond the range of other imaging technologies such as MRI. In a rather short period of time, because of the impact on clinical management, FDG PET has moved from being a research tool to a clinical tool. And recently PET/CT has moved rapidly to being a clinical tool without which it is not possible to practice optimal cancer therapy. Subsequent chapters of this book will present many examples of the clinical utility of PET and PET/CT. These developments could not have happened except for the remarkable ability of cancer cells to accumulate FDG as FDG 6-phosphate.

Although many metabolic alterations are present in cancers but not in normal tissues, and can be targeted with PET, this clinical atlas focuses mainly on the excessive glucose metabolism seen in many cancers. The observation that tumors have increased rates of glycolysis compared with most normal tissues was first made by Warburg over 60 years ago, and has been shown to be true in most human cancers. ^{18}F has a 109 min half-life and is generally cyclotron produced. FDG was first used in humans for brain imaging in the mid 1970s. In 1980, Som and colleagues demonstrated that FDG accumulated in rodent tumors following intravenous administration, apparently due to metabolic trapping. In 1982, the first imaging of human tumors was reported, both in brain tumors and colorectal cancer metastatic to the liver (Patronas et al., 1982; Yonekura et al., 1982).

KEY DEVELOPMENTS	
1930	Raised aerobic glycolysis in tumor cells (Warburg, 1930)
1974	First human PET tomograph built by Phelps and Hoffmann (Phelps *et al.*, 1976)
1978	FDG synthesized by Wolf and Fowler (Ido *et al.*, 1978)
1979	FDG for cerebral glucose metabolism (Reivich *et al.*, 1979)
1980	FDG for tumors in animals (Som *et al.*, 1980)
1982	FDG in brain tumor (Patronas *et al.*, 1982)
1982	FDG in colon cancer (Yonekura *et al.*, 1982)
1991	FDG for primary and metastatic breast cancer (Wahl *et al.*, 1991; Shields, 1998)

METABOLIC DIFFERENCES BETWEEN NORMAL TISSUE AND CANCER

Cancer tissue has:

  increased glycolysis
  increased protein synthesis
  more anoxic and hypoxic cells
  increased or decreased receptors
  increased DNA synthesis
  increased blood flow
  increased amino acid transport
  increased membrane synthesis and choline accumulation
  altered neo vasculature with altered integrin expression profile
  and increased vascular permeability

THE USE OF FDG

Although a rather wide range of biochemical alterations are present in cancer cells, the one studied most often in clinical PET has been the relative overconsumption of glucose by tumor cells. FDG, the ^{18}F-labeled analog of 2-deoxy-D-glucose, is transported into the cancer cells like glucose by facilitative glucose transporter molecules (often Glut 1), and is phosphorylated to FDG 6-phosphate by hexokinase (often hexokinase type II, see Fig. 3.1). FDG 6-phosphate is polar and does not cross cell membranes well, i.e. it is trapped in cancer cells. FDG 6-phosphate can be dephosphorylated to FDG by glucose-6-phosphatase, but this reaction occurs relatively slowly, particularly in cancer cells, which commonly lack glucose-6-phosphatase or have relatively low levels of it.

In the past several years, there has been rapid growth in the use of FDG for cancer imaging. This is because, in a wide variety of human cancers, a high tumor/background uptake ratio develops just 0.5–2 h after intravenous injection (Larson et al., 1981; Wahl et al., 1991b). The mechanisms for this increased FDG 6-phosphate accumulation in many cancer cells has been shown to be due to:

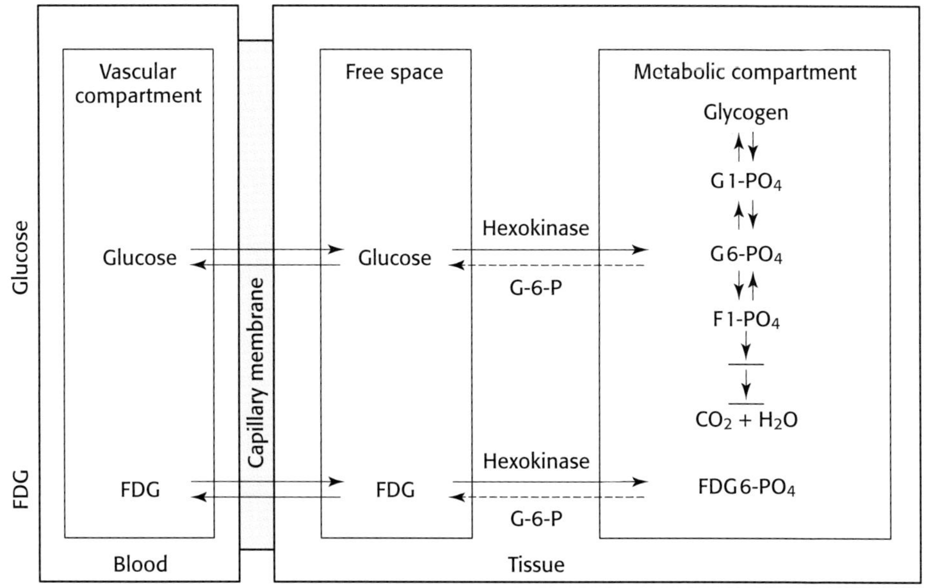

PET imaging is generally successful in cancer imaging because cancers differ from normal tissues in several ways. There are multiple alterations in cancer physiology, which can be detected using positron-emitting tracers. Tumors commonly grow more rapidly than normal tissues, and thus have higher rates of glucose metabolism, DNA synthesis, amino acid transport, and membrane synthesis. Tumors often express qualitatively or quantitatively different antigenic phenotypes from many normal tissues, as well as increased numbers of receptors, such as the estrogen receptor on some breast cancers. In addition, tumors commonly have different blood vessels than normal tissues.

Figure 3.1 *Compartmental model for glucose and FDG ([^{18}F]2-fluoro-2-deoxy-D-glucose)*

- increased expression of glucose transporter molecules at the tumor cell surface
- increased levels/activity of hexokinase (and other glycolytic enzymes)
- reduced levels of glucose-6-phosphatase compared with most normal tissues (Wahl, 1996) and in some instances increased blood flow
- hypoxia in many tumors which is known to upregulate FDG uptake (Brown *et al.*, 1993).

Autoradiographic studies have shown that there is much more FDG uptake into areas of viable tumor than into areas of frank necrosis, but studies in some rodent tumor models and in humans have shown that the uptake of FDG can be into areas where inflammatory cells are present or into areas of infection (Kubola *et al.*, 1992; Brown *et al.*, 1993). Thus, FDG is not a tumor-specific tracer and other disease processes can accumulate FDG, such as inflammatory arthritis, sarcoidosis, and tuberculosis among others.

The major tracer used to trace glucose metabolism is FDG, which is transported into cancer cells like glucose and phosphorylated like glucose, but is not substantially moved beyond this point in the intracellular glucose metabolic pathway.

BASIS OF FDG USE IN ONCOLOGY

Increased aerobic and anaerobic glycolysis:
  increased glucose transport
  increased hexokinase
  decreased glucose-6-phosphatase
FDG accumulation is greater in conditions of hypoxia
Cell surface glucose transporter molecules (Glut 1–5) (and others)
Activation of gene coding for synthesis of Glut 1 in tumors
Overexpression of Glut 1 and 3 demonstrated

Cancers often overexpress glucose transporter molecules such as Glut 1, and thus transport excess glucose; cancers often have elevated levels of hexokinase activity (especially hexokinase type II) and phosphorylate glucose faster than normal tissues; finally some tumors also have slower rates via loss of glucose-6-phosphatase than normal tissues, accentuating the accumulation of phosphorylated glucose analogs in tumors. The quantitative level of alterations in these metabolic pathways will often be greater in the more aggressive than the less aggressive tumors, leading to the potential for characterizing the aggressiveness of human tumors noninvasively. However, in several studies FDG uptake is more related to viable cell number than to proliferative rate.

WHY IS FDG SO USEFUL?

Long half-life for a PET tracer, but not too long to have unfavorable dosimetry
Availability; regional distribution possible
High uptake (T/NT) in most human cancers
'Reflects' glycolysis
Broad downstream marker of tumor activity

The normal human '*in vivo*' distribution of FDG includes the brain, heart, kidneys, bowel, and urinary tract, at 1 h after tracer injection (see Cases 2.1 and 2.2). Myocardial uptake is variable, and highly dependent on the dietary status of the patient, as the heart expresses insulin-sensitive glucose transporters (Glut 4) and myocardial uptake is thus enhanced in the presence of insulin, though in the fasting state there is little uptake of FDG in muscle. Serum fatty acid levels also influence FDG uptake in the myocardium. Prolonged fasting and low insulin levels are associated with the lowest levels of FDG uptake in the myocardium. Similarly, skeletal muscle has increased uptake of FDG in the presence of insulin. In general, at least 4 h of fasting is recommended before FDG PET studies in cancer, as fasting lowers insulin levels and also generally reduces blood sugar levels compared with the postprandial state (Wahl *et al.*, 1991b). Uptake within the myocardium can be variable.

High blood glucose levels can interfere with tumor targeting owing to competitive inhibition of FDG uptake by D-glucose. The latter phenomenon has been shown in preclinical and clinical series, although diabetes does not preclude the possibility of PET imaging of cancer in many patients. At present, the optimal method for handling diabetic patients for PET imaging is uncertain; but many centers have the patients fast and do not administer additional insulin (despite serum glucose level elevations), and obtain useful diagnostic information. Standardized uptake values (SUVs) can be lower than expected in diabetic patients, however, as well as tumor/background uptake ratios. Giving insulin just before tumor imaging with FDG in a diabetic patient can be counterproductive as the FDG may all go to skeletal muscle due to the effects of insulin, lowering diagnostic accuracy.

The exact meaning of the 'signal' seen during PET imaging of cancers remains a matter of active investigation. FDG does not precisely trace glucose metabolism despite its structural similarity to D-glucose: FDG has somewhat more uptake into tumors than would be expected for a tracer of glucose metabolism alone. This may be due to differences in transport of FDG and D-glucose, or possibly due to altered affinity of hexokinase for FDG rather than D-glucose, as their metabolism is clearly not identical. Although initial studies in brain tumors suggested that FDG uptake was strongly related to the proliferative activity of tumor cells, this has been questioned. *In vitro*, several groups have found a strong correlation between the number of viable cancer cells and the extent of FDG uptake. This relation between FDG uptake and the number of viable cancer cells also been shown *in vivo* in several animal models, e.g. in breast cancer (Brown *et al.*, 1996). This area remains under intense study, but there seems little question that high levels of FDG uptake are most consistent with a substantial number of viable cancer cells being present. Recent patient data in breast cancer have shown a consistent relation between FDG uptake and the number of Glut 1 positive viable cancer cells (Bos). It is clearly a multifactorial process, however, and careful *in vitro* studies have shown FDG uptake to be well correlated in single cells with the extent of mitochondrially bound hexokinase. The *in vivo* situation is complicated by issues of tracer delivery.

While FDG is an excellent tumor tracer, it has clear limitations. Many prostate cancers, renal cancers, and hepatomas have low levels of FDG uptake and can be undetectable when using FDG PET. So other tracers are needed for these conditions. The biologic reasons for these disparities in FDG uptake by different tumor types are under evaluation. Some tumors do induce a major host response and part of the signal seen on PET may be due to FDG accumulation in inflammatory cells as well as in the tumor cells themselves. While the clinical specificity of PET scanning with FDG is generally high, it should also be noted that FDG is by no means a specific tracer for tumors. Rather it traces glucose utilization, and benign conditions such as sarcoidosis and some infections can have intense FDG uptake *in vivo*. It is apparent that several factors govern FDG uptake into tumors, but clinical studies generally show that high FDG uptake is associated with tumors which are aggressive. Clinical studies, in several types of cancer, consistently show that with effective cytotoxic treatments, FDG uptake declines rapidly, often in days to weeks, and that rapid and continuing declines in FDG uptake are indicative of a good treatment response, whereas failure of FDG uptake to decline in a lesion in predicts a poorer response and reduced survival compared with responding patients.

ADDITIONAL CLINICAL TRACERS FOR CANCER

Glycolysis, while of tremendous importance in clinical PET imaging of cancer, is only one of several processes, which may be targeted for PET imaging. The transport and utilization of several amino acids is typical of many cancers. [^{11}C]L-Methionine, a tracer with a 20 min half-life has been used to a moderate extent in clinical PET imaging, especially in Japan where, in some centers with cyclotrons, its use is more common than that of FDG. This agent is more restricted in availability than FDG, because of its much shorter half-life (20 min for ^{11}C vs. 109 min for ^{18}F), but can be very helpful in imaging brain and other tumors. Use of ^{11}C]L-methionine in cancer imaging is based on this experience and the increased activity of the transmethylation pathways in some cancers. There is normally substantial uptake of this tracer in the pancreas, salivary glands, liver, bone marrow, and kidneys. [11]C]L-Methionine is a natural amino acid, so some metabolism occurs in the bloodstream and there is some limited uptake of ^{11}C into the normal brain, though the uptake is much lower there than with FDG. This tracer has been used in brain tumor imaging (including pituitary adenomas), in head and neck cancer imaging, in lymphomas and in lung cancers (Bergstrom *et al.*, 1983; Kubota *et al.*, 1985). The study of amino acid transport may be all that is possible if ^{11}C, with its 20 min half-life, is chosen as the tracer, as even with ^{11}C]L-methionine much of the early imaging is of the transport process, with relatively less of the protein synthetic process. This agent and ^{18}F-labeled amino acids may be of particular relevance in brain tumor imaging.

Other alterations in tumor physiology may be more tumor specific than general, allowing for the development of very specific PET radiopharmaceuticals. As an example, radioligands with specificity for the estrogen receptor expressed on many well-differentiated breast cancers are quite specific for their uptake into tissues rich in estrogen receptor (Mintun *et al.*, 1988). Similarly, PET tracers specific for monoamine uptake pathways are quite specific for adrenergic tissues such as pheochromocytomas (Shulkin *et al.*, 1993, 1999). Choline, both with ^{11}C and with ^{18}F labels has shown excellent capabilities for imaging prostate cancer, among others (Hara *et al.*, 1998, 2002; DeGrado *et al.*, 2000).

Other PET tracers of interest, currently showing potential in the research setting include:

- [11]C] thymidine and [^{18}F], FLT, tracers measuring tumor proliferation (Shields *et al.*, 1998)
- [11]C- and ^{18}F-labelled choline, which image prostate cancer well in some studies (DeGrado *et al.*, 2000; Hara *et al.*, 2002)
- [11]C] acetate, which can image some prostate cancers (Kato *et al.*, 2002; Oyama *et al.*, 2002)
- [18]F] sodium fluoride for imaging bone remodeling and metastases (Schirrmeister *et al.*, 1999, 2001)
- labeled receptor or antigen binding ligands such as agents binding to integrin targets in blood vessels (Haubner *et al.*, 2001)
- agents which trace tumor hypoxia such as fluoromisonidazole (Rajendran *et al.*, 2002) and possibly copper-labeled ATSM (Lewis *et al.*, 1999).

Although beyond the scope of this clinical atlas, such agents have considerable potential for expanding the clinical applications of PET and are likely to grow in importance in the coming years, especially as fluorinated analogs are made available.

HOW PET CAN BE USED CLINICALLY

		Examples
1	Diagnosis and lesion characterization	Benign vs. malignant in the solitary pulmonary nodule Prognostic grading of primary brain tumor
2	Extent of disease (staging), local and distant	Nonsmall cell lung cancer; Hodgkin disease, melanoma
3	Localization of primary disease	Unknown primary, e.g. head and neck
4	Treatment response, early and late	Lymphoma (with or without residual mass) Neoadjuvant therapy of esophageal or lung cancer
5	Suspected relapse of disease localization of raised serum markers, clinical features, or radiological changes	Head and neck cancer, colorectal cancer
6	Guiding biopsy	Brain, lung cancer, soft tissue sarcoma
7	Planning and guiding therapy	Lung cancer radiotherapy planning

REFERENCES AND FURTHER READING

Bergstrom M, Collins VP, Ehras E *et al.* (1983) Discrepancies in brain tumor extent as shown by CT and PET using ^{68}Ga-EDTA, ^{11}C-glucose and ^{11}C-methionine. *J Comput Assist Tomogr* **6**, 1062–6.

Brown RS, Fisher SJ, Wahl RL (1993) Autoradiographic evaluation of the intra-tumoral distribution of 2-deoxy-D-glucose and monoclonal antibodies in xenografts of human ovarian adenocarcinoma. *J Nucl Med* **34**, 75–82.

Brown RS, Leung JY, Fisher S *et al.* (1996) Intratumoral distribution of tritiated-FDG in breast carcinoma: correlation between glut-1 expression and FDG uptake. *J Nucl Med* **37**, 1042–7.

DeGrado TR, Coleman RE, Wang S *et al.* (2000) Synthesis and evaluation of 18F-labeled choline as an oncologic tracer for positron emission tomography: initial findings in prostate cancer. *Cancer Res* **61**, 110–17.

Hara T, Kosaka N, Kishi H (1998) PET imaging of prostate cancer using carbon-11-choline. *J Nucl Med* **39**, 990–5.

Hara T, Kosaka N, Kishi H (2002) Development of 18F-fluoroethylcholine for cancer imaging with PET: synthesis, biochemistry, and prostate cancer imaging. *J Nucl Med* **43**, 187–99.

Haubner R, Wester H-J, Burkhart F *et al.* (2001) Glycosylated RGD-containing peptides: tracer for tumor targeting and angiogenesis imaging with improved biokinetics. *J Nucl Med* **42**, 326–36.

Ido T, Wan CN, Casella JS *et al.* (1978) Labeled 2-deoxy-D-glucose analogs: 18F labeled 2-deoxy-2-fluoro-D-glucose, 2-deoxy-2-fluoro-D-mannose and 14C-2-deoxy-2-fluoro-D-glucose. *J Labeled Compds Radiopharmacol* **14**, 175–83.

Kato T, Tsukamoto E, Kuge Y *et al.* (2002) Accumulation of [11C]acetate in normal prostate and benign prostatic hyperplasia: comparison with prostate cancer. *Eur J Nucl Med Mol Imaging* **29**, 1492–5.

Kubota K, Matsuzawa T, Ito M *et al.* (1985) Lung tumor imaging by positron emission tomography using ^{11}C-L-methionine. *J Nucl Med* **26**, 37–42.

Kubota R, Yamada S, Kubota K *et al.* (1992) Intratumoral distribution of fluorine-18 fluorodeoxyglucose in vivo: High accumulation in macrophages and granulation tissues studied. *J Nucl Med* **33**, 1972–80.

Larson SM, Weiden PL, Grunbaum Z *et al.* (1981) Positron imaging feasibility studies. II: Characteristics of 2-deoxyglucose uptake in rodent and canine neoplasms. Concise communication. *J Nucl Med* **22**, 875–9.

Lewis JS, McCarthy DW, McCarthy TJ, Fujibayashi Y, Welch MJ (1999). Evaluation of 64Cu-ATSM in vitro and in vivo in a hypoxic tumor model. *J Nucl Med* **40**, 177–83.

Mintun MA, Wlech MJ, Siegel BA *et al.* (1988) Breast cancer: PET imaging of estrogen receptors. *Radiology* **169**, 45–8.

Oyama N, Akino H, Kanamaru H *et al.* (2002) 11C-acetate PET imaging of prostate cancer. *J Nucl Med* **43**, 181–6.

Patronas NJ, DiChiro G, Brooks RA *et al.* (1982) Work in progress: 18F fluorodeoxyglucose and PET in the evaluation of radiation necrosis of the brain. *Radiology* **144**, 885–9.

Phelps ME, Hoffman E, Mullani N *et al.* (1976) Design considerations for a positron emission transaxial tomograph (PET III). *IEEE Trans Biomed Eng* NS-23, 516–22.

Phelps ME, Huong SC, Hoffman EJ *et al.* (1979) Tomographic measurement of local cerebral glucose metabolic rate in humans with 18F2-fluoro-2-deoxy-D-glucose: validation of method. *Ann Neurol* **5**, 371–88.

Rajendran JG, Mankoff DA, O'Sullivan F *et al.* (2004) Hypoxia and glucose metabolism in malignant tumors: evaluation by [18F]fluoromisonidazole and [18F]fluorodeoxyglucose positron emission tomography imaging. *Clin Cancer Res* **10**, 2245–52.

Reivich M, Kuhl D, Wolf A *et al.* (1979) The [18F] fluorodeoxyglucose method for the measurement of local cerebral glucose utilization in man. *Cir Res* **44**, 127–37.

Schirrmeister H, Guhlmann A, Kotzerke J *et al.* (1999) Early detection and accurate description of extent of metastatic bone disease in breast cancer with fluoride ion and positron emission tomography. *J Clin Oncol* **17**, 2381–9.

Schirrmeister H, Kuhn T, Guhlmann A *et al.* (2001) Fluorine-18 2-deoxy-2-fluoro-D-glucose PET in the preoperative staging of breast cancer: comparison with the standard staging procedures. *Eur J Nucl Med* **28**, 351–8.

Shields AF, Grierson JR, Dohmen BM *et al.* (1998) Imaging proliferation in vivo with [F-18]FLT and positron emission tomography. *Nat Med* **4**, 1334–6.

Shulkin BL, Koeppe RA, Francis IR *et al.* (1993) Pheochromocytomas that do not accumulate metaiodobenzylguanidine: Localization with PET and administration of FDG. *Radiology* **186**, 711–15.

Shulkin BL, Thompson NW, Shapiro B, Francis IR, Sisson JC (1999) Pheochromocytomas: imaging with 2-[fluorine-18]fluoro-2-deoxy-D-glucose PET. *Radiology* **212**, 35–41.

Som P, Atkins HL, Bandoypadhyay D *et al.* (1980) A fluorinated glucose analogue 2-fluoro-2-deoxy-D-glucose. Non toxic tracer for rapid tumour detection. *J Nucl Med* **21**, 670–5.

Wahl RL (1996) Targeting glucose transporters for tumor imaging: 'sweet' idea, 'sour' result. *J Nucl Med* **37**, 1038–41.

Wahl RL, Cody R, Hutchins GD, Midgett E (1991a) Primary and metastatic breast carcinoma: Initial clinical evaluation with PET with the radiolabelled glucose analog 2-[^{18}F]-fluoro-deoxy-2-D-glucose (FDG). *Radiology* **179**, 765–70.

Wahl RL, Hutchins GD, Buchsbaum DJ *et al.* (1991b) ^{18}F-2-deoxy-2-fluoro-D-glucose uptake into human tumor xenografts. Feasibility studies for cancer imaging with positron-emission tomography. *Cancer* **67**, 1544–50.

Warburg O (1930) *The Metabolism of Tumors*, trans. F Dickens. Constable, London, pp. 129–69.

Yonekura Y, Benau RS, Brill AB *et al.* (1982) Increased accumulation of 2-deoxy-2–^{18}F fluoro-D-glucose in liver metastases from colon cancer. *J Nucl Med* **12**, 1133–7.

USEFUL WEBSITES AND SOURCE

Cancer Prevention and Control. http://apps.nccd.cdc.gov/uscs
Cancer Research UK. www.cancerresearchuk.org
Cancer Facts & Figures 2005. American Cancer Society, 2005.

CHAPTER 4
LUNG CANCER

INTRODUCTION AND BACKGROUND

Lung cancer is the most frequent and the most lethal of cancers in both men and women in the Western world. Most lung cancers are caused by smoking; however, smoking appears to be a somewhat less important factor in adenocarcinoma, which is also on the increase. Lung cancer makes up 16 percent of all cancers in men and 13 percent of all cancers in women. Although early lung cancers (nonsmall cell T1, T2 N0 cancers) are curable by surgery with a 60–80 percent 5-year survival, only 6 percent of all patients with lung cancer survive for 5 years.

The basic treatment for nonsmall cell lung cancer (NSCLC) remains surgical, although only approximately one in five patients are operable at the time of presentation. The remainder of the patients receive palliative chemotherapy or radiation therapy. Pilot screening programs for lung cancer using computed tomography (CT) screening can identify lung cancers at an earlier, more resectable stage, but these programs have not yet been shown to improve survival and suffer from the presence of many false-positive examinations with nonmalignant nodules more commonly identified than malignancies. Some patients can be converted from inoperable to 'operable' through the use of preoperative (neoadjuvant) chemotherapy. Recently, agents binding to surface receptor molecules such as the epidermal growth factor receptor have been shown to have some therapeutic activity in patients with nonsmall cell lung cancers. Patients with small cell lung cancer (SCLC) respond well initially to chemotherapy and radiation therapy and are generally not treated surgically.

Mesotheliomas are increasing in frequency with an incidence of 7.4 per 100 000 population in the UK and a lower incidence of 1.5–2.2 per 100 000 population in the USA. There tend to be geographic clusters of this type of tumor related to past occupational exposure. Cases occur 30–40 years after exposure and in the UK and other parts of western Europe the mortality of mesothelioma is expected to peak at around 2000 deaths per year between 2011 and 2015.

> *More people die of lung cancer than any other type of cancer. This is true for men and women.*

EPIDEMIOLOGY	
Annual incidence	
Men	83 new cases per 100 000/ 23 456 cases UK
	77 new cases per 100 000/ 93 010 cases USA
Women	49 new cases per 100 000/ 14 737 cases UK
	58 new cases per 100 000/ 79 560 cases USA
Male/female ratio	M>F but approaching 1:1
13% all new cancers	
30% all cancer deaths	

There are significant differences in frequency in different countries, the most noteworthy being the high and increasing incidence of adenocarcinoma in women in the USA. Deaths from NSCLC are reducing in men but have remained stable in women over the last 10 years. Small cell carcinoma appears to be declining in frequency. Mesotheliomas are quite commonly seen in patients with asbestos exposure, often occupational, and the incidence is rising.

The key issue is the spread to mediastinum, which usually renders the patient inoperable. While minimal tumor burden mediastinal disease can sometimes be operated upon – especially after chemotherapy – contralateral nodal metastases and bulky mediastinal disease are clear contraindications to surgery. CT backed up by mediastinoscopy and biopsy has historically been the basis of mediastinal staging. Unfortunately CT has poor sensitivity and specificity as nodal size criteria are not particularly robust indicators of the presence or absence of disease and consequently many patients have been inappropriately operated on when the disease has already spread and some denied potential cures because of false-positive results. The important goal is to decrease the number of patients undergoing surgical treatment unnecessarily.

PATHOLOGY

Tumor type	UK (%)	USA (%)
SCLC	25	20
NSCLC		
Adenocarcinoma	15	40
Large cell	10	10
Squamous cell	50	30
Mesothelioma	<2	<2

STAGING

Tumor (T)

T0   No evidence of primary tumor

T1   Tumor ≤ 3 cm

T2   Tumor >3 cm in greatest dimension
     Tumor involving main bronchus and is ≥2 cm distal to the carina
     Tumor invading the visceral pleura

T3   Any size tumor invading chest wall, diaphragm, mediastinal pleura, parietal pericardium
     Tumor in the main bronchus <2 cm distal to the carina
     Tumor with associated atelectasis/pneumonitis of the entire lung

T4   Any size tumor invading mediastinum, heart, great vessels, trachea, esophagus, vertebral body, carina
     Separate tumor nodules in the same lobe
     Tumor with a malignant pleural effusion

Regional lymph nodes (N)

NX   Regional lymph nodes cannot be assessed

N0   No regional lymph node metastasis

N1   Metastasis to ipsilateral peribronchial and/or ipsilateral hilar lymph nodes, and intrapulmonary nodes including involvement by direct extension of the primary tumor

N2   Metastasis to ipsilateral mediastinal and/or subcarinal lymph node(s)

N3   Metastasis to contralateral mediastinal, contralateral hilar, ipsilateral or contralateral scalene, or supraclavicular lymph node(s)

Distant metastasis (M)

MX   Distant metastasis cannot be assessed

M0   No distant metastasis

M1   Distant metastasis present. (Note: M1 includes separate tumor nodule(s) in a different lobe (ipsilateral or contralateral)

STAGE GROUPING AND PROGNOSIS

Stage	TNM description	5-year overall survival (%)
Stage IA	T1 N0 M0	80 (if operable)
Stage IB	T2 N0 M0	60 (if operable)
Stage IIA	T1 N1 M0	
Stage IIB	T2 N1 M0	25–50
T3	N0 M0	
Stage IIIA	T1/2 N2 M0	
	T3 N1/2 M0	5–30
Stage IIIB	Any T N3 M0	
	T4 any N M0	
Stage IV	Any T any N M1	2

Generally lung cancer carries a poor prognosis, less than 10 percent survival overall. However, a young person with a small peripheral NSCLC and no spread has a very good outlook if treated properly. Given the limited probability of cure in more advanced lung cancers, surgery can have greater immediate risks than long-term benefits. Thus, patients with lung cancer must be carefully evaluated before a choice of treatment is made.

PREFERENTIAL LOCAL SPREAD

Tumor site	
Lower lobe	→ Posterior mediastinal nodes, subcarinal nodes
Right upper lobe	→ Superior mediastinal nodes
Left upper lobe	→ Anterior mediastinal nodes, superior mediastinal nodes
Peripheral lesions	→ Pleura, chest wall or diaphragm

Knowledge of the likeliest early site of spread is helpful in getting the best results from staging procedures. Positron emission tomography (PET) can detect both locoregional and systemic metastases with high accuracy, thus better selecting patients for initial resectability.

COMMON METASTATIC SITES

Bone
Liver
Adrenal
Brain

At presentation, some patients will have distant metastatic disease: at the time of death, most will have distant disease.

KEY MANAGEMENT ISSUES

KEY MANAGEMENT ISSUES

Characterization of a lung nodule or lung mass
Staging of NSCLC
Assessment of recurrence
Monitoring therapy
Assessment of pleural malignancy

[¹⁸F]2-fluoro-2-deoxy-D-glucose (FDG) PET imaging for a solitary pulmonary nodule has >90 percent accuracy in separating malignant from benign disease. PET can replace biopsy, and is appropriate in many patients. FDG PET is preferred to biopsy in settings in which the risks of biopsy are increased, such as patients with severe emphysema, bleeding disorders, and where there has been failure of biopsy. Although FDG PET sensitivity is high, it is not 100 percent and follow-up anatomic imaging is usually recommended if FDG PET is negative in a pulmonary nodule, to assure there is not interval tumor growth.

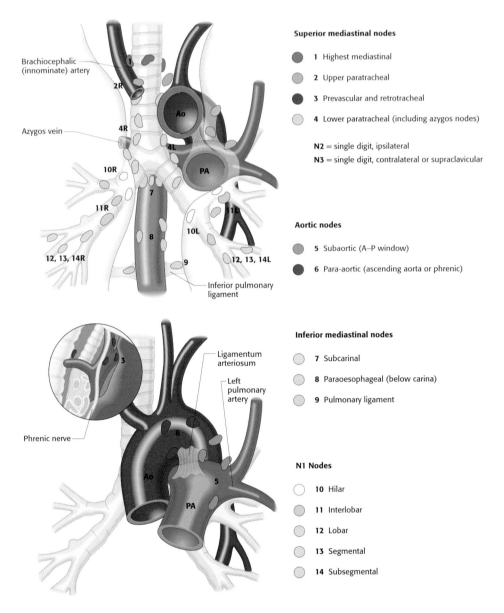

Figure 4.1 *Lymph node drainage from the lung. Reproduced from Mountain, CF, Dresler, CM (1997) Regional lymph node classification for lung cancer staging.* Chest **111**(b): 1719.

Role of PET in lung cancer

FDG PET has an important role in the differential diagnosis of focal pulmonary abnormalities, in the locoregional and systemic staging of proved lung cancers and in the follow-up of lung cancer therapies. Nearly all histological types of NSCLC are FDG avid and thus well imaged with FDG PET. SCLC and mesothelioma are normally FDG avid in their untreated states. Both FDG and [¹¹C]L-methionine have been used in imaging, but there are far more data for FDG. Many studies of the use of FDG PET in evaluating solitary pulmonary nodules (SPN) have been performed. The prospective PIOPLIN study showed a sensitivity of 92 percent, specificity of 90 percent for standardized uptake value (SUV) determinations in characterizing SPNs of >7 mm in diameter, though most SPNs were larger than this size. Qualitative and quantitative analyses were comparable in accuracy. A meta-analysis of the world FDG PET SPN literature was reported by Gould *et al.* (2001) and confirmed an overall joint operating sensitivity of 91.2 percent.

Most interpreters err on the side of sensitivity, so that to achieve a higher sensitivity for cancer detection a somewhat lower specificity is acceptable, with the test operating at 96.8 percent sensitivity and 77.8 percent specificity. False-negative results are sometimes seen in bronchioloalveolar carcinomas and some neuroendocrine tumors and might be seen in patients with high serum glucose levels who have lower tumor SUV levels. Occasionally false-negative PET imaging may occur in small (<1 cm) SPNs, especially in the lower zones where there is more respiratory movement, so follow-up of some small negative lesions may be indicated. Recently, respiratory gating has been shown to be promising in this setting, but is currently under study. Some benign inflammatory processes accumulate FDG, such as tuberculomas, aspergillomas, sarcoidosis, rheumatoid nodules, and active inflammation. Thus FDG is clearly not specific for cancer. Currently, FDG PET is the most accurate noninvasive method available for assessing SPNs, avoiding the morbidity of fine-needle biopsy or surgery.

For staging of the mediastinum, FDG PET has been shown in many studies series to be considerably more accurate than CT, as PET can detect cancer in normal sized lymph nodes as well as excluding cancer from enlarged nodes. An early series in 23 patients showed PET to be 82 percent accurate, whereas CT was only 52 percent accurate in mediastinal staging. Two meta-analyses of the literature have confirmed PET to be more accurate than CT for staging lung cancer. Dwamena *et al.* (1999) showed a sensitivity and specificity of PET of 79 percent and 91 percent, respectively, versus a 60 percent sensitivity and 77 percent specificity for CT (p<0.001). A more recent analysis by Gould *et al.* (2001) showed PET to have an overall operating sensitivity of 85 percent with specificity of 90 percent while CT was 61 percent sensitive and 79 percent specific.

False-positive uptake of FDG in the mediastinum can occur, particularly in areas of the USA where granulomatous disease such as histoplasmosis is endemic, meaning that biopsy confirmation of such nodal involvement is generally preferable to presumptive treatment. In Europe, false-positive FDG PET scans in the mediastinum are much less common. Excellent staging results have been seen in smaller studies using [^{11}C]L-methionine, but the literature is far larger using FDG PET. FDG PET/CT offers the clear advantage of displaying anatomy and functional information together which appear to increase diagnostic certainty. Lardinois *et al.* (2003) reported that PET/CT provided additional information compared with visual correlation of PET and diagnostic CT in 20/49 of patients (41 percent) referred for lung cancer staging. PET/CT was more accurate in tumor staging, nodal staging, and in detection of metastases. Antoch *et al.* (2003) also reported that PET/CT was more accurate than PET or CT alone in the staging of lung cancer. The correct TNM staging was made in 20/27 patients using PET, 19/27 patients using CT and 26/27 patients using PET/CT in their study. Changes to the PET report compared with PET/CT resulted in a change in management in four patients and changes to the CT report compared with PET/CT resulted in a change in management in five patients.

PET also has an important role in staging the whole body. A paper by one of our group (Lewis *et al.*, 1994) showed that additional malignant lesions were found in 41 percent of 34 patients, with management altered in 29 percent. Of greatest importance was a change to nonsurgical management, found in 18 percent of cases. The economic consequences of eliminating a thoracotomy are considerable. A recent prospective randomized trial (PLUS Trial) compared, in patients with newly diagnosed lung cancer randomized to PET plus anatomic versus anatomic staging, the frequency of futile thoracotomy, that is, thoracotomy which was performed in a patient who was found to be truly inoperable. In this multicenter study, the PET group had a 51 percent reduction in the number of inappropriate thoracotomies without a significant reduction in the number of appropriate thoracotomies (from a 41 percent surgery rate to a 21 percent thoracotomy rate).

PET appears helpful in assessing the early response of lung cancers to therapy and is useful for detecting residual disease post treatment when anatomic imaging is confusing due to distortions due to surgery/radiation. More recently, PET and PET/CT have been used for planning external beam irradiation treatments of lung cancer. PET and PET/CT plans have been shown to differ markedly from plans based only on anatomy. In most PET centers, known or suspected lung cancer is the most common indication for PET or PET/CT imaging.

EXAMPLES TO ILLUSTRATE KEY ISSUES

CASE 4.1	Diagnosis: Solitary pulmonary nodule

Clinical history:

This patient presented with left-sided pneumonia. Follow-up chest radiograph showed residual scarring on the left, so a CT scan was done. The CT demonstrated an SPN in the **right** lower lobe close to the diaphragm, inaccessible to biopsy. PET/CT was requested to characterize the SPN.

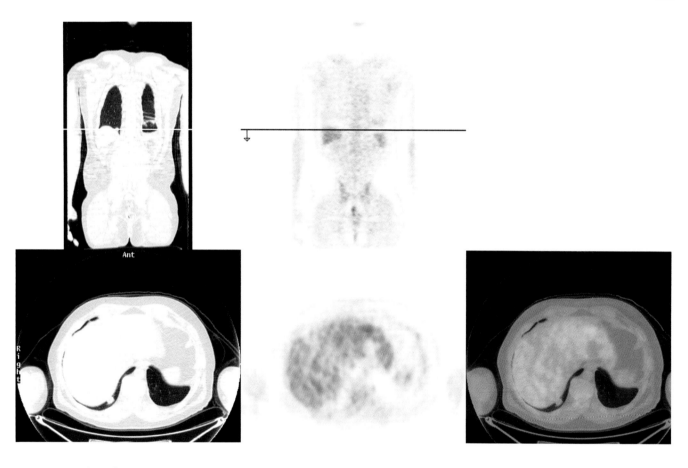

PET/CT findings:

There was no uptake of FDG in the nodule, indicating a benign etiology. Inflammatory changes were seen at the left lung base. Clinical follow-up has not shown malignant disease.

Key points:

1 PET/CT can distinguish benign from malignant disease in SPN.
2 Sensitivity of FDG PET for malignancy is reduced in the lower lobes with lesions smaller than 1 cm because of respiratory motion.
3 Radiological follow-up is therefore recommended for small PET 'negative' lesions.

| **CASE 4.2** | **Diagnosis: Solitary pulmonary nodule** |

Clinical history:

This patient had a solitary pulmonary nodule in the right upper lung. PET/CT was requested to characterize the lesion.

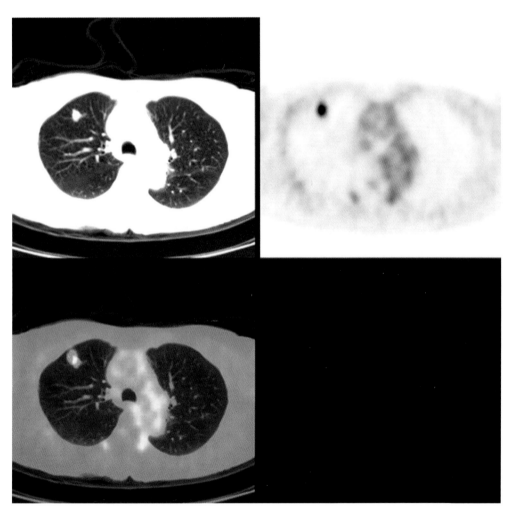

Reproduced with kind permission of Springer Science and Business Media from Cohade C, Osmand M, Marshall LN, Wahl RL (2003) PET-CT: accuracy of PET and CT spatial registration of lung lesions. Eur J Nucl Med Mol Imaging **30**, *721–6*

PET/CT findings:

There was high uptake in the lesion consistent with cancer.

Key point:

PET/CT can characterize SPN. High uptake of FDG in a lesion indicates there is a high probability of cancer.

| CASE 4.3 | Diagnosis: Inflammatory lung disease |

Clinical history:

This patient was referred with a right pulmonary opacity, which had been enlarging in size over 12 months on serial chest radiographs. Bronchoscopy was normal. Percutaneous biopsy revealed inflammatory cells only. The patient developed a pneumothorax post procedure. PET was requested to further characterize the pulmonary opacity.

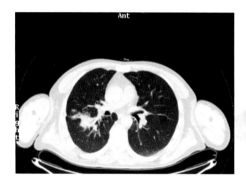
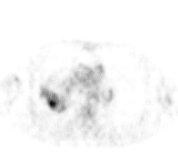
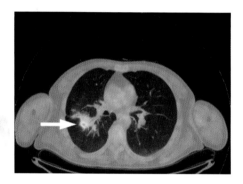

PET findings:

There was moderately intense FDG uptake within the mass. The maximum SUV was 7.0, suggestive of cancer. The patient proceeded to surgery with frozen section and removal of the mass. Histologic examination revealed fibrosis and inflammation only with type II pneumocyte hyperplasia.

Key point:

There can be high uptake of FDG in active inflammation. Other causes of false-positive FDG uptake include granulomatous disease (including tuberculosis, sarcoidosis), pneumoconiosis, amyloidosis, and rheumatoid nodules.

CASE 4.4	Diagnosis: Lung cancer – lesion characterization

Clinical history:

This patient was referred with a left hilar mass visible on chest radiograph and at bronchoscopy, however only necrotic material was obtained at biopsy. PET/CT was requested to characterize the lesion which was thought likely to be cancer and to direct biopsy.

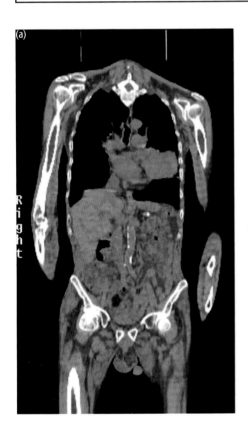
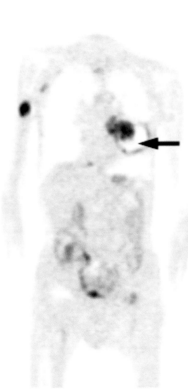
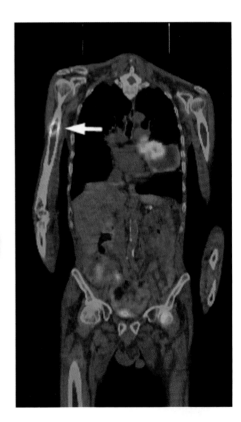

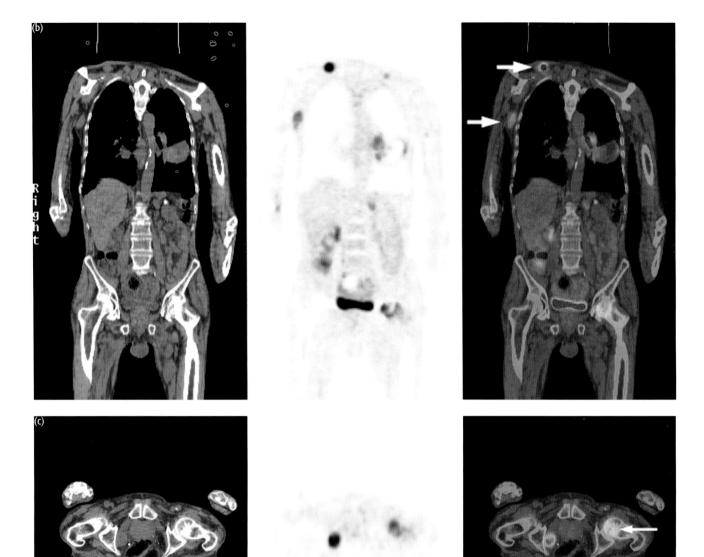

PET/CT findings:

There was extensive uptake in a large mass at the left hilum. The more distal parts of the tumor had increased uptake around a central photopenic area, from which the biopsy sample had presumably been taken (black arrow in a). Further focal uptake was seen in left hilar lymph nodes and in bone. Note the uptake in the right humerus (white arrow in a). There was uptake in multiple soft tissue nodules including a nodule superior to the right scapula (b) and a large nodule in the right axilla (b). There was further abnormal soft tissue which was FDG avid in the right pelvic side wall (c). This image also shows a metastasis in the left femoral head. A small left adrenal lesion was also suspicious for a metastasis (not shown).

The features were those of extensive metastatic disease. The right axillary lesion was biopsied revealing large cell poorly differentiated carcinoma.

Key points:

1 Large pulmonary masses are commonly malignant.
2 There is discordance between anatomic and metabolic tumor volume accounting for the initial false negative biopsy.
3 PET should be performed in any patient with lung cancer in whom curative surgery or radiotherapy is considered.

CASE 4.5	Diagnosis: Lung cancer – diagnosis

Clinical history:

This patient was referred with one pulmonary nodule in the left upper lobe and a second nodule in the right middle lobe. There was a history of emphysema, hypertension, renovascular disease, and peripheral vascular disease placing her at high risk for biopsy or surgery. PET was requested to characterize the lesions.

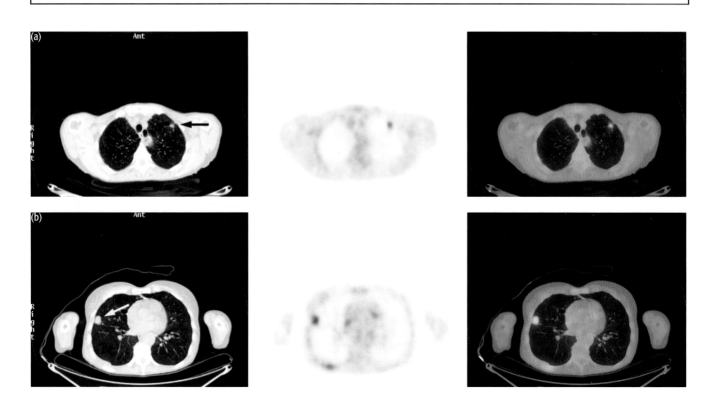

PET/CT findings:

There was intense uptake in the nodules (a, b) consistent with bilateral malignancy. Uptake associated with a pleural plaque was considered likely to be benign (b). There was no definite evidence of metastases. Given the risks associated with biopsy and poor lung function that precluded surgery, chemoradiotherapy was initiated.

Key point:

In patients at high risk of complications from biopsy PET provides a 'metabolic' biopsy to guide treatment.

| CASE 4.6 | Diagnosis: Lung cancer – lesion characterization |

Clinical history:

This patient was referred with two lesions in the left upper lobe of the lung on CT and enlargement of the left adrenal gland. PET was requested to characterize the pulmonary lesions and to determine operability if malignant.

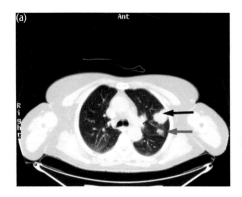
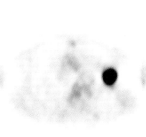
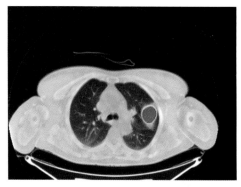
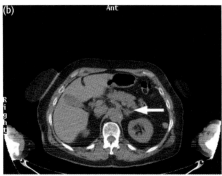

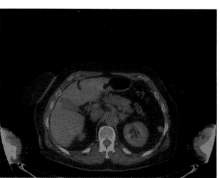

PET/CT findings:

The PET/CT scan showed high uptake in a spiculated mass in the left upper lobe (black arrow in a), but no uptake in a smaller mass posterior to this (red arrow in a). There was no uptake in the left adrenal gland (b). The patient proceeded to surgery, and a left upper lobectomy was performed. The resection specimen revealed a well-defined 3 cm squamous cell carcinoma corresponding to the FDG avid lesion. No cancer was identified in the smaller lesion. Resection margins were clear of tumor and 7/7 lymph nodes removed were also clear of tumor. Clinical follow-up has not shown metastatic disease.

Key points:

1 PET/CT can characterize pulmonary nodules.
2 PET/CT can characterize adrenal masses.

| CASE 4.7 | Diagnosis: Lung cancer and chronic lymphatic leukemia |

Clinical history:

The patient was referred with a history of chronic lymphatic leukemia (CLL) and good performance status. A 5 cm lesion in the right lower lobe of the lung had been found on CT with mediastinal, abdominal, iliac, and inguinal lymphadenopathy making assessment difficult. An enlarged right adrenal gland was also present. PET/CT was requested to determine whether the lung mass was malignant, if the mediastinal nodes were involved by CLL or lung cancer and whether the enlarged adrenal gland represented an adenoma or metastasis.

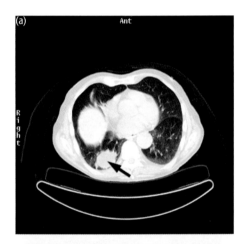

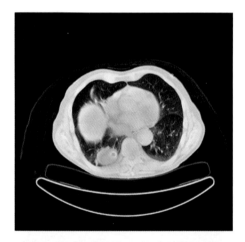
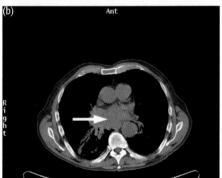
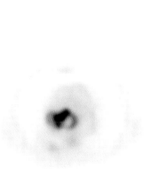
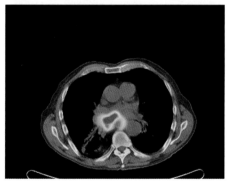

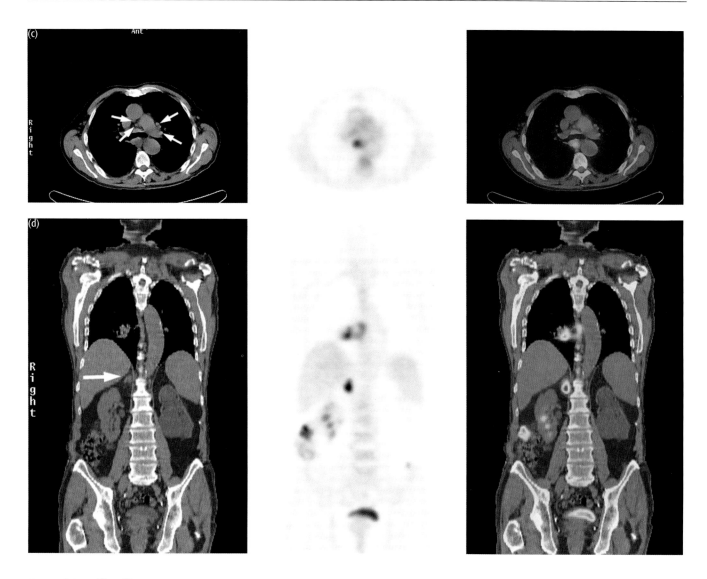

PET/CT findings:

PET/CT showed increased uptake associated with the lesion in the right lower lobe (a). Note that there is some misregistration between PET and CT. This axial slice shows the mass on the CT component of the scan better than the FDG uptake. There was high uptake in the subcarinal (b) and paraesophageal regions (c) indicating these areas were lymph nodes involved by lung cancer. Histologic examination confirmed poorly differentiated NSCLC. Lymphadenopathy elsewhere did not take up FDG and was presumed to represent inactive nodes associated with CLL. Note that there are multiple small nodes in the mediastinum not taking up FDG (c). There was high uptake in the right adrenal gland indicating an adrenal metastasis (d).

Key points:

1 PET enabled separation of low metabolic activity within nodes involved by CLL from those involved by lung cancer.
2 PET can differentiate benign adrenal adenoma from metastasis.

CASE 4.8	Diagnosis: Lung cancer – characterization of lesion/staging

Clinical history:

This patient was referred with a 3 cm spiculated mass in the right middle lobe on CT scan. PET/CT was requested to characterize the lesion and to determine operability if malignant.

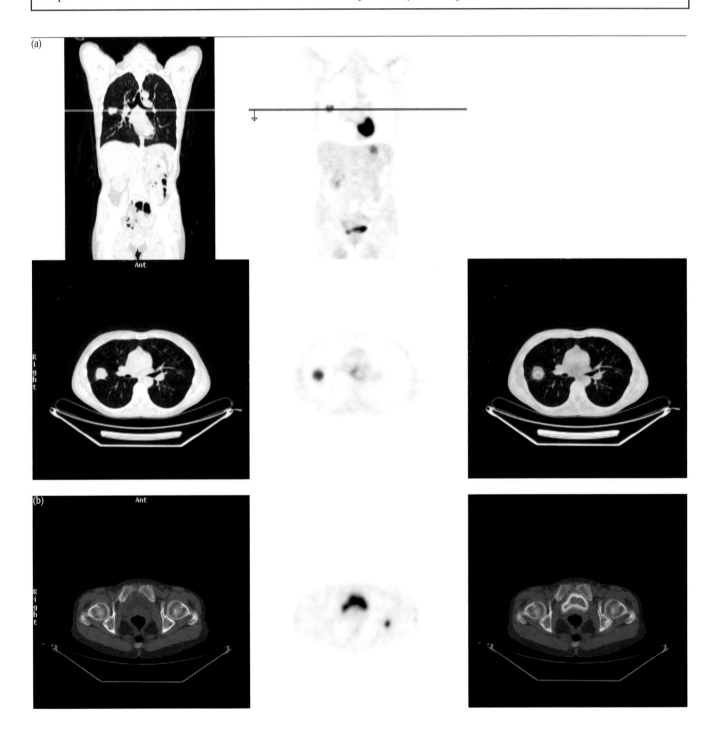

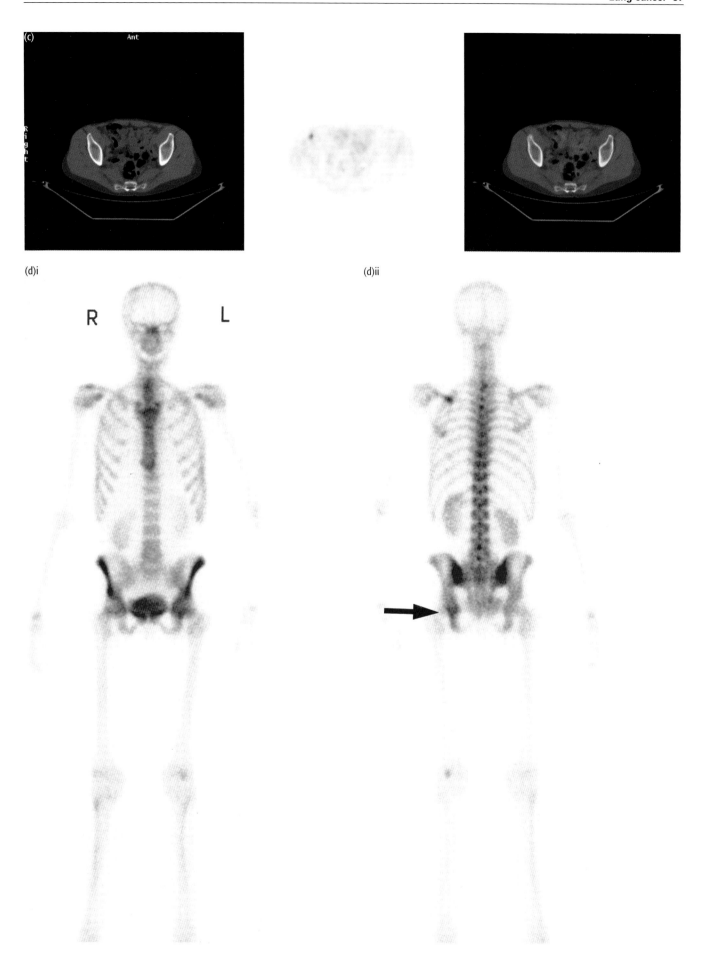

(c)

(d)i

(d)ii

R L

PET/CT findings:

There was intense uptake within the mass in the right middle lobe of the lung (a). Small intense foci were also seen corresponding to lytic lesions in the pelvis, in the left side of the ischium posterior to the acetabulum (b) and in the right anterior iliac crest (c), consistent with primary lung cancer and early bone metastases. A bone scan of these areas was reported as normal but correlation with PET showed increased uptake in the left ischium on the bone scan but no abnormality in the right anterior iliac crest (d).

Key points:

1 PET can reduce the number of 'futile thoracotomies' by 50 percent by detecting metastases.
2 PET with FDG is more sensitive for metastases than bone scanning.

CASE 4.9	Diagnosis: Lung cancer – staging

Clinical history:

This patient was referred with right upper lobe adenocarcinoma. There was a small nodule in the right lower lobe in the CT, the significance of which was uncertain. PET/CT was requested to stage the cancer.

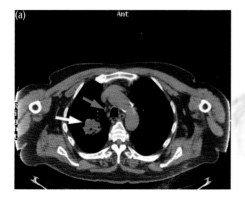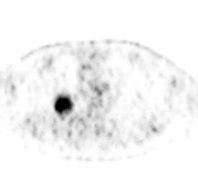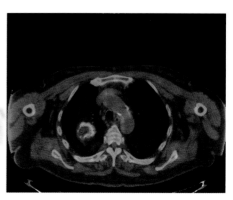

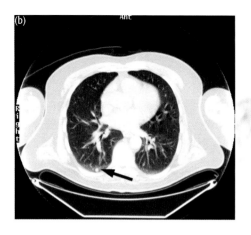

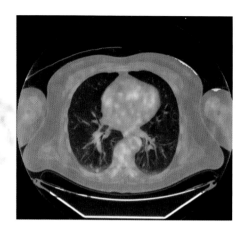

PET/CT findings:

There was high uptake in a cavitating mass in the right upper lobe consistent with adenocarcinoma (white arrow in a). Small volume lymph nodes present in the right paratracheal region did not take up FDG (grey arrow in a). There was no uptake in the small (0.6 cm) nodule in the right lower lobe (b), although the sensitivity of PET for cancer in small nodules in the lower lobes is reduced. The patient underwent surgery. A poorly differentiated adenocarcinoma was removed from the right upper lobe. Enlarged nodes in stations 4 (lower paratracheal) and 10 (hilar) were removed and did not contain cancer. The right lower lobe nodule was removed by wedge resection and was a benign chondroid hamartoma.

Key point:

The resolution of PET limits the sensitivity for detecting cancer in small nodules, especially in the lower lobes due to respiratory motion, however, in this case the small nodule which was FDG-negative turned out to be benign.

CASE 4.10 | Diagnosis: Lung cancer – staging

Clinical history:

This patient was referred with collapse of and consolidation in the right upper lobe of the lung with suspected tumor. Bronchoscopic biopsy revealed squamous cell carcinoma. There were minimally enlarged subcarinal and right hilar lymph nodes in CT. The tumor was anatomically staged as T3 N2 M0 and was therefore likely to be inoperable on CT criteria. PET/CT was requested for nodal and systemic staging.

(a)

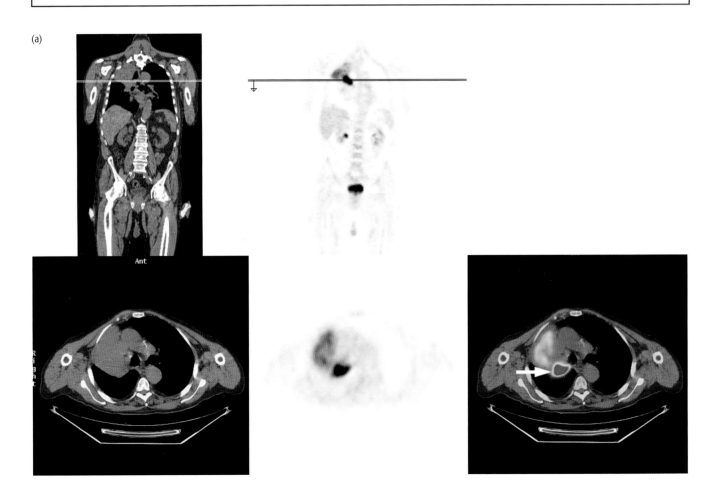

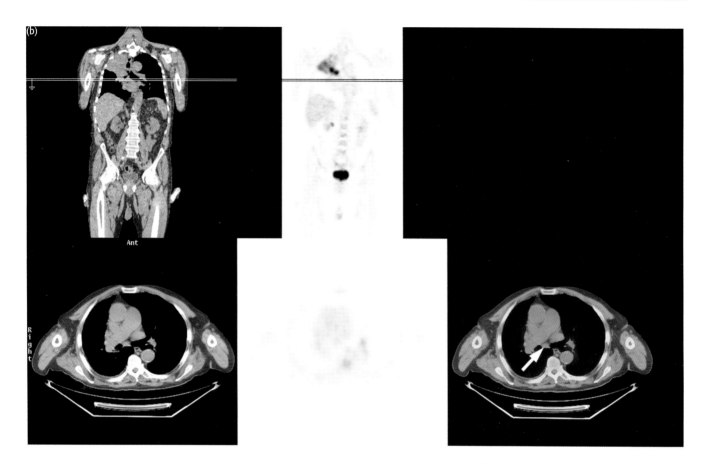

PET/CT findings:

There was intense uptake of FDG in the central tumor with lower grade uptake distally within consolidated lung (a). No uptake was seen in the subcarinal (b) or hilar lymph nodes. The tumor was restaged as T3 N0 M0.

Key points:

1. PET/CT defined the area of central active tumor separating it from consolidation.
2. PET/CT differentiated reactive change from cancer in enlarged mediastinal nodes, showing the tumor to be operable.

CASE 4.11	Diagnosis: Lung cancer – staging

Clinical history:

This patient was referred with squamous cell carcinoma of the left main bronchus. There was a history of tuberculosis and the CT findings of multiple small lung nodules were difficult to interpret. PET/CT was requested to determine whether the nodules represented old tuberculosis or metastases and to stage the patient.

(a)

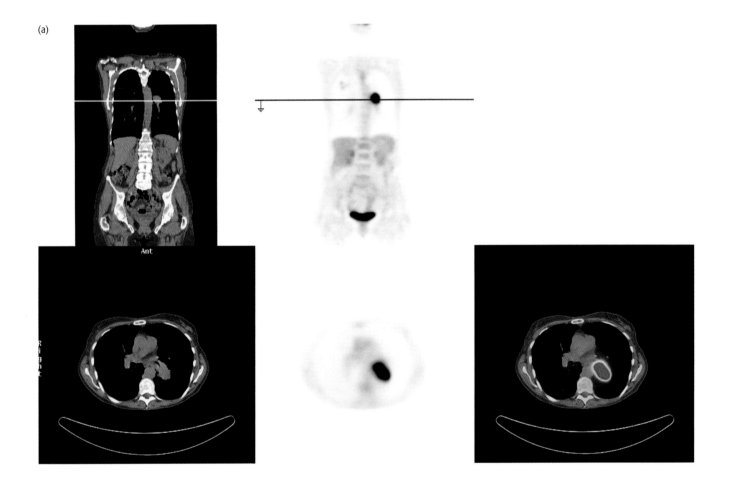

(b)

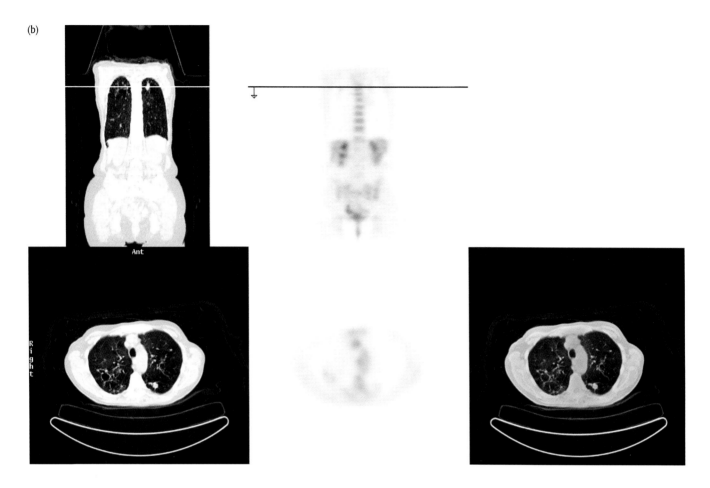

PET/CT findings:

There was high uptake in the primary cancer (a) with low-grade uptake in the nodules consistent with old tuberculosis (b). However, on PET/CT the tumor was considered to be too close to the left pulmonary artery and therefore not resectable (a). The patient was referred for chemoradiotherapy.

Key points:

1 In this case the lung nodule in the left upper lobe was of sufficient size to assume that the low-grade uptake within it meant benign disease. However, low-grade uptake if associated with nodules smaller than 1 cm may indicate low-volume metastases.
2 PET alone cannot determine direct mediastinal involvement by tumor (T4 disease) but PET/CT may be more informative.

CASE 4.12	Diagnosis: Lung cancer – staging

Clinical history:

This patient was referred with known squamous cell carcinoma in the right upper lobe. PET/CT was requested for staging.

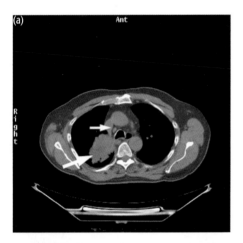

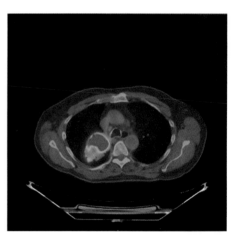

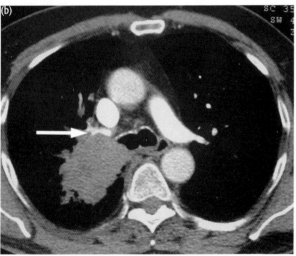

(a) PET/CT (b) CT only

PET/CT findings:

There was intense uptake in the primary cancer (a) and low uptake in the collapsed lung distally. No increased uptake was associated with a minimally enlarged right paratracheal lymph node on the CT scan. It was unclear whether there was direct mediastinal invasion on the noncontrast CT scan. A contrast-enhanced CT scan showed the tumor was invading the mediastinum (b) and the patient was referred for chemotherapy.

Key points:

1 In this case the noncontrast CT as part of the PET/CT was not as informative as the CT scan with contrast, which clearly showed mediastinal vascular invasion.
2 PET and CT are complementary to one another.

CASE 4.13	Diagnosis: Bronchioloalveolar carcinoma – restaging

Clinical history:

This patient was referred with a history of bronchioloalveolar carcinoma treated with right lower lobectomy. Two years later she developed radiological findings suggestive of relapse in the right upper lobe. PET was requested to confirm recurrence and restage.

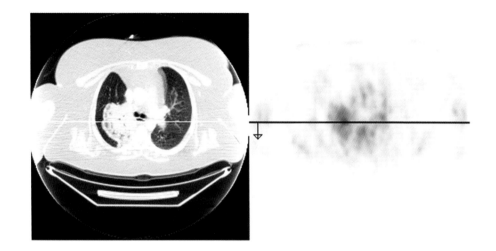

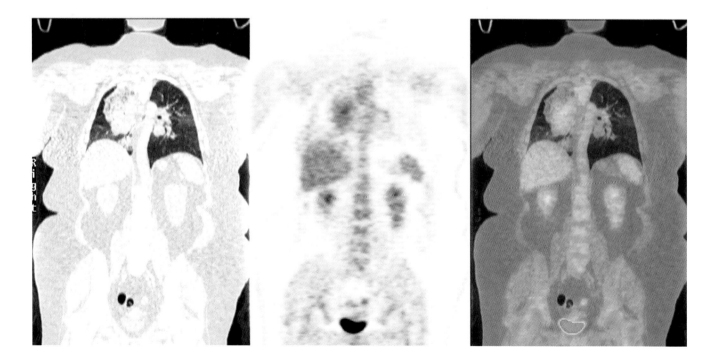

PET/CT findings:

There was low-grade heterogeneous uptake in the right upper lobe tumor typical of bronchioloalveolar carcinoma but no evidence of local or distant spread. The patient proceeded to completion pneumonectomy.

Key points:

1 Bronchioloalveolar carcinomas may have low uptake of FDG.
2 Other lung cancers, e.g. carcinoid and some well-differentiated adenocarcinomas, including those arising within scar tissue, may have low FDG uptake.

| CASE 4.14 | Diagnosis: Lung cancer – recurrence? |

Clinical history:

This patient was referred 12 months after chemoradiotherapy for lung cancer in the left lower lobe. CT scan performed because of worsening fatigue demonstrated residual soft tissue in the posterior left lower lobe and a new nodule in the right upper lobe. PET/CT was requested to determine whether there was disease recurrence.

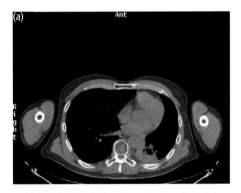

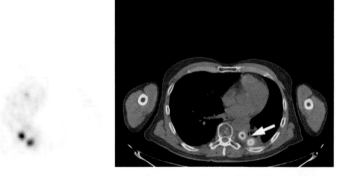

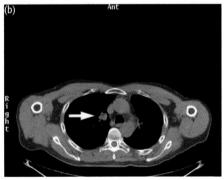

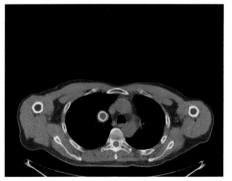

PET/CT findings:

There was high-grade focal uptake within the consolidated left lower lobe close to the site of treatment confirming recurrent malignancy (a). Increased uptake was also seen in the right upper lobe most consistent with a new primary cancer (b).

Key points:

1 PET/CT can distinguish treatment effect from recurrent cancer.
2 Patients with one lung cancer are at increased risk of developing an additional lung cancer.

| CASE 4.15 | Diagnosis: Lung cancer – recurrence? |

Clinical history:

This patient presented with SCLC in the left upper lobe and hilum infiltrating the left atrium. She received chemoradiotherapy with complete response. On routine follow-up a new nodule was noted in the left upper lobe of the lung, which was not accessible via bronchoscopy or percutaneous biopsy. PET/CT was requested to characterize the lesion.

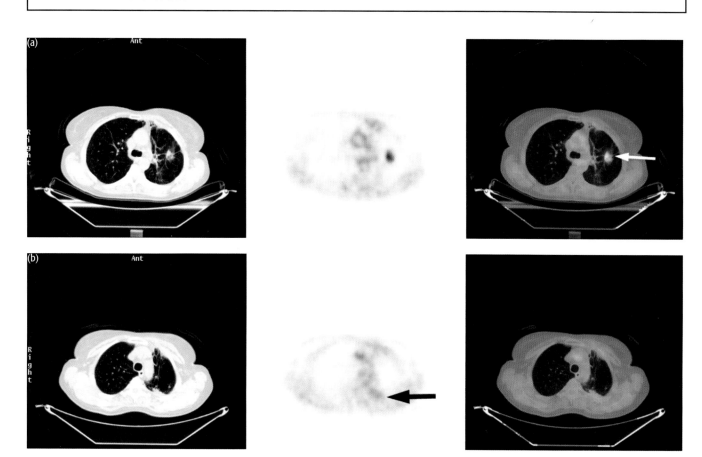

PET/CT findings:

There was high uptake in the left upper lobe nodule suggestive of recurrent disease or a new primary cancer (a). Open biopsy however revealed inflammatory changes with the presence of foreign body granuloma, probably in response to treatment. There was low-grade uptake in the left upper lobe attributable to post radiotherapy change (b).

Key point:

FDG is not specific for cancer and high uptake can be seen with active inflammation, including granulomatous conditions.

| CASE 4.16 | Diagnosis: Small cell lung cancer and breast cancer |

Clinical history:

This patient had known SCLC. PET/CT was requested to stage the tumor.

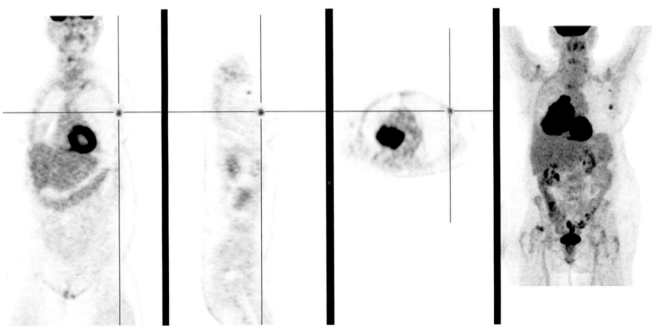

*Reproduced by kind permission from Ishimori T, Patel PV, Wahl RL. (2005) Detection of unexpected additional primary malignancies with PET/CT. J Nucl Med. **46**(5), 752–7.*

PET/CT findings:

There was high uptake in multiple sites consistent with extensive stage SCLC. Focal uptake was also present in the left breast which turned out to be a primary breast cancer.

Key points:

1 There are few indications for PET scanning in SCLC as there is usually extensive disease at presentation. Occasionally it can be used for lesions that present as 'solitary' lesions that may be considered for surgical treatment.
2 Patients with cancer may have second primaries.

| CASE 4.17 | Diagnosis: Lung cancer – treatment response |

Clinical history:

This patient was referred with adenocarcinoma in the left lung following neoadjuvant chemotherapy. PET/CT scan was requested to determine if there was active residual disease treatable with radical radiotherapy.

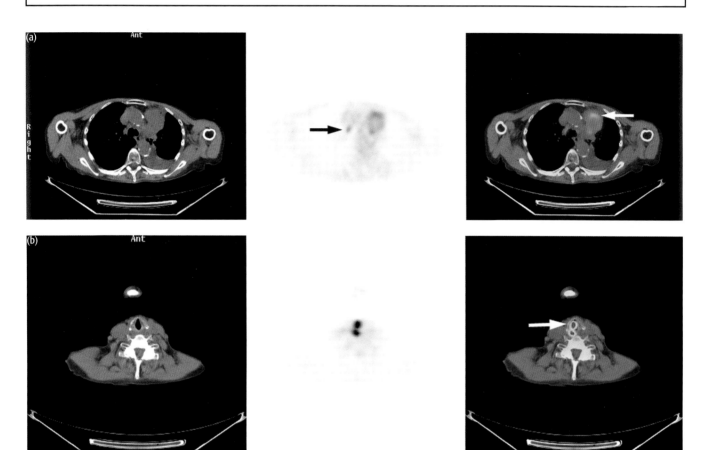

PET/CT findings:

There were foci of low-grade uptake within the residual mass in the left upper lobe consistent with residual cancer (a). A further focus of uptake was seen in a right paratracheal lymph node consistent either with low-volume disease post treatment or reactive change (a). Asymmetric uptake was seen in the larynx with compensatory increased uptake on the right side secondary to left vocal cord palsy because of compression of the left recurrent laryngeal nerve by the tumor in the mediastinum (b).

Key points:

1 PET/CT demonstrates residual malignancy following chemotherapy. Uptake may be low grade following treatment and it was impossible to determine in this case whether the uptake in the right paratracheal region was partly treated cancer or not. The most appropriate time to scan after chemotherapy is not known with certainty. In our centers we prefer to wait a minimum of 4–6 weeks.
2 Asymmetric uptake in the larynx can indicate vocal cord palsy.

| CASE 4.18 | Diagnosis: Lung cancer – radiotherapy planning |

Clinical history:

This patient was treated with right middle and lower lobectomy for squamous cell carcinoma (T2 N1). There was residual tumor within the bronchial stump after surgery and the patient received chemotherapy. Following treatment CT was unable to differentiate post treatment change from residual fibrosis. The PET/CT scan was requested for planning of radical radiotherapy.

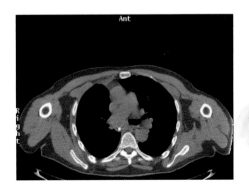 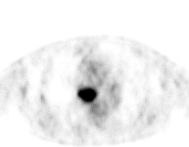 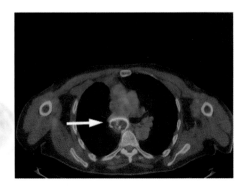

PET/CT findings:

There was intense uptake in abnormal soft tissue posterior to the right mainstem bronchus adjacent to the surgical clips, consistent with residual active cancer.

Key points:

1 PET/CT can differentiate active tumor from treatment effect.
2 PET/CT can assist in radiotherapy planning.

CASE 4.19 | Diagnosis: Mesothelioma

Clinical history:

This patient was referred with pleural thickening in the left hemithorax and subaortic and left lower paratracheal adenopathy on CT. There was previous asbestos exposure. PET/CT was requested to direct biopsy of suspected mesothelioma and to stage the patient for possible surgery.

(a)

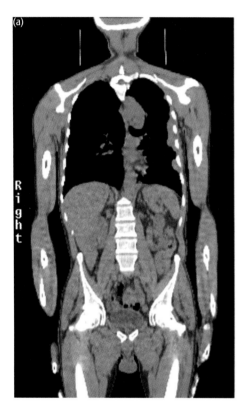

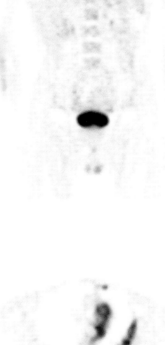

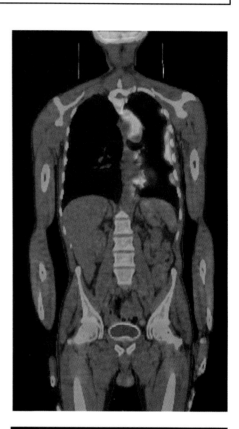

(b)

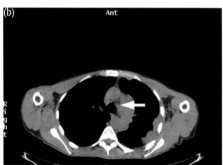

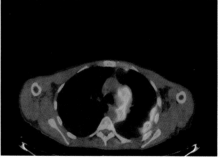

PET/CT findings:

There was high uptake of FDG in multiple pleural-based lesions in the left lung including large areas of abnormal tissue abutting the aortic arch and extending into the aortopulmonary window (b). This uptake did not involve the enlarged lymph nodes. The patient underwent extrapleural pneumonectomy and no lymph nodes were involved by tumor.

Key points:

1 Mesothelioma usually has high uptake of FDG although some lower-grade epithelioid tumors may have low FDG uptake.
2 High uptake of FDG occurs after talc pleurodesis but there had been no pleurodesis in this case. Contrast this with Case 4.20.

CASE 4.20 | Diagnosis: Talc pleurodesis

Clinical history:

This patient with amelanotic melanoma was treated with chemotherapy followed by resection of a right lung mass which contained residual melanoma. Postoperatively talc pleurodesis was performed to treat a persistent chylothorax. PET/CT was performed 6 months after pleurodesis to determine if apical pleural thickening present on CT was likely to represent tumor progression.

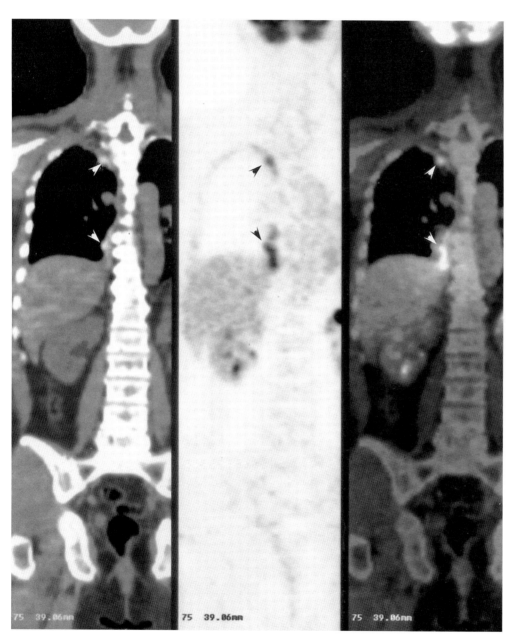

*These figures are published by kind permission from Weiss N, Solomon SB (2003) Talc pleurodesis mimics pleural metastases: differentiation with positron emission tomography/computed tomography. Clin Nucl Med **28**, 811–14 © 2003 Lippincott Williams & Wilkins, Inc.*

PET/CT findings:

There was high uptake associated with the pleural changes consistent with an inflammatory reaction to previous talc pleurodesis. At 21 months after the scan there was no clinical or radiological evidence of progression.

Key point:

Inflammatory uptake occurs after talc pleurodesis – contrast this case with Case 4.19. It is crucial to determine if talc pleurodesis has been performed in patients with suspected mesothelioma.

CASE 4.21 | Diagnosis: Mesothelioma – recurrence?

Clinical history:

This patient had mesothelioma in the right hemithorax and was treated with extrapleural pneumonectomy and radiotherapy. He subsequently developed weight loss, abdominal pain, and ascites. PET was requested to help differentiate between radiation-induced hepatitis and malignancy.

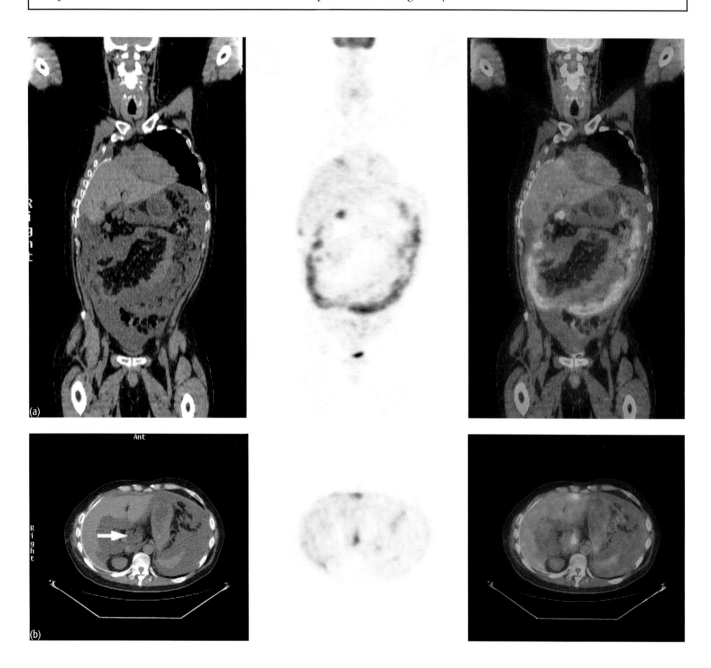

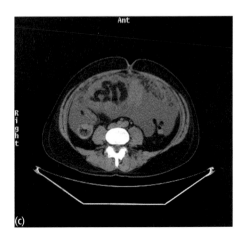

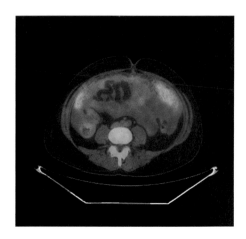

PET/CT findings:

There were multiple peritoneal deposits taking up FDG (a–c) and uptake in the celiac axis (b) indicative of recurrent mesothelioma.

Key points:

1 Mesothelioma can occur in the peritoneal cavity as well as in the pleural cavity.
2 PET imaging should not be limited to the thorax in mesothelioma cases.

CONCLUSIONS

CURRENT CLINICAL INDICATIONS
1 Evaluation of SPN and lung masses
2 Staging of NSCLC
3 Assessing for recurrent tumor where anatomic imaging unhelpful
4 Monitoring response to treatment
5 Staging of mesothelioma

EMERGING INDICATIONS
1 Measuring and prediction of response to chemotherapy
2 Surveillance for early relapse
3 SCLC staging and treatment monitoring
4 Evaluation of pleural thickening to direct biopsy in suspected mesothelioma

A possible algorithm for the use of FDG PET in the evaluation of an SPN or staging lung cancer is shown in Figure 4.2.

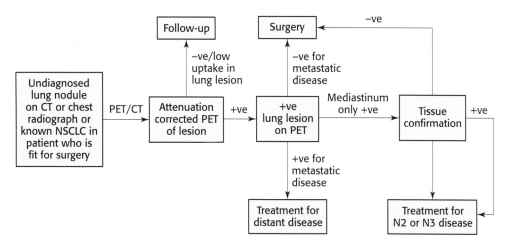

Figure 4.2 *Solitary pulmonary nodule and staging of nonsmall cell lung cancer – clinical algorithm*

REFERENCES AND FURTHER READING

Antoch G, Stattaus J, Nemat AT *et al.* (2003) Non-small cell lung cancer: dual-modality PET/CT in preoperative staging. *Radiology* **229**, 526–33.

Bradley JD, Dehdashti F, Mintun MA *et al.* (2004) Positron emission tomography in limited-stage small-cell lung cancer: a prospective study. *J Clin Oncol* **22**, 3248–54.

Bury T, Dowlati A, Paulus P *et al.* (1996a) Evaluation of the solitary pulmonary nodule by positron emission tomography imaging. *Eur Respir J* **9**, 410–14.

Bury T, Paulus P, Dowlati A *et al.* (1996b) Staging of the mediastinum: value of positron emission tomography imaging in non-small cell lung cancer. *Eur Respir J* **9**, 2560–4.

Cheran SK, Nielsen ND, Patz EF Jr (2004) False-negative findings for primary lung tumors on FDG positron emission tomography: staging and prognostic implications. *Am J Roentgenol* **182**, 1129–32.

Dwamena BA, Sonnad SS, Angobaldo JO, Wahl RL (1999) Metastases from non-small cell lung cancer: mediastinal staging in the 1990s – meta-analytic comparison of PET and CT. *Radiology* **213**, 530–6.

Gambhir SS, Hoh CK, Phelps ME *et al.* (1966) Decision tree sensitivity analysis for cost-effectiveness of FDG PET in the staging and management of non-small-cell carcinoma. *J Nucl Med* **37**, 1428–36.

Gerbaudo VH (2003) 18F-FDG imaging of malignant pleural mesothelioma: scientiam impendere vero. *Nucl Med Comm* **24**, 609–14.

Gerbaudo VH, Sugarbaker DJ, Britz-Cunningham S *et al.* (2002) Assessment of malignant pleural mesothelioma with 18F-FDG dual-head gamma-camera coincidence imaging: comparison with histopathology. *J Nucl Med* **43**, 1144–9.

Gould MK, Maclean CC, Kuschner WG, Rydzak CE, Owens DK (2001) Accuracy of positron emission tomography for diagnosis of pulmonary nodules and mass lesions: a meta-analysis. *JAMA* **285**, 914–24.

Gould MK, Kuschner WG, Rydzak CE *et al.* (2003) Test performance of positron emission tomography and computed tomography for mediastinal staging in patients with non-small-cell lung cancer: a meta-analysis. *Ann Intern Med* **139**, 879–92.

Gupta NC, Frank AR, Dewan NA *et al.* (1992) Solitary pulmonary nodules: Detection of malignancy with PET with 2-[^{18}F]-fluoro-2-deoxy-D-glucose. *Radiology* **184**, 441–4.

Haberkorn U (2004) Positron emission tomography in the diagnosis of mesothelioma. *Lung Cancer* **45**(Suppl 1), S73–6.

Hain SF, Curran KM, Beggs AD *et al.* (2001) FDG-PET as a 'metabolic biopsy' tool in thoracic lesions with indeterminate biopsy. *Eur J Nucl Med* **28**, 1336–40.

Kubota K, Matsuzawa T, Ito M *et al.* (1985) Lung tumor imaging by positron emission tomography using ^{11}C L-methionine. *J Nucl Med* **26**, 37–42.

Kubota K, Yamada S, Ishiwata K *et al.* (1993) Evaluation of the treatment response of lung cancer with positron emission tomography and L-[methyl-^{11}C] methionine: A preliminary study. *Eur J Nucl Med* **20**, 495–501.

Lardinois D, Weder W, Hany TF *et al.* (2003) Staging of non-small-cell lung cancer with integrated positron-emission tomography and computed tomography. *N Engl J Med* **19**, 2500–7.

Lewis P, Griffin S, Marsden P *et al.* (1994) Whole-body ^{18}F-fluorodeoxyglucose positron emission tomography in preoperative evaluation of lung cancer. *Lancet* **344**, 1265–6.

Lowe VJ, Duhaylongsod FG, Patz EF *et al.* (1997) Pulmonary abnormalities and PET data analysis: a retrospective study. *Radiology* **202**, 435–9

Lowe VJ, Fletcher JW, Gobar L *et al.* (1998) Prospective investigation of positron emission tomography in lung nodules. *J Clin Oncol* **16**, 1075–84.

Nolop KB, Rhodes CG, Brudin LH *et al.* (1987) Glucose utilization in vivo by human pulmonary neoplasms. *Cancer* **60**, 2682–9.

Patz EF Jr, Lowe VJ, Hoffman JM *et al.* (1993) Focal pulmonary abnormalities: Evaluation with ^{18}F fluorodeoxyglucose PET scanning. *Radiology* **188**, 487–90.

Schneider DB, Clary-Macy C, Challa S *et al.* (2000) Positron emission tomography with F18-fluorodeoxyglucose in the staging and preoperative evaluation of malignant pleural mesothelioma. *J Thorac Cardiovasc Surg* **20**, 128–33.

Shon IH, O'Doherty MJ, Maisey MN (2002) Positron emission tomography in lung cancer. *Semin Nucl Med* **32**:240–71.

Steinert HC, Hauser M, Allemann F *et al.* (1997) Non-small cell lung cancer: nodal staging with FDG PET versus CT with correlative lymph node mapping and sampling. *Radiology* **202**, 441–6.

van Tinteren H, Hoekstra OS, Smit EF *et al.* (2002) Effectiveness of positron emission tomography in the preoperative assessment of patients with suspected non-small-cell lung cancer: the PLUS multicentre randomised trial. *Lancet* **359**, 1388–93.

Wahl RL, Quint LE, Greenough RL *et al.* (1994) Staging of mediastinal non small cell lung cancer with FDG-PET, CT and fusion images: Preliminary prospective evaluation. *Radiology* **191**, 371.

CHAPTER 5
LYMPHOID NEOPLASMS

INTRODUCTION AND BACKGROUND

Hodgkin disease (HD) and non-Hodgkin lymphoma (NHL) are common and important malignancies which are increasing in frequency. Although they have many features in common and share some common treatments, there are significant differences between the two conditions, which must be appreciated for both diagnosis and treatment. A significant fraction of lymphomas are curable but only if appropriate treatment is given.

- **Hodgkin disease** starts as a unifocal disease involving a single group of malignant lymph nodes and spreads to adjacent associated lymph node groups. Limited stage disease is often treated appropriately with radiation therapy, which results in a complete cure in a high proportion of patients. Even after recurrence, treatment with systemic chemotherapies can result in a cure. Patients with bulky disease and stage III–IV disease have poorer prognosis and usually require treatment with chemotherapy in addition to radiotherapy. Disease that is resistant to chemotherapy and/or radiotherapy may be managed with bone marrow or stem cell transplantation. There are several histologic subtypes of Hodgkin lymphoma and treatment results vary somewhat by histology.
- **Non-Hodgkin lymphoma** normally presents (>90 percent frequency) with disseminated disease, usually requiring combined chemotherapy, sometimes radiotherapy, and in some instances high-dose chemotherapy with bone marrow transplantation. The vast majority of NHLs are of B cell origin, with about 15 percent of T cell origin. Classification of these tumors histologically and by molecular methods is the key to optimal treatment, which can be curative. Radioimmunotherapy also plays a role in the management of this tumor type and has been applied in the low-grade tumors more extensively. Low-grade NHL is ultimately fatal in most patients but long remissions can be induced. In intermediate- and higher-grade NHLs, cure can be achieved using aggressive chemotherapy including, in some settings, stem cell transplantation. Low-grade NHL, although carrying a better prognosis untreated, fails to respond as well to chemotherapy and consequently may, paradoxically, have a worse prognosis than some higher-grade tumors.

Many patients, with lymphomas (up to 25 percent) have systemic symptoms including fever, weight loss, and night sweats, which often indicates a poorer prognosis. Disease outside the lymph nodes occurs in 10–20 percent and is more common in patients with NHL. Conventional staging includes clinical examination and computed tomography (CT) of the chest, abdomen, and pelvis, and is more critical in management of patients with Hodgkin disease than with NHL.

The incidence of lymphoma is increasing in industrialized countries, with significant differences in incidence and age peaks between HD and NHL.

EPIDEMIOLOGY

		HD	NHL
Incidence per 100 000			
Men	UK	3	17
	USA	3	19.4
Women	UK	2.1	14.5
	USA	2.4	16.8
Peak age		< 40 years	> 40 years
		M > F	M > F

There are several systems of classifying lymphoma in current use for pathologic classification and they continue to evolve. As the biology of these tumors is better understood, staging systems based on cell of origin, in addition to morphology, are growing in importance.

CLASSIFICATION OF LYMPHOMAS

	Percentage	Usual behavior
Common NHL entities (based on WHO classification)		
Diffuse large B cell lymphoma (DLBCL)	31	Aggressive
Follicular lymphoma (FL)	22	Indolent
Mucosa-associated lymphoid tissue (MALT)	8	Indolent
Peripheral T cell lymphoma (PTCL)	7	Aggressive
Chronic lymphocytic lymphoma (CLL)/small lymphocytic lymphoma (SLL)	6	Indolent
Mantle cell lymphoma (MCL)	6	Intermediate
Angioimmunoblastic T cell lymphoma	4	Aggressive
Anaplastic large T cell lymphoma	2	Aggressive
Lymphoblastic lymphoma (T or B cell)	<1	Aggressive
Burkitt lymphoma	<1	Aggressive
Hodgkin disease		
Nodular lymphocyte-predominant HD	4–5	
Classical HD		
Nodular sclerosis HD	60–70	
Mixed cellularity HD	15–30	
Lymphocyte-depleted HD	<1	
Lymphocyte-rich HD	5–6	

Hodgkin disease, if localized and effectively treated has high rates of cure. Non-Hodgkin lymphoma is more likely to be fatal, but there is a great deal of variation. 'Low-grade' NHL is paradoxically very hard to cure, whereas 'intermediate- and high-grade' NHLs can be cured in a substantial fraction of cases with aggressive chemotherapy, sometimes including stem cell transplantation.

PROGNOSIS (%)

Hodgkin disease		
Limited disease (stage Ia–IIa)	≥80	
Advanced disease (stage IIb–IVb)	≤70	
NHL	5-year OS	10-year OS
Follicular lymphoma*		
Good	91	71
Intermediate	78	51
Poor	53	36
Diffuse large B cell lymphoma†		
Good	73	
Good/intermediate	51	
Intermediate/poor	43	
Poor	26	

*Prognosis based on the presence of poor prognostic features, i.e. age over 60, hemoglobin <12 g/dL, lactate dehydrogenase above the normal level, stage III or IV and more than four nodal sites.
†Prognosis based on the presence of poor prognostic features, i.e. older age, advanced stage, poor performance status, high lactate dehydrogenase and number of extranodal sites of disease.
OS, overall survival.

STAGING OF HD AND NHL

Stage[a/b]	Description
Stage I	Single lymph node region or localized (unifocal) extralymphatic site
Stage II	Two or more lymph node regions on same side of diaphragm or localized extralymphatic organ/site and its regional nodes (± other lymph node regions on same side of diaphragm)
Stage III	Lymph node regions on both sides of the diaphragm ± involvement of an associated extralymphatic organ/site or spleen or both
Stage IV	Multifocal involvement of one or more extralymphatic organ/sites

[a/b]Suffix, absence or presence of constitutional symptoms (i.e. fever, night sweats, and/or loss of more than 10 percent of body weight over 6 months).

OTHER NONNODAL METASTATIC SITES (FREQUENCY)

	HD	NHL
Marrow	−	++
Spleen	+	+
Liver	−	+
Central nervous system	−	+
Skin	−	+
Gastrointestinal tract	−	++
Testes	−	+
Bone	+	+

Generally staging is more important in HD than NHL as it is more likely to determine the therapeutic regimen. It should be indicated whether the staging is clinical only or based on pathology (P). The stages are divided into: A (no systemic symptoms) or B (systemic symptoms: weight loss, fever, night sweats). Gallium has been used for staging but has reduced sensitivity with low-grade lymphoma and in the detection of abdominal disease because of marked physiologic bowel uptake. Computed tomography has generally been used but suffers from a low sensitivity. Positron emission tomography (PET) is being applied much more commonly in initial staging of lymphomas.

Non-Hodgkin lymphoma is a multifocal disease rather than a spreading nodal disease. Patients with NHL are much more likely to develop non-nodal metastatic sites than patients with HD.

KEY MANAGEMENT ISSUES

KEY MANAGEMENT ISSUES

Staging prior to treatment
Treatment response:
- Early (e.g. interim assessment of chemotherapy)
- Late (e.g. residual masses)
Detection of relapse/restaging
Prognosis assessment

Role of PET in lymphoma

Both HD and NHL can be imaged well with PET using either [^{18}F]2-fluoro-2-deoxy-D-glucose (FDG) or [^{11}C]L-methionine. Far more work has been done with FDG than [^{11}C]L-methionine and, in many centers, the standard work-up of patients with lymphoma requires FDG PET at diagnosis for staging and at multiple time points during the course of the illness to monitor therapy. The earliest human PET imaging of lymphoma was with planar gamma cameras and FDG. In this early work, FDG was shown to detect more foci of NHL than were seen with gallium-67 (^{67}Ga). In most centers, FDG has totally replaced ^{67}Ga in lymphoma imaging. There is an abundant literature demonstrating the sensitivity of FDG PET in detecting most types of untreated lymphoma. Most studies do not have surgical confirmation of results, but it is clear FDG PET will detect nearly all 1 cm and larger foci of untreated lesions in a wide variety of histologic types. When PET/CT is directly compared with CT, about 25 percent of lesions identified by PET are found to correspond to lesions of <1 cm in diameter on CT. Thus, PET with FDG is more sensitive than CT. False-negative results in untreated NHL are infrequent, but can occur in MALT (mucosa-associated lymphoid tissue) lymphomas of the gastrointestinal tract and in some low-grade NHLs, though these are rare. Some studies have suggested PET can noninvasively stage the bone marrow as well, however PET will clearly fail to detect some small tumor foci and cannot detect microscopic, low-volume disease. There is a weak, but significant, relation between the proliferative rate (S phase fraction) and FDG uptake in untreated NHL. However, FDG uptake is normally high enough in the 'low-grade' NHLs for these to be quite easily visible with PET imaging.

A major challenge in managing lymphomas with anatomic imaging is that sometimes lymphoma masses are very large at the time of diagnosis, 10 cm or larger. With effective treatment, these often do not shrink to a normal size. Thus, 'residual masses' after therapy are a common diagnostic problem in up to 50 percent of cases of NHL or HD. ^{67}Ga was previously shown to have superior diagnostic performance (in comparison with CT) in terms of providing prognostic information about the ultimate behavior of these residual masses. However, ^{67}Ga suffers in performance in the abdomen and single photon emission computed tomography (SPECT) has lower resolution than PET. PET is accurate in characterizing the residual mass. Several studies have shown a markedly better disease-free survival period for FDG PET-negative residual masses than for FDG-positive masses, the latter of which almost always represent recurrent tumor. PET certainly can fail to detect microscopic or low tumor volume disease posttreatment, but this is a general limitation of PET imaging. Thus, a negative PET cannot exclude completely the possibility of tumor recurrence after treatment has been completed.

Tumor glucose metabolism falls very rapidly with effective chemotherapy. In some studies, FDG uptake can decline within a single day. In both HD and NHL, significant declines in tumor FDG uptake should be apparent after one or two cycles of treatment. Indeed, the 'mid treatment' FDG PET has been shown to have greater prognostic significance than at the end of treatment. If the PET remains 'positive' half way through planned chemotherapy, tumor control and long-term survival are far less likely than if the scan is negative. Indeed, in some studies, a virtually 100 percent failure rate for therapies is seen if PET images remain positive midway through chemotherapy of lymphoma (Fig. 5.1). A negative PET scan does not mean therapy can be stopped, but it predicts a superior outcome to a positive PET at mid treatment. Investigative studies are now under way in which additional aggressive therapy is being administered to the patients at highest risk of failure based on PET. It is anticipated that PET imaging with quantitation of treatment response at early time posttreatment will grow in frequency and be capable of providing a therapeutic strategy tailored to risk for an individual patient. It is envisaged that more aggressive treatment might be adopted for the patient with limited or no response on PET, but shorter duration and less aggressive treatment could be given for patients with very rapid responses on PET.

While PET is very useful, there are pitfalls in lymphoma imaging. As discussed in Chapter 16, thymic rebound after treatment with intense FDG uptake can be problematic. Similarly, uptake in the normal thymus can be confusing. Colony-stimulating factors can also increase the normal marrow FDG signal and can make interpretation of PET of the marrow and skeleton difficult. Coincident viral

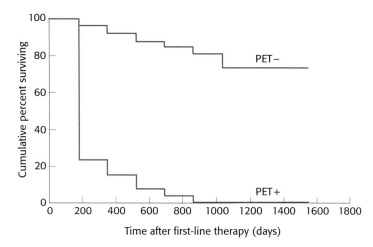

Figure 5.1   *Kaplan–Meier estimate of progression-free survival in 26 patients with a positive [¹⁸F]FDG PET after first-line chemotherapy compared with 67 patients with a negative [¹⁸F]FDG PET after therapy. Reproduced with kind permission from Spaepen K, Stroobants S, Dupont P, et al. (2001) Prognostic value of positron emission tomography (PET) with fluorine-18 fluorodeoxyglucose ([¹⁸F]FDG) after first-line chemotherapy in non-Hodgkin's lymphoma: is [¹⁸F]FDG-PET a valid alternative to conventional diagnostic methods?* J Clin Oncol **19**, 414–19

infections can cause increased FDG uptake without tumor, so that biopsy may still be appropriate in lymphomas if apparent 'recurrence' is atypical in appearance.

In some centers, PET imaging of lymphoma patients, because it is performed at many times through the history of the illness, has become the single most common indication for which clinical FDG PET imaging is performed. We anticipate that patient individualized treatment of lymphomas using PET will grow in acceptance in the coming years and that FDG PET (or PET/CT) will be the only imaging test required for management of most lymphomas.

EXAMPLES TO ILLUSTRATE KEY ISSUES

CASE 5.1	Diagnosis: Hodgkin disease – staging

Clinical history:

This patient presented with an enlarged lymph node in the right side of the neck. Biopsy revealed HD. PET/CT was requested for staging and as a baseline for treatment response.

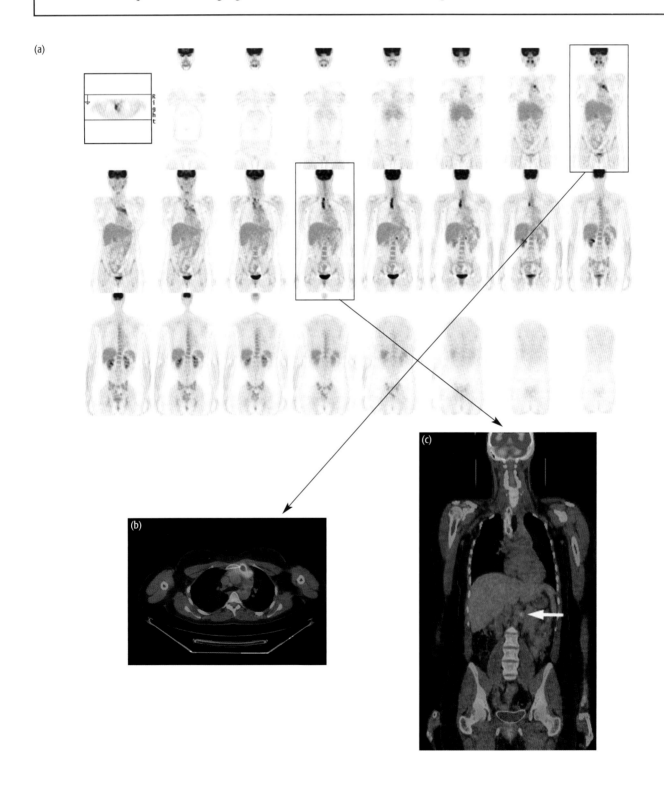

PET/CT findings:

Increased FDG uptake was seen in multiple lymph nodes (a) including the superior mediastinum, the right paratracheal region (b, c) and within a soft-tissue mass in the left anterior mediastinum (d). In the abdomen there was a single area of increased uptake fusing to a small left para-aortic lymph node (c).

Key points:

1 PET can detect disease in lymph nodes that are not enlarged by CT criteria.
2 PET is more accurate than CT staging alone. In this case PET detected disease below the diaphragm not seen on CT. This altered the staging in this patient who was treated with chemotherapy.

CASE 5.2	Diagnosis: Burkitt lymphoma – staging

Clinical history:

This patient was referred with Burkitt lymphoma diagnosed on liver biopsy. She had presented with jaundice and pruritus. The patient had received a renal transplant 9 years prior to diagnosis. PET was requested for initial staging.

(a)

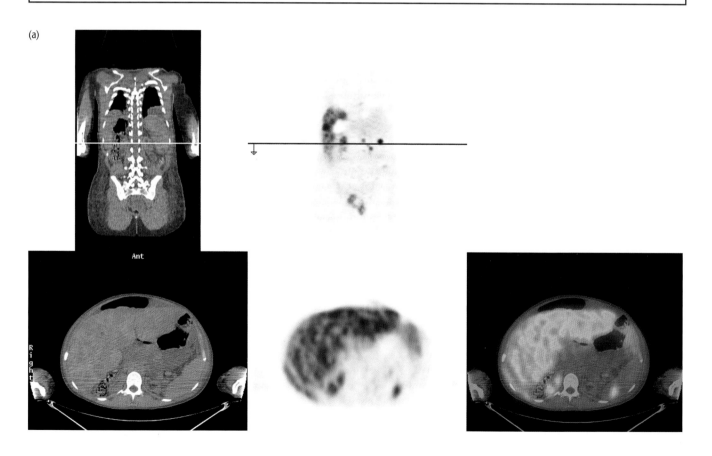

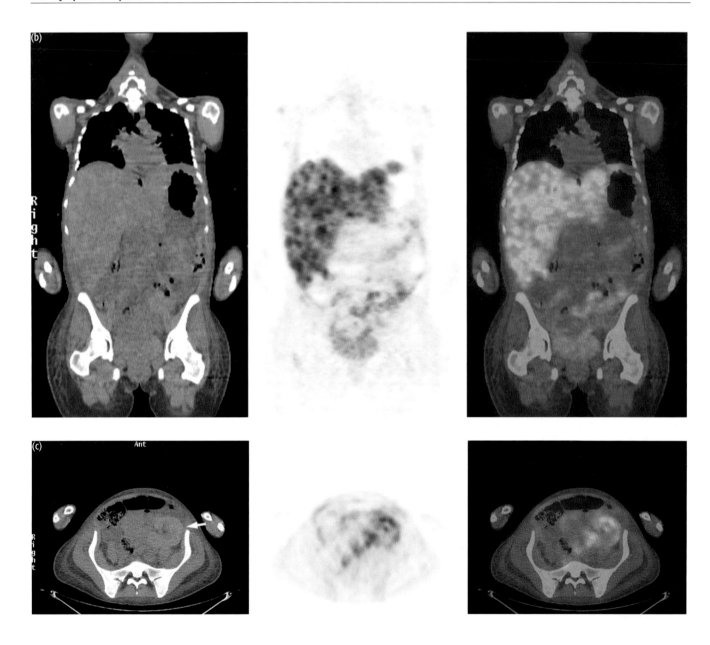

PET/CT findings:

There was extensive disease in the liver (a,b) and focal disease in the spleen (a). FDG uptake in the left lower abdomen corresponds to a renal transplant (c).

Key points:

1 PET can be useful in extranodal as well as nodal disease assessment.
2 A scan prior to treatment is valuable both for staging and as a baseline for treatment response.
3 Increased FDG uptake can be seen in normal structures such as renal transplants and should not be confused with disease.
4 Lymphoma occurs at increased frequency in immunosuppressed patients with transplants.

| CASE 5.3 | Diagnosis: Hodgkin disease – staging |

Clinical history:

This patient presented with a cough and feeling unwell. Lymph node biopsy of an enlarged axillary node revealed mixed cellularity HD. PET/CT was requested for staging and baseline assessment.

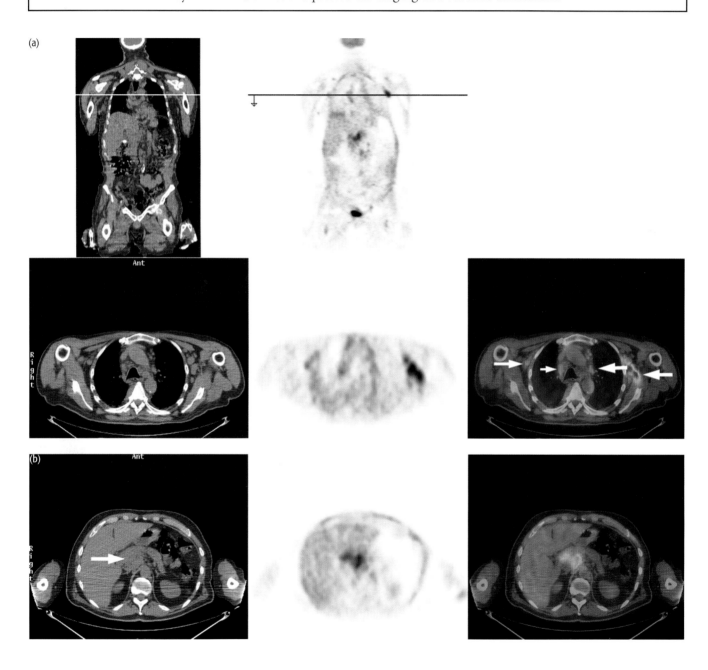

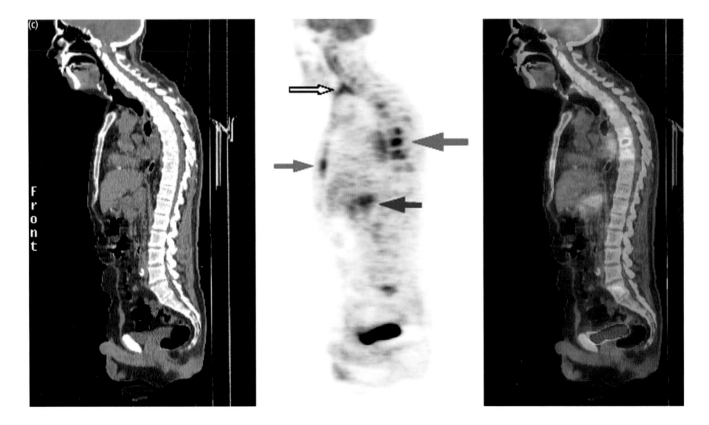

PET/CT findings:

There was uptake of FDG in multiple lymph node groups above and below the diaphragm including both axillae, right paratracheal, para-aortic, and aortopulmonary nodes in the chest (a) and celiac nodes in the abdomen (b, blue arrow in c). The scan also indicated widespread bone involvement: note uptake in the sternum and multiple vertebrae (red arrows in c). Also note that the physiologic uptake is seen within laryngeal muscles (white arrow in c). The laryngeal muscles often have an inverted 'V' shape on sagittal images. (Not shown is uptake in subcarinal aortocaval and bilateral para-aortic nodes as well as bone involvement in left sacroiliac joint, sacrum, and femora.)

Key points:

1 PET is sensitive for the detection of lymphoma, both nodal and extranodal disease.
2 Where there is patchy bone involvement, PET can be used to direct biopsy.

| CASE 5.4 | Diagnosis: Hodgkin disease – staging |

Clinical history:

This patient was referred with newly diagnosed nodular sclerosing HD for initial staging.

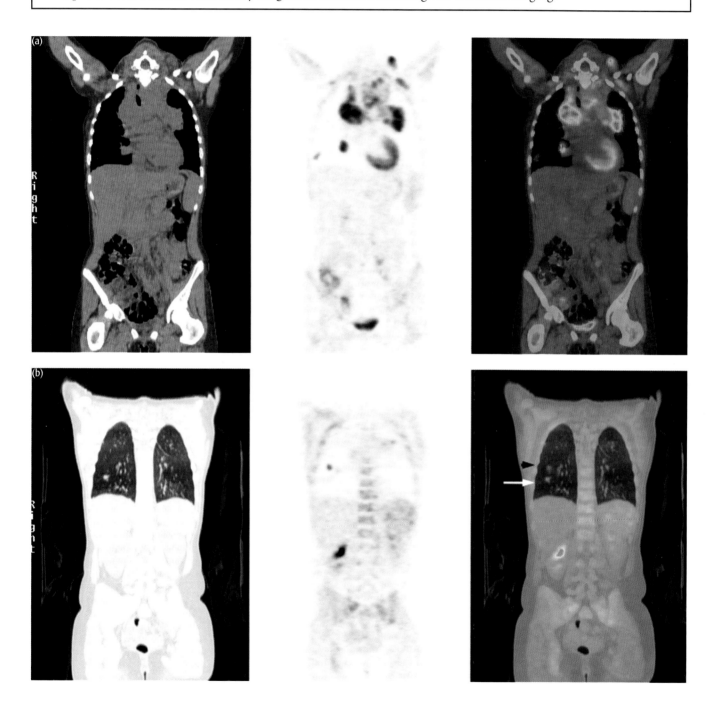

PET/CT findings:

PET showed uptake in multiple lymph node groups above the diaphragm. Uptake in left cervical, left axillary, mediastinal, and paracardiac nodes is shown (a) as well as uptake in lung nodules (a, b).

Note that there is some misregistration between the PET and the CT images in the cranio–caudal direction (b), with the PET uptake lying superior to the nodule position in the lung on CT. There is also a pericardial effusion, which does not appear to be taking up FDG (a). Marked physiologic uptake is also seen in the myocardium (b).

Key points:

1 This represents stage IV disease because of multifocal lung involvement.
2 Misregistration between PET and CT is not uncommon in the thorax due to respiratory motion.

CASE 5.5	Diagnosis: Burkitt lymphoma – treatment response

Clinical history:

This patient was referred for PET scanning on the first occasion for staging of Burkitt lymphoma. The patient was treated with chemotherapy and rescanned after a single cycle.

(a)

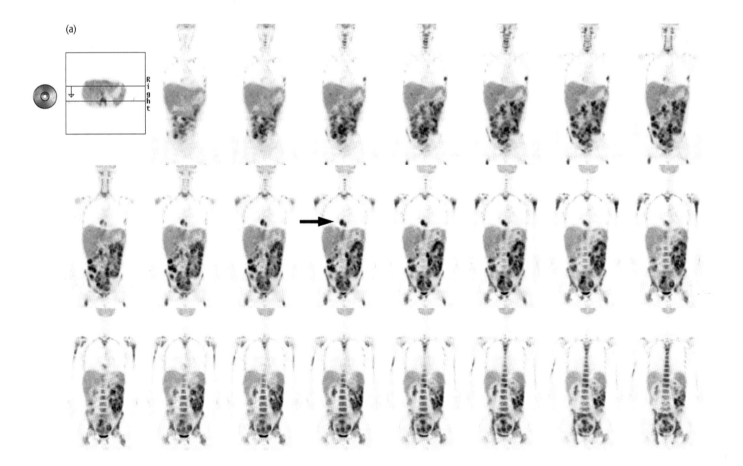

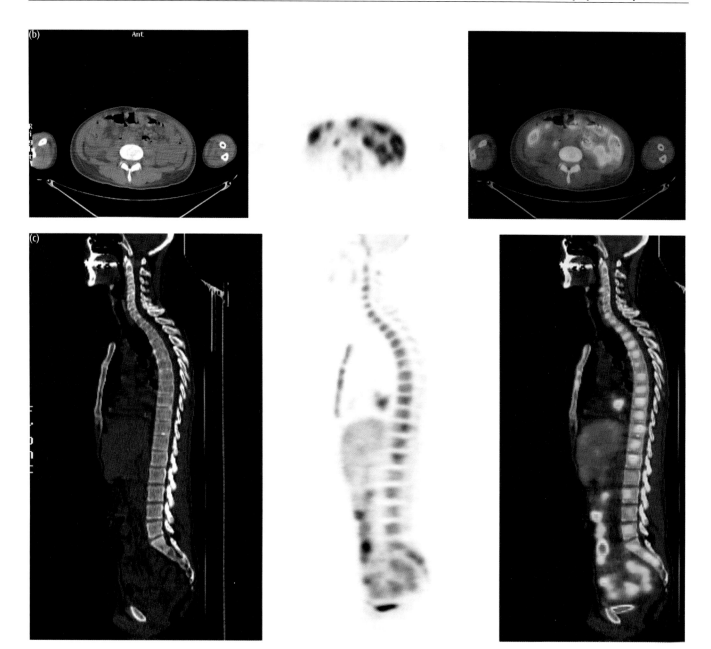

(d)

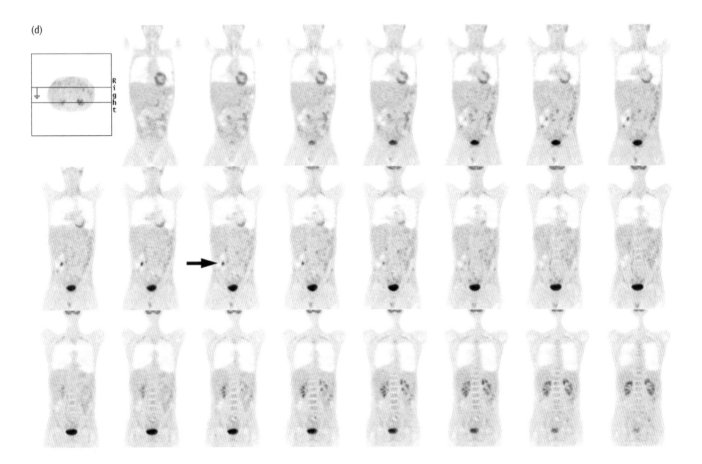

PET/CT findings:

The initial scan showed extensive uptake in the bone marrow (a, c), small bowel/mesentery (a, b), and in paracardiac lymph nodes (arrowed in a). After a single cycle the PET scan showed almost complete resolution of disease with the exception of a small area of increased uptake in the abdomen (d), within small bowel. The low-grade uptake seen elsewhere corresponded to large bowel and was physiologic.

The patient subsequently presented with uncontrolled gastrointestinal bleeding. Resection of small bowel revealed cytomegalovirus rather than residual Burkitt lymphoma.

Key points:

1 PET can be used to assess early response to treatment.
2 When assessing response to treatment, if there are findings that are not easily explained, it is worth considering alternative pathology including infection. Such findings might include unexpected 'new' disease at a site not involved at presentation or disease at a single site with almost complete response elsewhere.

Case 5.6	Diagnosis: Hodgkin disease – treatment response

Clinical history:

This patient was diagnosed with HD, with multiple small lymph nodes above and below the diaphragm at presentation on CT and with marrow involvement on bone marrow biopsy. PET was requested for baseline assessment and again following two cycles of chemotherapy to assess treatment response.

(a)

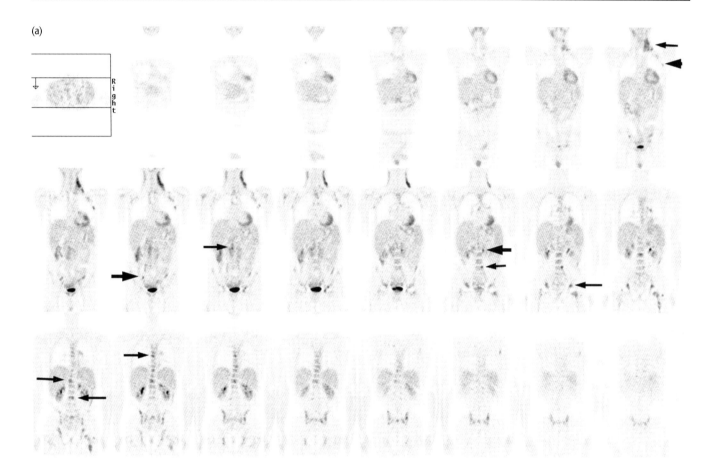

(b)

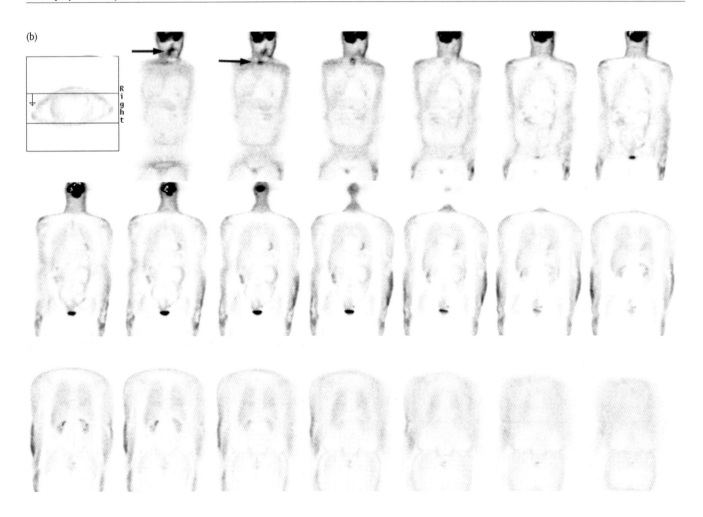

PET/CT findings:

The initial PET scan showed abnormal uptake in multiple lymph nodes including left cervical, left supraclavicular, left axillary, bilateral para-aortic and right external iliac nodes (a). Uptake was also seen in bone including left femoral head and thoracic and lumbar spine (a).

Following two cycles of chemotherapy all abnormal uptake had completely resolved indicating complete response (b). Note: this scan was performed on an older scanner and nonattenuation corrected scans are shown. Physiologic uptake is seen within the larynx and within the tonsils, which are asymmetric because of head rotation on this scan (b).

Key points:

1 Rapid response to treatment on PET predicts a good outcome.
2 Although PET/CT is useful, PET alone is highly accurate in lymphoma management.

CASE 5.7	Diagnosis: Hodgkin disease – treatment response

Clinical history:

This patient presented with bilateral cervical and axillary lymphadenopathy and a widened mediastinum on chest radiograph. Biopsy of a neck node had revealed HD. PET was requested for baseline assessment and again following two cycles of chemotherapy for treatment response.

(a)

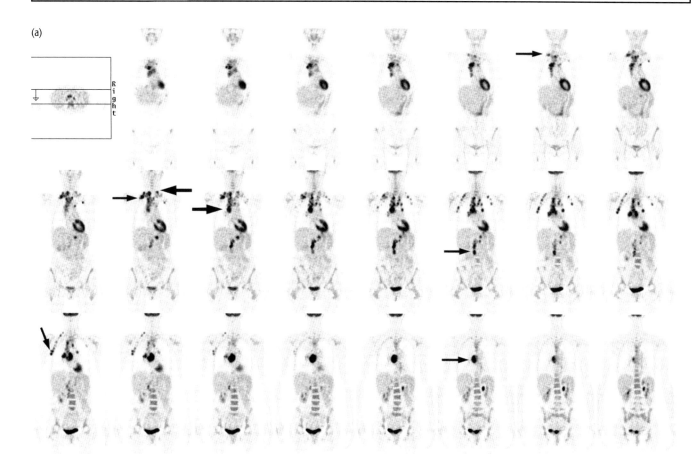

(b)

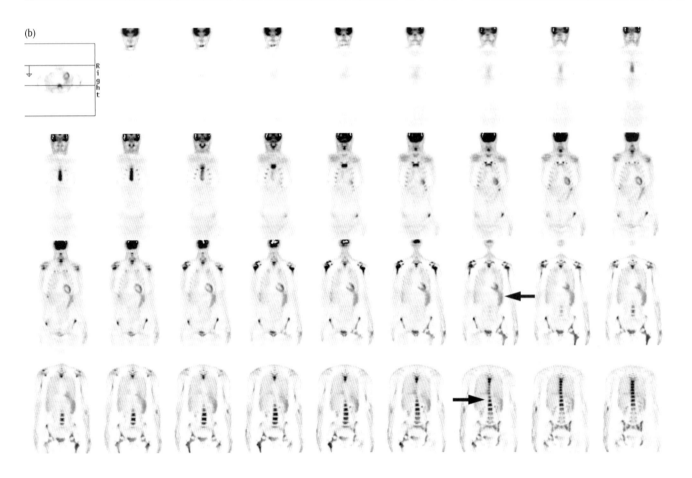

PET/CT findings:

The initial PET scan showed abnormal uptake in multiple lymph nodes including both cervical and supraclavicular regions, the mediastinum, right axilla, and right para-aortic nodes (a).

Following two cycles of chemotherapy all abnormal uptake had completely resolved indicating complete response (b). The markedly increased uptake within marrow and spleen reflects marrow activation due to treatment. Note: this scan was performed on an older scanner and nonattenuation corrected scans are shown.

Key points:

1 Metabolic changes precede structural changes. PET can be used as an early indicator of treatment response.
2 PET scanning after two cycles gives an accurate response assessment.

CASE 5.8 | Diagnosis: NHL – treatment response

Clinical history:

This patient with B cell follicular lymphoma was scanned at the end of eight cycles of chemotherapy to assess response. He complained of persisting pain in the anterior right chest wall.

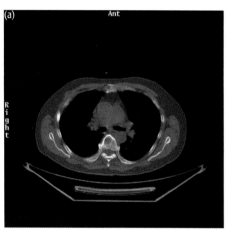

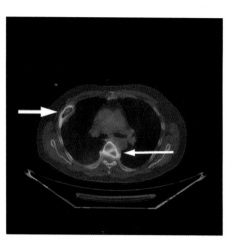

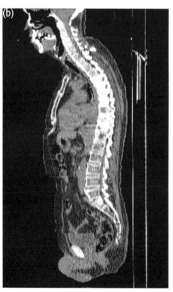
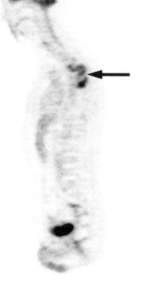

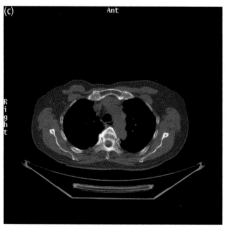
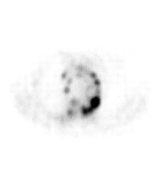
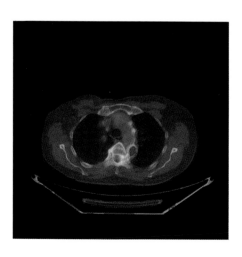

PET/CT findings:

There were multiple lesions within bone and in the chest wall with high FDG uptake (a). Note the uptake in the thoracic vertebra between T5 and T7 (arrowed in b). Extensive nodal disease was also seen in the mediastinum (c). The findings were those of widespread disease, resistant to treatment.

Key points:

1 PET is very sensitive in lymphoma and has the ability to show both nodal and extranodal disease.
2 Note in the sagittal image (b) that not all the abnormal sclerotic vertebral bodies on the CT show FDG uptake. The PET shows only those areas with active disease posttreatment.

| CASE 5.9 | Diagnosis: Lymphoma – treatment response |

Clinical history:

This patient was scanned after six cycles of chemotherapy with residual active lymphoma identified in both axillary regions on PET. The patient proceeded to further high-dose chemotherapy and autologous bone marrow transplant. PET/CT was requested to assess whether the patient would be suitable for mantle radiotherapy or if disease could not be encompassed within the radiotherapy field if allograft transplantation should be considered.

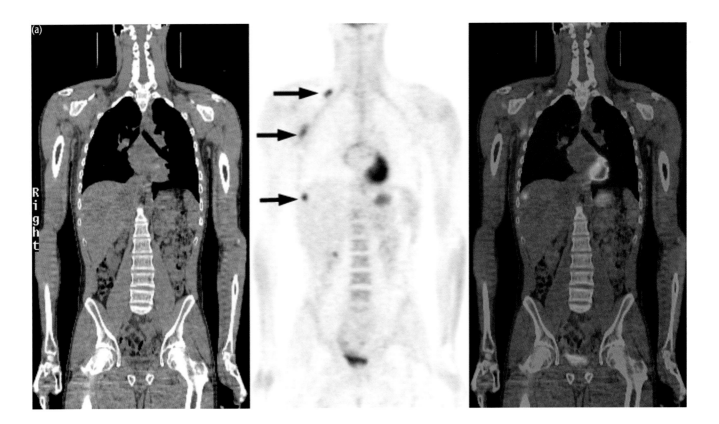

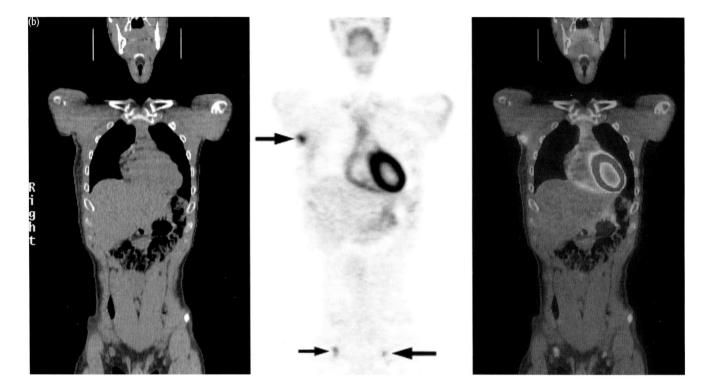

PET/CT findings:

There was residual active disease in the right axilla (a, b) as well as uptake in the right supraclavicular region, liver (a), and in both inguinal regions (b), indicating that radiotherapy was not the appropriate treatment.

Key point:

PET can identify tumor that would be missed in radiation ports planned anatomically.

| CASE 5.10 | Diagnosis: Lymphoma – residual mass post treatment |

Clinical history:

This patient with nodular sclerosing HD was treated with chemotherapy. There was resolution of enlarged neck nodes and partial anatomic response in a large mediastinal mass. However, there was concern that the mass remained enlarged and a PET/CT scan was requested to determine whether viable tumor remained.

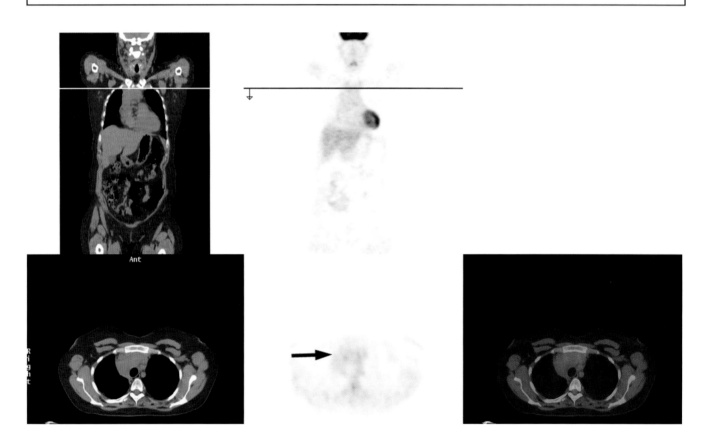

PET/CT findings:

There was no uptake of FDG associated with the anterior mediastinal mass, representing residual fibrosis. On the basis of this, high-dose chemotherapy and stem cell transplantation were avoided.

Key points:

1 PET/CT can accurately differentiate active tumor from fibrosis in residual masses after treatment of lymphoma.
2 A negative PET predicts a longer disease-free survival.

| CASE 5.11 | Diagnosis: Non-Hodgkin lymphoma – residual mass |

Clinical history:

This patient presented with renal impairment secondary to perirenal lymphadenopathy due to NHL. At the end of eight cycles of chemotherapy there was residual lymphadenopathy at the left renal hilum. PET/CT was requested to determine if this represented residual disease or fibrosis.

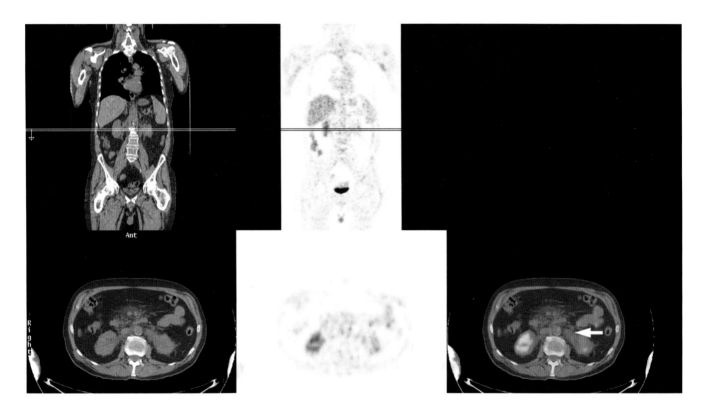

PET/CT findings:

There was no uptake at the site of the residual mass, which represented fibrosis and not active tumor.

Key point:

High-grade NHL usually takes up FDG but some types of lymphoma including low-grade lymphomas, mantle cell lymphoma, and MALTomas may have variable uptake of FDG, and it is preferable to scan patients at baseline. A posttreatment 'negative' scan with a baseline scan that shows that the lymphoma is FDG avid gives greater confidence that there is complete response to treatment.

| CASE 5.12 | Diagnosis: Non-Hodgkin lymphoma – residual mass |

Clinical history:

This patient was referred following six courses of chemotherapy for diffuse large B cell lymphoma of the abdomen and pancreas. There was resolution of much of the abdominal lymphadenopathy but a 3.5 cm × 3.8 cm residual mass remained near the head of the pancreas. PET was requested to determine if the mass contained active tumor.

(a)

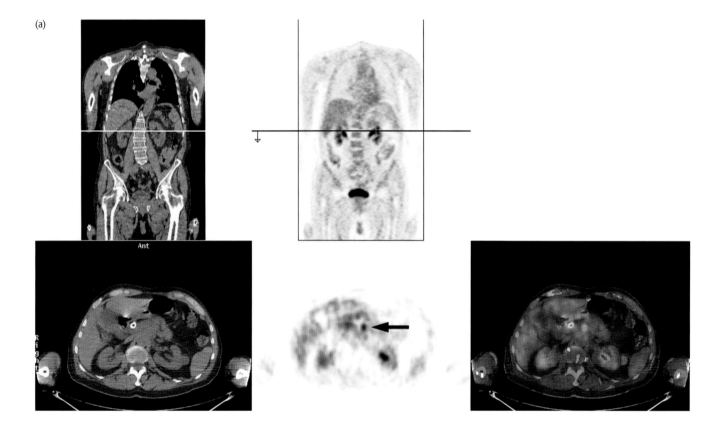

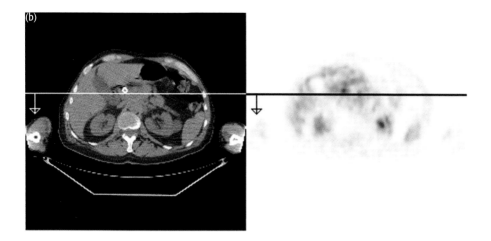

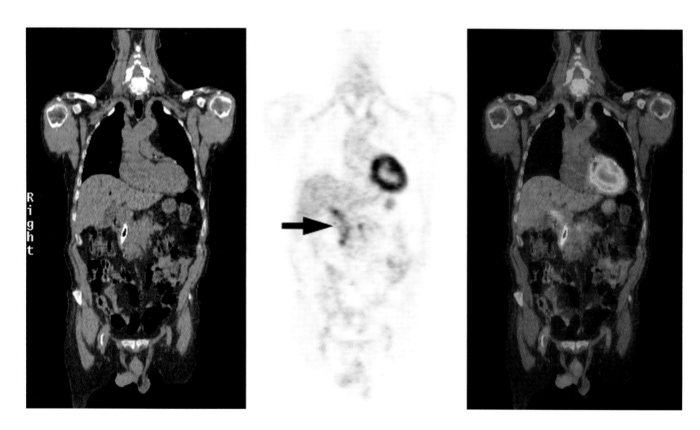

PET/CT findings:

There was a small but intense focus of uptake within the peripancreatic nodal mass adjacent to the biliary stent suggestive of active residual disease. Curvilinear uptake related to the stent was also identified.

Key points:

1 Uptake along stents is common and this does not necessarily represent active tumor.
2 A focus of uptake remote from the stent is most consistent with active NHL.

CASE 5.13	Diagnosis: Castleman disease

Clinical history:

This 60-year-old gentleman with multicentric Castleman disease was treated with stem cell transplantation and chemotherapy. CT showed stable disease with residual lymphadenopathy in the mediastinum and in axillary and inguinal lymph nodes. PET/CT was requested to determine if there was active disease in the mediastinum that would require radiotherapy.

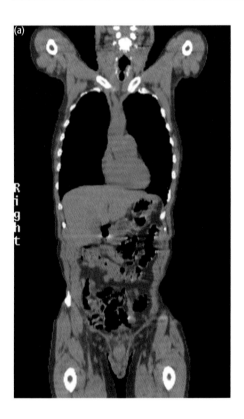
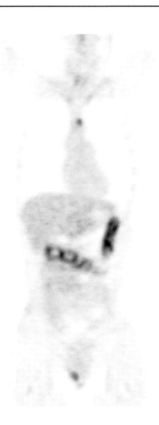
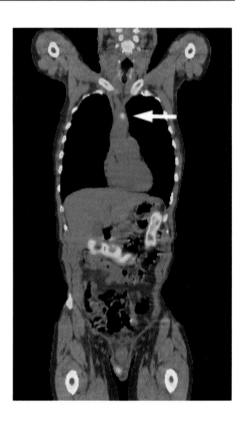

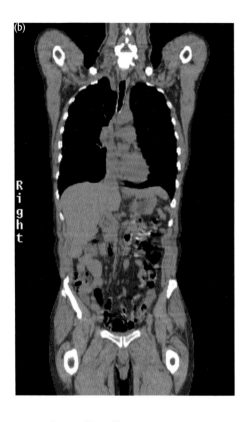 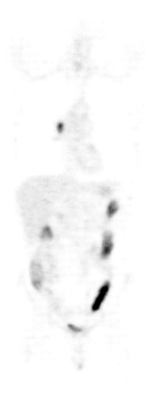 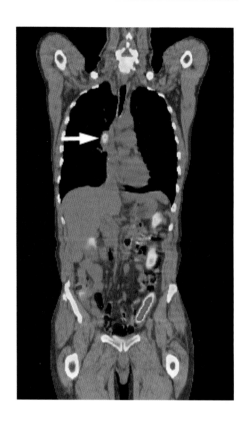

PET/CT findings:

There was intense uptake in the left side of the superior mediastinum and at the right hilum indicative of active residual disease. The right hilar lesion was biopsied and revealed plasmacytic change in keeping with multicentric Castleman disease. Interestingly the peripheral nodes that did not take up tracer had been biopsied previously but did not show plasmacytic change, and they may have represented more 'benign' changes that can be seen in association with Castleman disease or sites of eradicated disease.

Key points:

1 Castleman disease is a lymph node disorder, the most common type of which is hyaline–vascular, which is associated with benign enlargement of lymph nodes and presents in the young.
2 The plasma cell type can present as multicentric disease associated with hepatosplenomegaly in older patients and is associated with systemic symptoms, infection, and lymphoma. The multicentric form of the disease is usually progressive despite treatment.
3 PET/CT can identify active lymph nodes for biopsy.

CASE 5.14	Diagnosis: MALToma – relapse/restaging

Clinical history:

This patient had a history of MALToma that affected the right middle lobe of the lung 6 years earlier. He complained of cough. A CT scan 8 weeks before PET showed consolidation in the right middle lobe. The patient was treated with antibiotics without any effect on his symptoms. PET/CT was requested to determine if there was relapse.

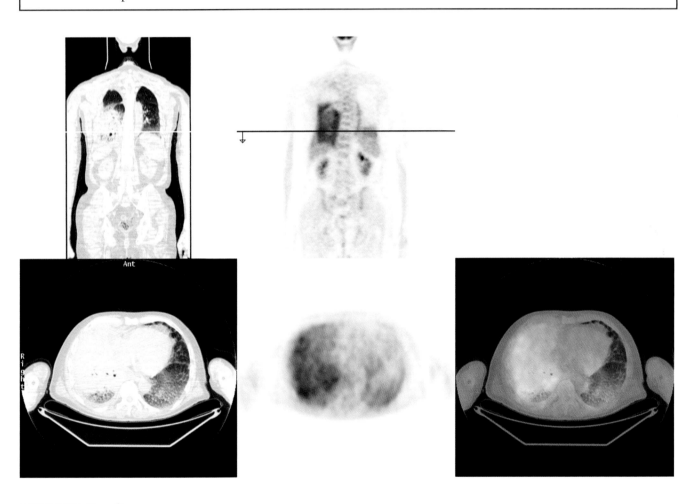

PET/CT findings:

There was diffuse increased uptake within much of the right lung as well as in the left lower lobe, with rapid progression of disease since the earlier CT scan. Transbronchial biopsy from the right lung revealed MALToma.

Key points:

1 Infection or tumor could give these appearances on PET, indeed the diffuse nature of the uptake might have favored infection. However, the patient was relatively well which would not have been in keeping with extensive infection and the biopsy confirmed tumor.
2 MALToma may have variable uptake with FDG and, along with low-grade follicular and lymphocytic lymphomas and mantle cell lymphoma, is one of the subtypes of lymphoma which may be FDG negative. In this case, however, there was extensive uptake.

CONCLUSIONS

CURRENT CLINICAL INDICATIONS

1 Staging
2 Early prediction of therapy response
3 Activity of residual masses
4 Remission assessment/suspected recurrence
5 Central nervous system: infection versus lymphoma in human immunodeficiency virus (HIV) disease
6 Assessment of prognosis

FURTHER READING

Barrington SF, O'Doherty MJ (2003) Limitations of PET for imaging lymphoma. *Eur J Nucl Med Mol Imaging* **30**(Suppl 1), S117–S127.

Carr R, Barrington SF, Saunders CAB, Maden B *et al.* (1998) Can FDG PET predict bone marrow involvement in patients with lymphoma? *Blood* **91**, 3340–6.

Goldberg MA, Lee MJ, Fischman AJ *et al.* (1993) Fluorodeoxyglucose PET of abdominal and pelvic neoplasms: potential role in oncologic imaging. *Radiographs* **13**, 1047–62.

Harris NL, Jaffe ES, Diebold J *et al.* (1999) World Health Organization classification of neoplastic diseases of the hematopoietic and lymphoid tissues: report of the Clinical Advisory Committee meeting – Airlie House, Virginia, November 1997. *J Clin Oncol* **17**, 3835.

Hoff JM, Waskin HA, Schifter T *et al.* (1993) FED-PET in differentiating lymphoma from nonmalignant central nervous system lesions in patients with AIDS. *J Nucl Med* **34**, 567–75.

Kasamon YL, Wahl RL, Swinnen LJ (2004) FDG PET and high-dose therapy for aggressive lymphomas: toward a risk-adapted strategy. *Curr Opin Oncol* **16**, 100–5.

Kostakoglu L, Coleman M. Leonard JP, Kuji I, Zoe H (2002) PET predicts prognosis after 1 cycle of chemotherapy in aggressive lymphoma and Hodgkin's disease. *J Nucl Med* **43**, 1018–27.

Lapela M, Leskinen S, Minn HRI *et al.* (1995) Increased glucose metabolism in untreated non-Hodgkin's lymphoma: a study with positron emission tomography and fluorine-18-fluorodeoxyglucose. *Blood* **86**, 3522–7.

Mikhaeel NG, Timothy AR, Hain SF, O'Doherty MJ (2000) 18-FDG-PET for the assessment of residual masses on CT following treatment of lymphomas. *Ann Oncol* **11**(Suppl 1), 147–50.

Mikhaeel NG, Timothy AR, O'Doherty MJ, Hain SF, Maisey MN (2000) 18-FDG PET as a prognostic indicator in the treatment of aggressive non-Hodgkin's lymphoma – comparison with CT. *Leuk Lymphoma* **39**, 543–53.

Newman JS, Francis IR, Kaminski MS, Wahl RL (1994) FDG-PET imaging in lymphoma: correlation with CT. *Radiology* **190**, 111–16.

No authors listed (1993) A predictive model for aggressive non-Hodgkin's lymphoma. The International Non-Hodgkin's Lymphoma Prognostic Factors Project [see comments]. *N Engl J Med* **329**, 987.

O'Doherty MJ, Hoskin PJ (2003) Positron emission tomography in the management of lymphomas: a summary. *Eur J Nucl Med Mol Imaging* **30**(Suppl 1), S128–S130.

O'Doherty MJ, Barrington SF, Cambell M *et al.* (1997) PET scanning and the HIV positive patient. *J Nucl Med* **38**, 1575–83.

Okada J, Yoshikawa K, Imazeki K *et al.* (1991) The use of FDG-PET in the detection and management of malignant lymphoma: correlation of uptake with prognosis. *J Nucl Med* **32**, 686–91.

Partridge, S, Timothy, AR, O'Doherty *et al.* (2000) 2-Fluorine-18-fluoro-2-deoxy-D glucose positron emission tomography in the pretreatment staging of Hodgkin's disease: influence on patient management in a single institution. *Ann Oncol* **11**, 1273–9.

Paul R (1987) Comparison of fluorine-18-2-fluorodeoxyglucose and gallium-67 citrate imaging for detection of lymphoma. *J Nucl Med* **28**, 288–92.

Rodriguez M, Rehn S, Ahlstrom H *et al.* (1995) Predicting malignancy grade with PET in non-Hodgkin's lymphoma. *J Nucl Med* **36**, 1790–6.

Solal-Celigny P, Roy P, Colombat P *et al.* (2004) Follicular lymphoma international prognostic index. *Blood* **104**, 1258–65.

Spaepen K, Stroobants S, Dupont P, Mortelmans L (2001) Prognostic value of positron emission tomography (PET) with fluorine-18 fluorodeoxyglucose ([18F]FDG) after first-line chemotherapy in non-Hodgkin's lymphoma: is [18F]FDG-PET a valid alternative to conventional diagnostic methods? *J Clin Oncol* **15**, 414–19.

Spaepen K, Stroobants S, Dupont P *et al.* (2003) Prognostic value of pretransplantation positron emission tomography using fluorine 18-fluorodeoxyglucose in patients with aggressive lymphoma treated with high-dose chemotherapy and stem cell transplantation. *Blood* **102**, 53–9.

Spaepen K, Stroobants S, Verhoef G *et al.* (2003) Positron emission tomography with [(18)F]FDG for therapy response monitoring in lymphoma patients. *Eur J Nucl Med Mol Imaging* **30**(Suppl 1), S97–S105.

CHAPTER 6

COLORECTAL AND HEPATOBILIARY TUMORS

INTRODUCTION AND BACKGROUND

Colorectal cancer is the second most common cause of death from cancer overall in industrialized Western countries. There are, however, great international variations – 20-fold variations in incidence rates. Some of the highest rates are found in Connecticut in the USA. A clear relation between the incidence of colorectal cancer and dietary fat content has been demonstrated. Primary treatment is surgical with approximately a 55 percent 5-year survival rate. Adjuvant chemotherapy is widely employed but chemotherapeutic response to recurrence is poor. Follow-up with serum carcinoembryonic antigen (CEA) levels is valuable for detecting recurrence, but CEA is only elevated with active disease in about 50 percent of patients. Resection of limited metastases to the liver has been shown to improve survival in carefully selected patients. Radiation therapy may be used for rectal carcinoma but less commonly for carcinoma of the colon. Only about 20 percent of patients who have recurrence are considered suitable for further resection and of these about half relapse early due to unsuspected metastatic sites elsewhere.

Hepatobiliary primary tumors are less common in the Western world than are metastases to the liver, but liver and bile duct cancers are more common in Asia. Hepatomas are the fifth most common cancer worldwide. Risk factors include aflatoxins, hepatitis B and C, and schistosomiasis. Cancers of the biliary ducts and of the gall bladder are less common, but can be diagnostically challenging. Since colon cancer can present with liver metastases, separating primary liver neoplasms from colon cancer metastases can be an important clinical question.

Colon cancer is more frequent than rectal cancer and is increasing in frequency in industrialized Western countries.

EPIDEMIOLOGY OF COLORECTAL CANCERS	
Incidence	
Men	66 new cases per 100 000/ 18 956 cases UK
	54 new cases per 100 000/ 71 820 cases USA
Women	54 new cases per 100 000/ 16 344 cases UK
	51 new cases per 100 000/ 73 470 cases USA
Male/female ratio	M >F but approaching 1:1
Peak age	Elderly (85% > 60 years)
~10% of all cancers	
10% of all cancer deaths	

The vast majority of colorectal cancers are adenocarcinomas, which may be ulcerating or fungating and cause large bowel obstruction if not discovered promptly. Screening colonoscopy allows detection of these tumors at earlier stages.

PATHOLOGY		
Histology	>90% adenocarcinoma	
Tumour site	Anorectal	31%
	Cecum/ascending colon	19%
	Sigmoid colon	18%
	Transverse/descending colon	10%

Although there are a number of predisposing factors the majority of colorectal cancers occur in patients with no currently obvious predisposing factors.

RISK FACTORS

Family history
Familial adenomatous polyposis (FAP)
Hereditary nonpolyposis colorectal cancer (HNPCC)
Ulcerative colitis
Crohn disease
Previous diagnosis of bowel cancer
Diet

The prognosis in general is worse for rectal than colon cancer but varies from 90 percent 5-year survival for early localized disease to less than 10 percent when the disease presents in an advanced form.
Approximately 25 percent of patients will have metastases at the time of presentation.

PROGNOSIS

Dukes stage	5-year survival (%)
A	85–95
B	60–80
C	30–60
D	<10

Approximately 45 percent of patients diagnosed as having colorectal cancer can be cured by effective surgical resection.

RESECTION

100 patients
- 70 resectable
  - 45 cured
  - 25 recur
- 30 advanced

Primary staging of colon cancer is usually surgical and pathological as most patients require resection to control local disease and prevent obstruction. PET systematically underestimates the number of lymph nodes involved with tumor as it cannot detect microscopic disease in nodes.

STAGING

TNM stage		Modified Dukes
Stage 0	Carcinoma *in situ*	A
Stage I	Tumor invades submusosa (T1)	A
	Tumor invades muscularis propria (T2)	
	No nodal/distant metastases	
Stage II	Tumor invades beyond muscularis propria (T3)	B
	Tumor invades into other organs (T4)	
	No nodal/distant metastases	
Stage III	1–3 regional lymph nodes involved (N1), any T	C
	4 or more regional lymph nodes (N2)	
	No distant metastases, any T	
Stage IV	Distant metastases (M1), any T, any N	D

SITES OF RECURRENCE AND METASTASES (%)	
Isolated local	20
Hepatic	30
Other abdominal	20
Pulmonary	20
Retroperitoneal	10
Ovarian	7
Peritoneal seedlings	3–6

Approximately 70 percent of patients who develop distant metastasis will also have a local recurrence.

KEY MANAGEMENT ISSUES

KEY MANAGEMENT ISSUES
Primary staging
Preresection assessment
Evaluating liver lesions
Response to treatment
Suspected recurrence and restaging

Role of PET in colorectal cancer

Colorectal cancer was the first noncentral nervous system neoplasm to be imaged with positron emission tomography (PET) in humans (in 1982). Although PET can detect primary colon cancers, there is substantial background [^{18}F]2-fluoro-2-deoxy-D-glucose (FDG) uptake in normal bowel, which serves to lower tumor/background uptake ratios. PET is therefore not generally used for primary diagnosis or screening, but focal intense FDG uptake in the colon may be indicative of an incidental colon cancer (or a cellular adenoma) and may be found in patients who have PET performed for other reasons.

PET can be used for the initial staging of colon cancer because it is able to detect locoregional and disseminated metastatic disease. In most centers, standard practice has been not to perform PET or PET/CT before primary surgery, as the primary tumor must be removed in most cases to avoid obstruction and since PET detects only about 30 percent of nodal metastases. In some instances, however, if multiple systemic metastases are present at diagnosis, the patient may be treated with systemic chemotherapy instead of surgical resection of the primary when a baseline PET may be useful. PET may be helpful in defining unusual sites of lymph node drainage, such as to the external iliac or inguinal nodes from tumors located near the anus, where lymphatic drainage differs from that seen with more proximal colon cancers. Thus, the use of PET in primary tumor staging is becoming more common, but is by no means the norm.

The best established use of PET in clinical practice has been for the detection of tumor recurrence in patients with rising levels of serum CEA and otherwise normal radiographic studies, or in the setting of what appears to be limited recurrent disease. Here PET is used to determine if a radiological abnormality is a resectable recurrence and what its true extent is, and the presence or absence of metastasis elsewhere. Many reports have shown FDG PET to be much more accurate than computed tomography (CT) for detection of intra-abdominal metastases from colorectal cancer. The largest series, with 76 patients, reported an accuracy of 95 percent for PET but only 65 percent for CT. Detection of liver metastases was also feasible and accurate. A comprehensive review of the literature (2244 patient studies) showed 94 percent sensitivity and 87 percent specificity of PET for recurrent colorectal cancer, which was higher than of CT (79 percent sensitivity and 73 percent specificity). A recent meta-analysis has confirmed FDG PET to be more accurate than CT, magnetic resonance imaging (MRI), or ultrasound for the detection of colorectal cancer metastases.

Tumors with mucinous histology have lower FDG uptake than those with other histologies because of the high ratio of mucin to cellular components, and these occasionally may be falsely negative on PET imaging. PET has been reported to have sensitivity in excess of 80 percent for the detection of recurrent colorectal carcinoma when CEA levels are rising and CT scans have not identified the source.

Detection of extrahepatic metastases of colorectal cancer dramatically changes management as that planned when metastasis is truly isolated to the liver. Major changes of management in 30–60 percent of such patients studied by PET have been reported. These changes in patient management can result in substantial cost savings by avoiding unnecessary therapeutic procedures. Patients with recurrent colorectal cancer selected by PET for resectability appear to have longer survival than patients selected without the use of PET. Limited reports to date on both chemotherapy and radiotherapy support the role of PET in assessing treatment response. With radiotherapy, response should be assessed several months or longer after treatment is completed, as the PET signal declines only slowly, even with effective treatment. However with chemotherapy, the fall in tracer uptake occurs much more promptly. PET may be of particular utility in monitoring treatment of liver metastases of colorectal carcinoma, as it appears to be able to define responders/nonresponders much earlier than anatomic means. This is of particular relevance now that patients are being treated with a variety of local therapies to the liver.

As with other parts of the body, knowledge of the normal patterns of tracer uptake is essential to allow differentiation of tumor uptake from that seen in normal tissues, such as colon or caecum. In this regard PET/CT is more accurate than PET alone in colorectal cancer, with the increase being achieved through much higher levels of reader confidence in lesion localization compared with PET alone. Overall, PET is assuming a growing role in the evaluation of recurrent colorectal carcinoma, although, to date, it is much more limited in the assessment of primary tumors.

Primary hepatic tumors, hepatomas, and cholangiocarcinoma are less commonly studied tumors in Western clinical PET centers, but are nonetheless important conditions globally. FDG uptake in hepatomas is lower than in many other cancers and about half of hepatomas have tracer uptake levels comparable with normal liver, and thus are undetectable using standard imaging times. Alternative tracers like [^{11}C]acetate have shown promise, but are not widely used at present. Cholangiocarcinomas and gall bladder cancers are generally FDG avid. Small-volume cholangiocarcinomas are commonly not detected on PET, but are detected when larger volumes of tumor are present or when there are nodal or organ metastases. PET with FDG is not particularly useful in screening patients with cirrhosis for development of tumor on a background of hepatocellular disease. Thus, while occasionally used in primary hepatic tumors, FDG PET is much more commonly applied in metastatic disease to the liver.

EXAMPLES TO ILLUSTRATE KEY ISSUES

CASE 6.1	Diagnosis: Colorectal cancer – staging

Clinical history:

This patient was referred with a primary tumor in the sigmoid colon. There was a lung nodule in the right lower lobe on CT of uncertain significance. PET/CT was requested to determine whether the colon cancer was operable.

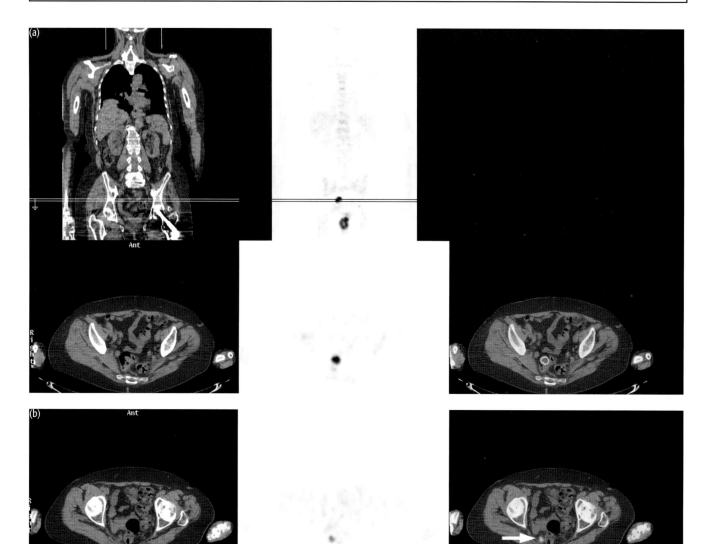

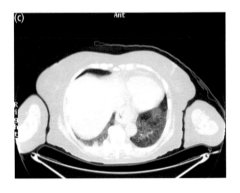

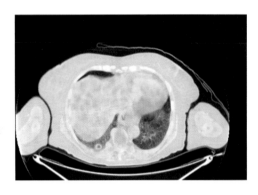

PET/CT findings:

There was uptake in the primary sigmoid cancer (a) with uptake in a small perirectal lymph node (b) and in the right lower lobe lung nodule (c) consistent with nodal and systemic metastases. The patient was treated with chemoradiotherapy.

Key point:

PET/CT may have a role in the primary staging of colorectal cancer, especially if there are suspicious findings on other tests or if the lesion is large and at increased risk of metastasis.

CASE 6.2	Diagnosis: Colorectal cancer – recurrence/restaging

Clinical history:

This patient had a right hemicolectomy and chemotherapy for carcinoma of the cecum. At follow-up his CEA was elevated to 8 mg/L. CT with contrast prior to PET (not shown) demonstrated no evidence of liver metastasis although there was some thickening close to the anastomotic site of uncertain significance. PET/CT was requested to determine if this was postoperative change or cancer and to restage the patient's disease.

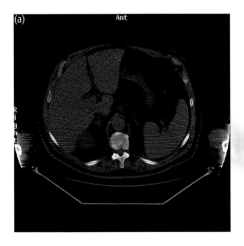
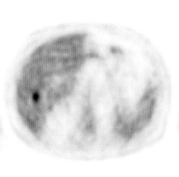
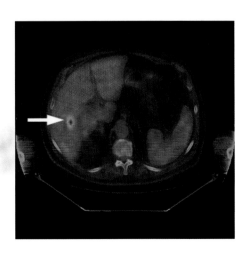

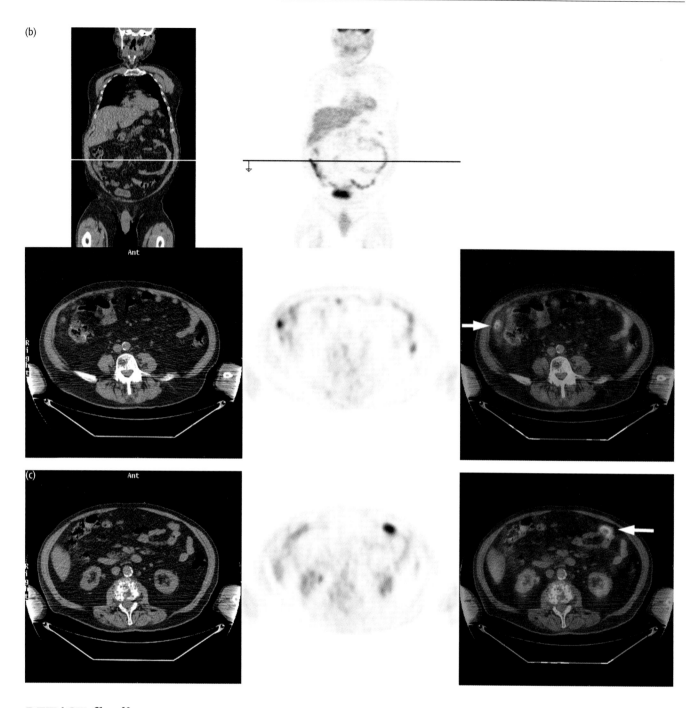

PET/CT findings:

There was high uptake in a liver metastasis (a) and multiple peritoneal deposits (b, c). Physiological uptake in the right ureter is also seen (c). (Not shown are non-FDG-avid left upper lung nodule and renal cyst and multiple additional peritoneal tumor deposits.)

Key points:

1 The combination of PET and CT helps to differentiate physiologic uptake within bowel from small adjacent peritoneal deposits. Note how difficult it is in the coronal images (b) to distinguish physiologic bowel uptake from disease. Remember that physiologic bowel uptake may be focal or diffuse.
2 PET can find liver metastases not visible on CT.

CASE 6.3	Diagnosis: Colorectal cancer – rising markers

Clinical history:

This patient had a history of Dukes C carcinoma of the colon, previously treated with surgery and chemotherapy. He had rising CEA tumor markers. PET/CT was requested to determine if there was recurrent disease.

(a)

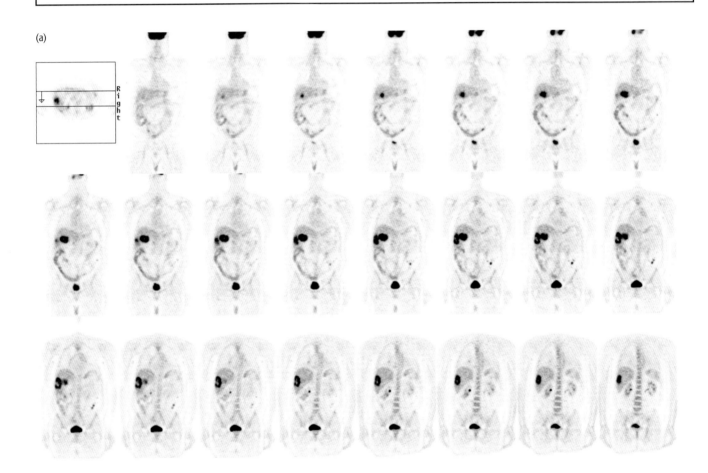

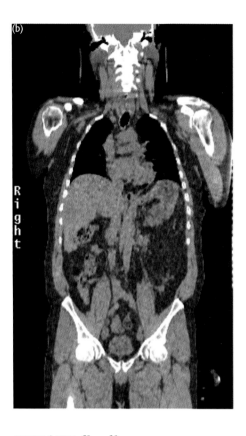
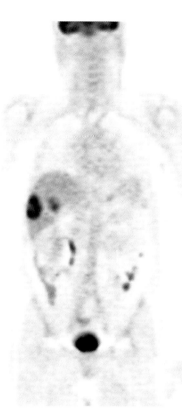
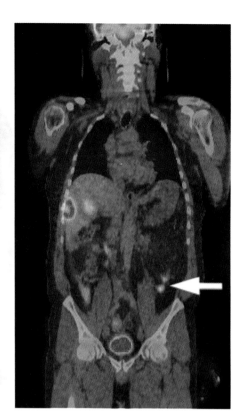

PET/CT findings:

There was uptake in two large liver metastases (a). There were also multiple foci of increased uptake present in the left side of the abdomen on the PET scan. On the CT scan these were seen to correspond to small intra-abdominal soft-tissue deposits (arrowed in b).

Key point:
PET/CT helps to differentiate FDG uptake, which is physiologic within bowel, from peritoneal deposits.

CASE 6.4	Diagnosis: Colorectal cancer – rising markers

Clinical history:

This patient was referred with a history of Dukes C carcinoma of the colon, which had been resected 1 year prior to PET. Postoperative anatomic imaging was unremarkable but her CEA markers continued to rise. PET/CT was requested to determine if there was tumor recurrence.

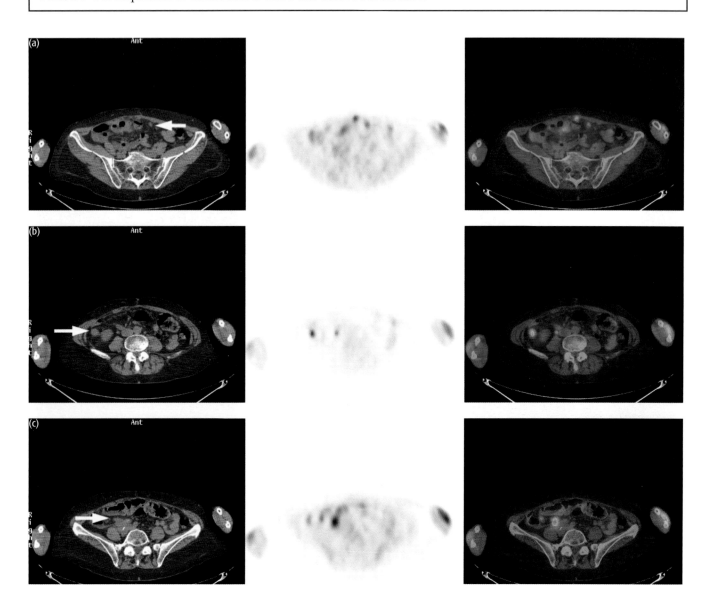

PET/CT findings:

There was increased tracer uptake within the abdomen corresponding to soft-tissue nodules in the peritoneum (a). Note uptake within a peritoneal nodule lying adjacent to the ascending colon (b) and a further nodule anterior to the right ureter at the level of the aortic bifurcation causing obstruction to the renal outflow tract at this level (c).

Key point:

PET/CT establishes the site of recurrent disease with rising tumor markers in patients with cancers that express markers.

CASE 6.5	Diagnosis: Colorectal cancer – recurrence and restaging

Clinical history:

This patient was referred with a history of T4 N1 rectal carcinoma, which had been treated with neoadjuvant chemoradiation, followed by surgery. Seven months postoperatively the patient developed renal failure with bilateral hydronephrosis. There was a large mass in the posterior pelvis on CT. Tumor markers were not raised and the PET was requested to differentiate between posttreatment fibrosis and recurrent local or disseminated tumor.

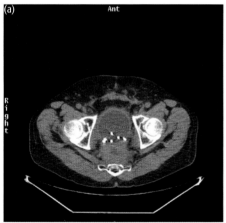
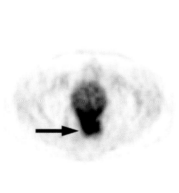
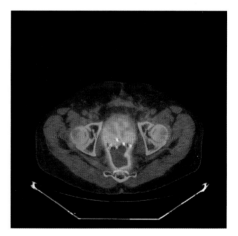
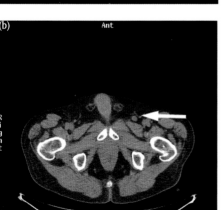
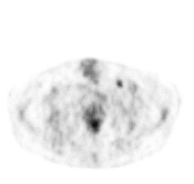
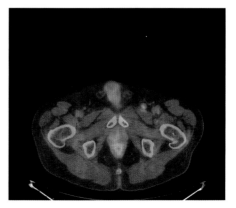

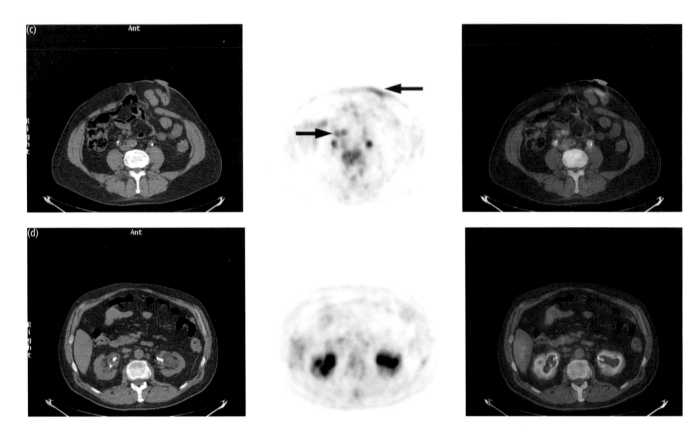

PET/CT findings:

There was intense uptake in the region of the rectal space/stump consistent with tumor (a). Increased uptake in both inguinal (left inguinal node shown in b) and right para-aortic nodes was indicative of nodal metastases (c). Note the stoma uptake (c), bilateral hydronephrosis (d) and ureteric stents (a, c, d).

Key points:

1 PET/CT can distinguish active tumor from the effects of treatment.
2 PET/CT can differentiate between local recurrence and nodal metastatic disease.
3 This scan was performed long enough after treatment that PET should be reliable in separating active tumor from inflammatory tissue associated with the scar.

CASE 6.6 | Diagnosis: Colorectal cancer – recurrence and restaging

Clinical history:

This patient had a history of rectal carcinoma treated with surgery and chemotherapy. Subsequently a partial hepatectomy had been performed for two liver metastases. He was referred with rising CEA. CT and MRI had failed to reveal evidence of disease apart from an equivocal area in the region of the hepatic resection margin. PET/CT was requested to determine if this was postoperative change or cancer.

(a)

(b)

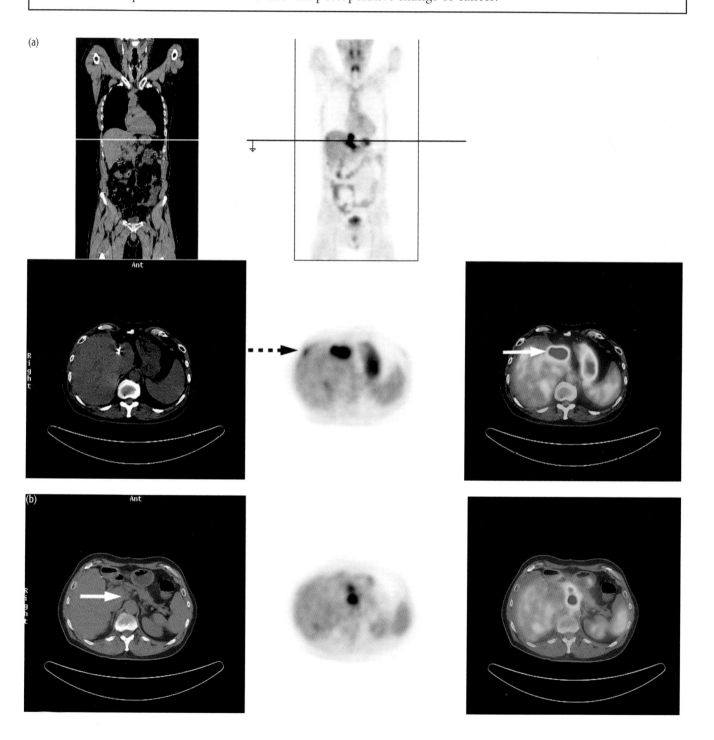

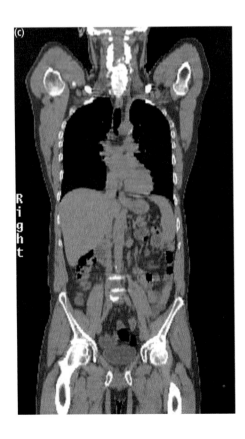 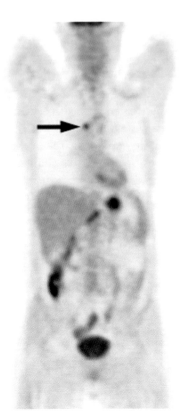 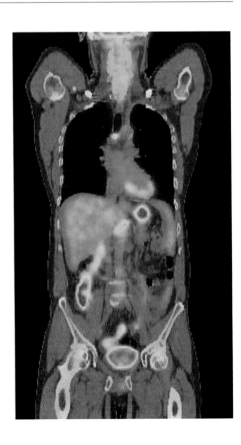

PET/CT findings:

There was recurrent disease within the liver adjacent to the resection margin (solid arrow in image a) with additional uptake in the lateral aspect of the liver (broken arrow in image a). Marked physiologic uptake was also seen within the stomach (a). Uptake was also seen outside the liver, in celiac nodes (b) and in a right paratracheal node (c) indicative of nodal metastases. (Not shown is non-FDG-avid apical lung scarring.)

Key points:

1 PET/CT establishes the presence of recurrent disease and its location. This can directly affect patient management.
2 Commonly patients with apparently solitary metastases may have undiagnosed metastatic disease elsewhere on PET.

CASE 6.7 | Diagnosis: Colorectal cancer – metastasectomy?

Clinical history:

This patient was referred after resection of rectal carcinoma. There was a right lower lobe lung nodule on CT scan, which had been increasing in size. PET/CT was requested to determine if this was a solitary metastasis suitable for surgery.

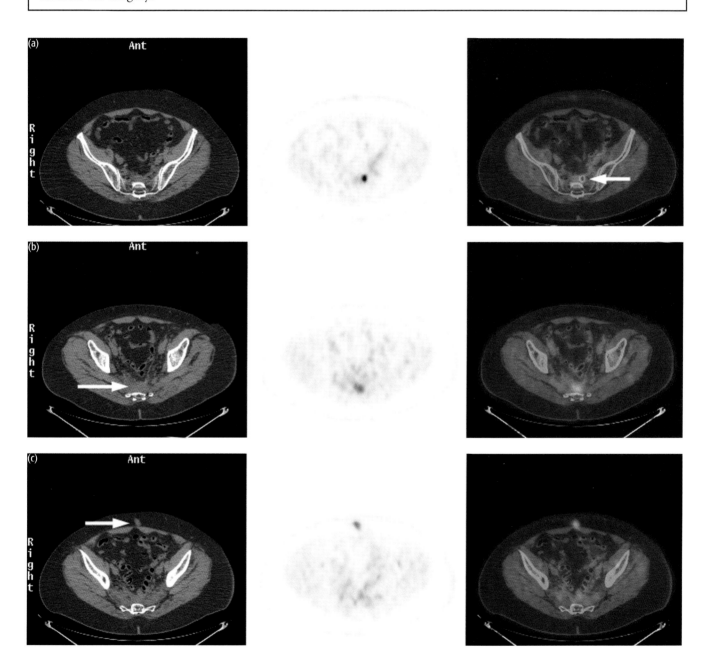

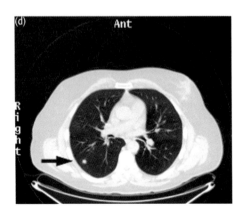
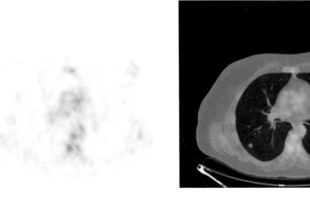

PET/CT findings:

There was increased uptake in abnormal soft tissue in the presacral region (a, b) indicating active malignancy. High-grade uptake was also present in a subcutaneous nodule in the lower abdomen in the midline, suspicious of malignancy (c). No increased uptake was associated with the nodule in the right lower lobe of the lung (d) but the size of the lesion was small and therefore may be below the size that can be resolved using PET. PET/CT showed that resection of the lung nodule was not appropriate, given the presacral recurrence.

Key points:

1 PET/CT can identify other sites of disease in patients with apparently solitary metastasis.
2 PET/CT changed disease management markedly.

CASE 6.8	Diagnosis: Colorectal cancer – metastasectomy?

Clinical history:

This patient was referred with known metastasis in the left lobe of the liver. PET/CT was requested to determine whether there was extrahepatic disease.

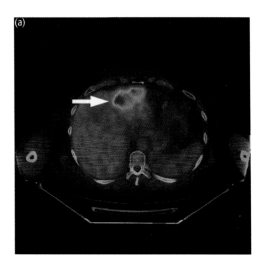

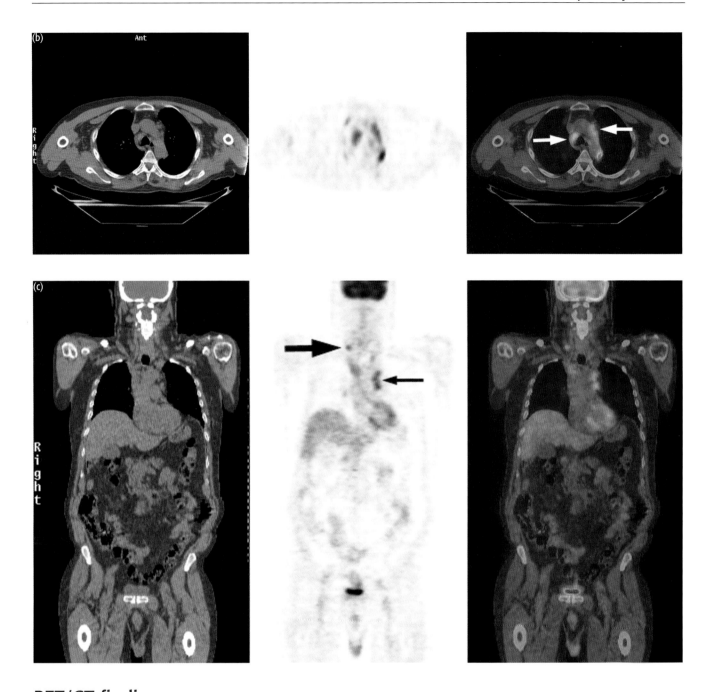

PET/CT findings:

There was uptake in the liver metastasis (a). Further metastatic disease was identified in multiple lymph node groups. Uptake was seen in the right paratracheal (b) and left para-aortic (b, c) regions. Focal increased uptake was also seen in a right lower cervical lymph node (level VB) (c).

Key point:

Patients with 'isolated' colorectal cancer by anatomic imaging often have additional tumor foci detected by PET/CT.

| CASE 6.9 | Diagnosis: Colorectal cancer – metastasectomy? |

Clinical history:

This patient was referred with liver metastases from rectal adenocarcinoma which had previously been treated with resection and radiotherapy. Small-volume mediastinal lymphadenopathy was seen on the chest CT scan and the patient was referred to determine whether this represented metastatic disease which would preclude liver resection.

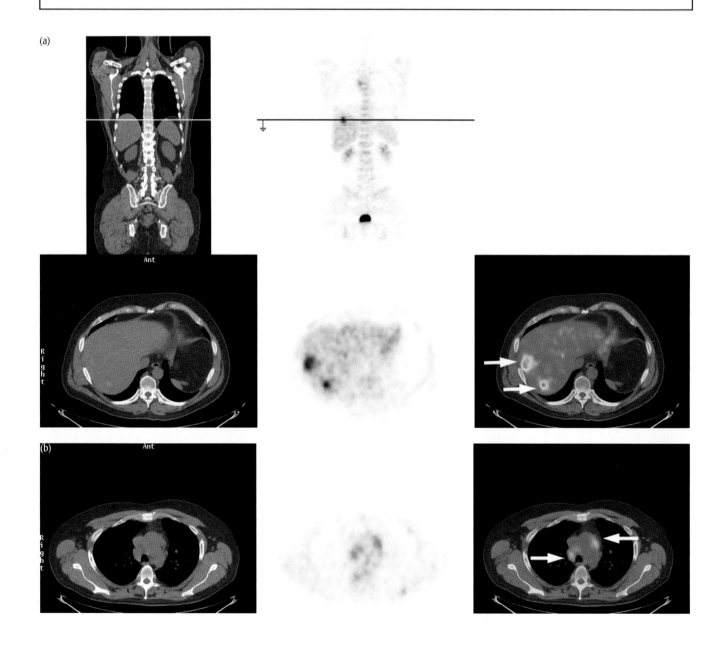

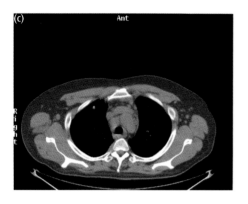  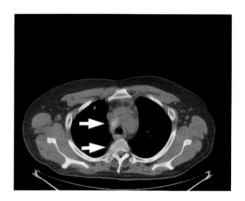

PET findings:

There was intense uptake in two liver metastases (a). There was lower-grade uptake in lymph nodes adjacent to the arch of the aorta (b) and in the right paratracheal region (b, c) and in the right paravertebral region (c). The lower-grade uptake was reported as suspicious for disease, but biopsy was recommended in view of the difference in intensity from the liver metastases and the slightly unusual distribution.

Follow-up

Mediastinoscopy and biopsy of the right paravertebral region revealed no definite evidence of malignancy. The patient proceeded to liver resection. Metastatic rectal cancer was present in the liver but there were also multiple abnormal lymphocytes identified in tissue removed from around the porta hepatis. The earlier biopsy specimens were reviewed and a diagnosis of low-grade lymphoma was made.

Key points:

1 When uptake is low grade, especially if the uptake is different in intensity from sites of known metastatic disease, biopsy should be taken where possible.
2 Patients may have more than one pathology, and if the findings are not easily explained by the disease process for which the patient has been referred, an alternative pathology should be considered. FDG is sensitive but not specific.

| CASE 6.10 | Scan 1 | Diagnosis: Colorectal cancer – treatment response |

Clinical history:

This patient was diagnosed with a primary carcinoma of the rectum. CT staging indicated possible lung metastases in the left lower lobe posteriorly. PET/CT was requested initially to characterize the lung lesions.

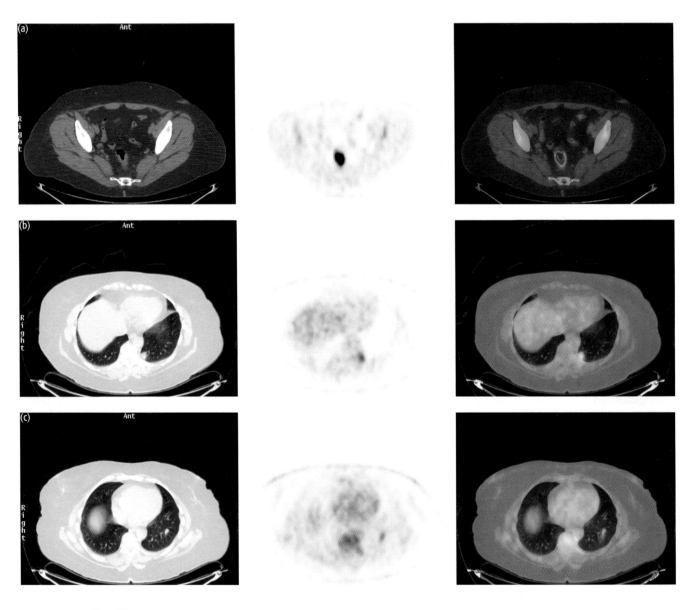

PET/CT findings:

There was uptake in the rectal cancer (a) and within two lung lesions indicative of metastatic disease in the left lower lobe (b, c).

Key point:

PET/CT can be used to stage primary colorectal cancer in selected cases.

CASE 6.10	Scan 2

Clinical history:

The patient underwent resection of the primary rectal cancer and received adjuvant chemotherapy for the metastatic disease in the left lung. PET/CT was requested to assess treatment response to determine suitability for resection of lung metastases.

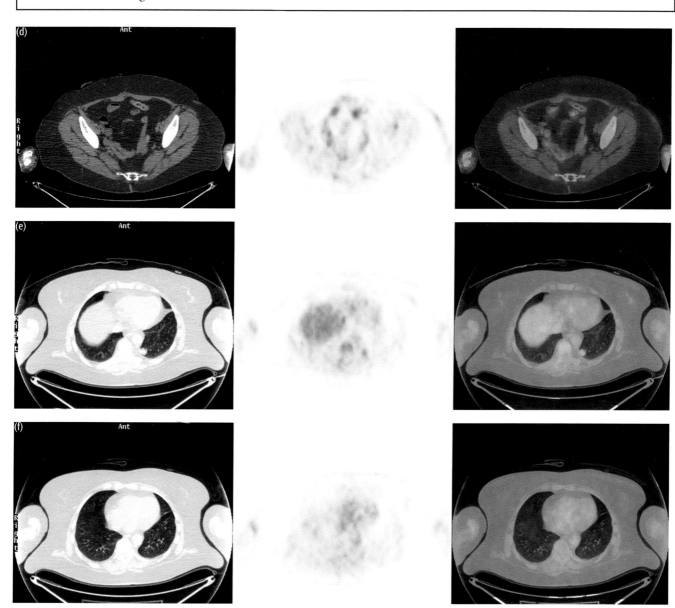

PET/CT findings:

There was partial response with significant reduction of FDG uptake in the larger lung lesion (e). The smaller lesion was no longer present (f). There was no residual disease in the pelvis (d). The patient underwent left lower lobectomy.

Key point:

PET/CT can be used to assess treatment response.

CASE 6.11	Scan 1	Diagnosis: Colorectal cancer – recurrence

Clinical history:

This patient had had previous recurrences of colorectal cancer, which had been treated. In this episode she presented with sacral nerve root pain and rising CEA levels suggestive of malignancy rather than post treatment fibrosis. CT scan had showed no definite sign of recurrence. PET/CT was requested so the patient could be offered palliative chemotherapy/radiotherapy if there was clear evidence of another recurrence.

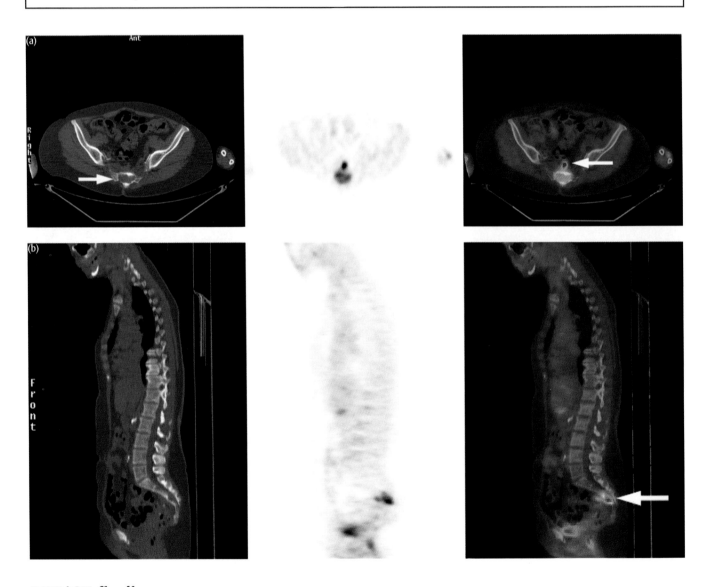

PET/CT findings:

Uptake was increased within the soft tissues in the presacral region (a, b) and within a large lytic lesion in the sacrum itself (a, b) confirming the presence of recurrent malignancy.

CASE 6.11	Scan 2

Clinical history:

The patient returned after treatment with chemotherapy for assessment of response.

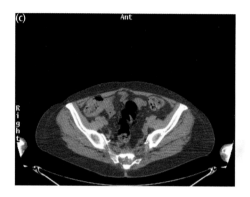  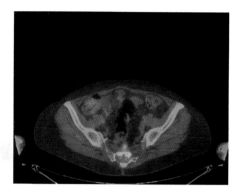

PET/CT findings:

There was resolution of uptake in the sacrum and reduction in size and intensity of the presacral uptake (c).

Key points:

1 PET/CT can differentiate cancer from fibrosis after treatment in presacral masses.
2 PET/CT can be used to assess metabolic response to treatment.

CASE 6.12	Diagnosis: Colorectal cancer – response to treatment

Clinical history:

This patient with primary colon cancer and liver metastasis was treated with embolization of the liver lesion. PET/CT was requested before and after treatment to monitor response.

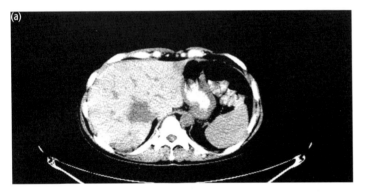
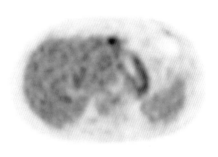
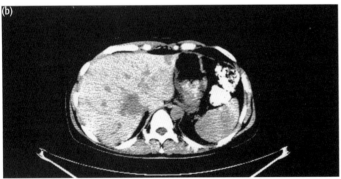
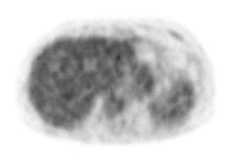

PET/CT findings:

There was high uptake in the metastasis in the left lobe of the liver (a) which resolved after treatment (b).

Key point:

Metabolic changes in response to treatment may be seen in advance of anatomic changes.

| CASE 6.13 | Diagnosis: Gastrointestinal stromal tumor (GIST) |

Clinical history:

This patient with known GIST was referred for PET/CT for staging of disease at diagnosis.

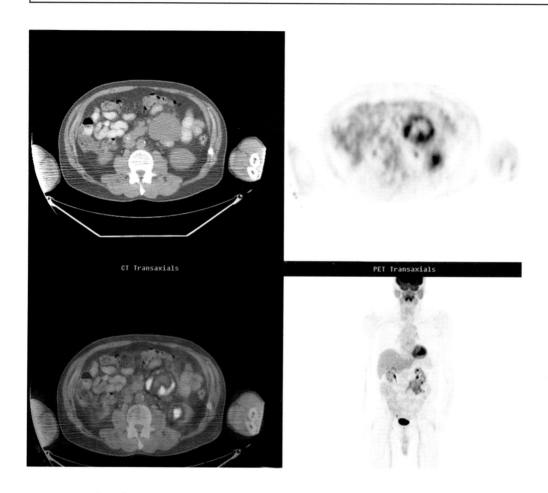

PET/CT findings:

There was increased uptake, associated with two large soft-tissue masses in the abdomen, consistent with the diagnosis of GIST.

Key point:

Avid uptake of FDG can be seen in GIST tumors.

CASE 6.14	Diagnosis: Hepatoma

Clinical history:

This patient with hepatoma was scanned prior to treatment for staging.

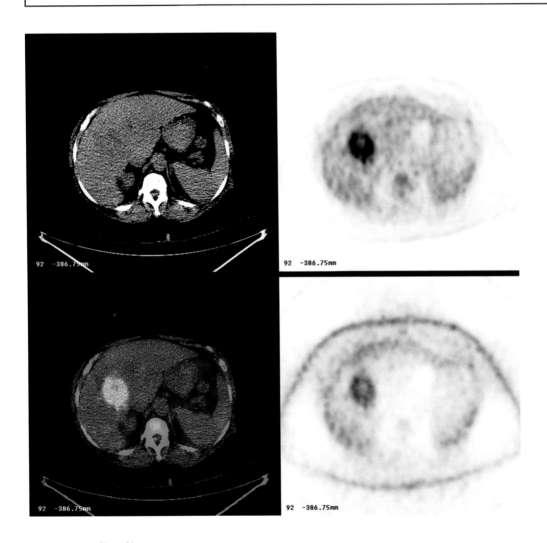

PET/CT findings:

High uptake was associated with the tumor, which was solitary. Attenutation-corrected images (top right) and nonattenuation-corrected images (bottom right) are shown.

Key point:

PET/CT demonstrated the hepatoma in this case but about half of primary liver tumors are not FDG avid because of the presence of glucose-6-phosphate dehydrogenase within some liver tumors.

| CASE 6.15 | Diagnosis: Pancreatic cancer – restaging |

Clinical history:

This patient underwent a Whipple operation 4 years previously for pancreatic carcinoma. CT scan showed a new lesion in the liver suggestive of metastasis. PET/CT was requested to restage the patient's disease.

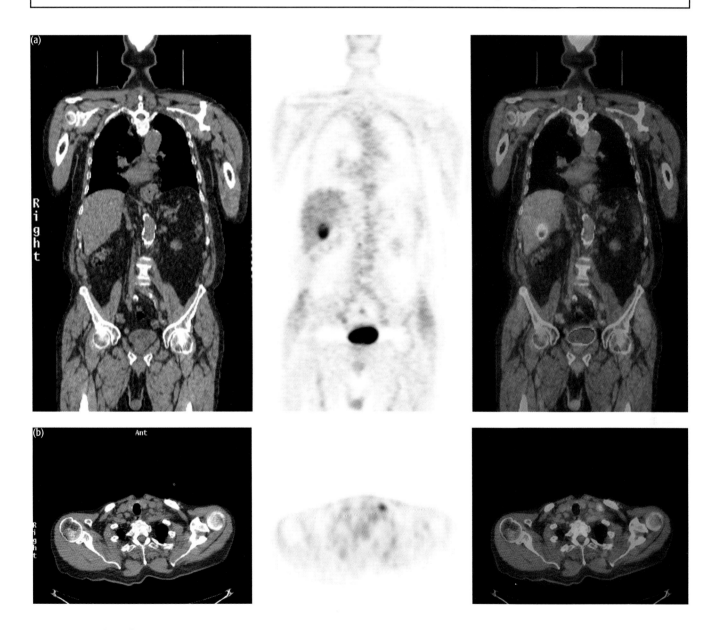

PET/CT findings:

There was high uptake in the liver lesion consistent with metastasis (a) and high uptake in a left supraclavicular lymph node consistent with a further metastasis (b).

Key point:

PET/CT detected extrahepatic disease in this patient requiring systemic treatment rather than local resection.

CASE 6.16	Diagnosis: Cholangiocarcinoma

Clinical history:

This patient with a history of cholangiocarcinoma was scanned to assess possible recurrence.

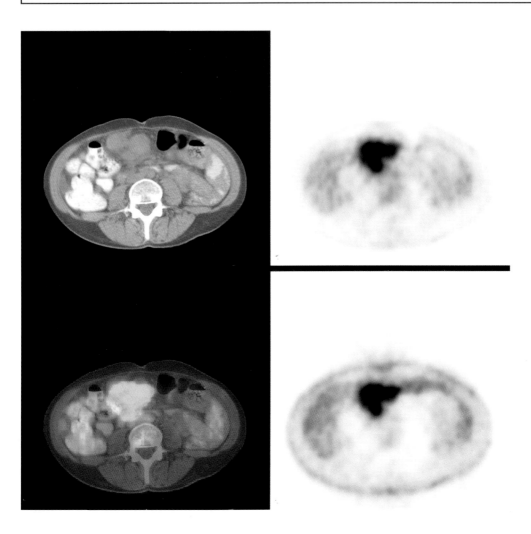

PET/CT findings:

This patient had high uptake associated with a soft-tissue mass in the anterior abdomen inferior to the liver, consistent with recurrent cholangiocarcinoma. Attentuation-corrected images (top right) and non attenuation-corrected images (bottom right) are shown.

Key point:
Cholangiocarcinomas usually have high uptake of FDG.

CONCLUSIONS

CURRENT CLINICAL INDICATIONS
1 Rising CEA after primary treatment
2 Prior to possible surgical resection of 'limited' recurrence
3 Systemic or local symptoms in patient with no CEA marker
4 Residual mass after abdominoperineal resection
5 Primary staging in selected cases
6 Evaluation of radiologic abnormalities

PET is better established in the management of recurrent than primary disease. PET does detect many primary cancers and can find distant or unexpected metastases in patients with untreated primary colon cancers. Far more PET is used, however, in the management of patients after surgery for recurrence as well as in the assessment of the effects of chemotherapy or locoregional therapies of metastases. While PET/CT is not as fully evaluated as is PET, when directly compared, PET/CT has been superior to PET in imaging accuracy. Figure 6.1 shows a possible algorithm that uses the known benefits of PET for patients with recurrent disease when surgery is contemplated.

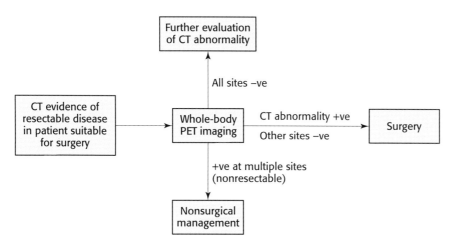

Figure 6.1   *Possible uses of PET in recurrent colorectal cancer*

FURTHER READING

Abdel-Nabi H, Doerr RJ, Lamonica DM *et al.* (1998) Staging of primary colorectal carcinomas with fluorine-18 fluorodeoxyglucose whole-body PET: correlation with histopathologic and CT findings. *Radiology* **206**, 755–60.

Bar-Shalom R, Yefremov N, Guralnik L *et al.* (2003) Clinical performance of PET/CT in evaluation of cancer: Additional value for diagnostic imaging and patient management. *J Nucl Med* **44**, 1200–9.

Bohdiewicz PJ, Scott GC, Juni JE *et al.* (1995) Indium-111 Oncoscint CR/OV and ^{18}F in colorectal and ovarian carcinoma recurrences: early observations. *Clin Nucl Med* **20**, 230–6.

Cohade C, Osman M, Leal J, Wahl RL. (2003) Direct comparison of (18F)-FDG PET and PET/CT in patients with colorectal carcinoma. *J Nucl Med* **44**, 1797–803.

Delbeke D, Martin WH (2004) PET and PET-CT for evaluation of colorectal carcinoma. *Semin Nucl Med* **34**, 209–23.

Fernandez FG, Drebin JA, Linehan DC *et al.* (2004) Five-year survival after resection of hepatic metastases from colorectal cancer in patients screened by positron emission tomography with F-18 fluorodeoxyglucose (FDG-PET). *Ann Surg* **240**, 438–47.

Gupta NC, Falk PM, Frank AL *et al.* (1993) Pre-operative staging of colorectal carcinoma using positron emission tomography. *Nebr Med J* **78**, 30–5.

Huebner RH, Park KC, Shepherd JE *et al.* (2000) A meta-analysis of the literature for whole-body FDG PET detection of recurrent colorectal cancer. *J Nucl Med* **41**, 1177–89.

Ito K, Kato T, Tadokoro M *et al.* (1992) Recurrent rectal cancer and scar: differentiation with PET and MR imaging. *Radiology* **182**, 549–52.

Jeng LB, Changlai SP, Shen YY *et al.* (2003) Limited value of 18F-2-deoxyglucose positron emission tomography to detect hepatocellular carcinoma in hepatitis B virus carriers. *Hepatogastroenterology* **50**, 2154–6.

Kalff V, Hicks RJ, Ware RE *et al.* (2002) The clinical impact of (18)F-FDG PET in patients with suspected or confirmed recurrence of colorectal cancer: a prospective study. *J Nucl Med* **43**, 492–9.

Kinkel K, Lu Y, Both M, Thoeni RF (2002) Detection of hepatic metastases from cancers of the gastrointestinal tract by using noninvasive imaging methods (US, CT, MR imaging, PET): a meta-analysis. *Radiology* **224**, 748–56.

Lai DTM, Fulham M, Stephens MS *et al.* (1996) The role of whole-body positron emission tomography with [18F] fluorodeoxyglucose in identifying operable colorectal cancer metastases to the liver. *Arch Surg* **131**, 703–7.

Meyer M (1995) Diffusely increased colonic 18F FDG uptake in acute enterocolitis. *Clin Nucl Med* **20**, 434–5.

Schiepers C, Penninckx F, DeVadder N *et al.* (1995) Contribution of PET in the diagnosis of recurrent colorectal cancer: comparison with conventional imaging. *Eur J Surg Oncol* **21**, 517–22.

Staib L, Schirrmeister H, Reske SN, Beger HG (2000) Is (18)F-fluorodeoxyglucose positron emission tomography in recurrent colorectal cancer a contribution to surgical decision making? *Am J Surg* **180**, 1–5.

Strauss LG, Clorius JH, Schlag P *et al.* (1989) Recurrence of colorectal tumors: PET evaluation. *Radiology* **170**, 329–32.

Tutt AN, Plunkett TA, Barrington SF, Leslie MD (2004) The role of positron emission tomography in the management of colorectal cancer. *Colorectal Dis* **6**, 2–9.

Valk PE, Abella-Columna E, Haseman MK *et al.* (1999) Whole-body PET imaging with [18F]fluorodeoxyglucose in management of recurrent colorectal cancer. *Arch Surg* **134**, 503–11.

Wudel LJ Jr, Delbeke D, Morris D *et al.* (2003) The role of [18F]fluorodeoxyglucose positron emission tomography imaging in the evaluation of hepatocellular carcinoma. *Am Surg* **69**, 117–24.

Yonkura Y, Benau RS, Brill AB *et al.* (1982) Increased accumulation of 2-deoxy-2-[18F] fluoro-D-glucose in liver metastases from colon carcinoma. *J Nucl Med* **23**, 1133–7.

CHAPTER 7
ESOPHAGEAL CANCER

INTRODUCTION AND BACKGROUND

Esophageal cancer is diagnosed in about 14 000 patients/year in the USA and 7364 patients/year in the UK, representing about 1–5 percent of all cancers. Unfortunately, the vast majority of patients ultimately die of their disease, with 5-year survivals of only about 10 percent. Both adenocarcinomas and squamous cell carcinomas occur, but the relative frequency of adenocarcinomas has been rapidly increasing, possibly related to gastric reflux disease. Patients who have localized disease are candidates for surgery, however, patients with systemic metastases are clearly not surgical candidates. Chemotherapy has an important role in esophageal cancer and a variety of protocols in which neoadjuvant chemotherapy is given have been applied. Patients responding well to neoadjuvant therapy, which may also include radiotherapy, may then undergo surgery and have a better prognosis than those who do not respond well to treatment.

Esophageal adenocarcinoma is increasing in frequency. Generally esophageal cancer carries a poor prognosis, less than 10 percent survival at 5 years. Patients with low-volume disease, no nodal or systemic metastases, and those who respond well to neoadjuvant chemotherapy followed by surgery appear to have the best prognosis.

EPIDEMIOLOGY

Annual incidence	
Men	15.7 new cases per 100 000/4485 cases UK
	7.4 new cases per 100 000/ 11 220 cases USA
Women	9.5 new cases per 100 000/ 2879 cases UK
	2.3 new cases per 100 000/ 3300 cases USA
Male/female ratio	~1.5:1 (UK) 3:1 (USA)
1–5% all new cancers	
1–5% all cancer deaths	
8% 5-year survival	

There are significant differences in frequency in different countries, the most noteworthy being the high and increasing incidence of adenocarcinoma relative to squamous histologies.

PATHOLOGY

Histology	
Adenocarcinoma	Rising incidence (>50%)
Squamous cell carcinoma	

The key issue is detection of systemic metastatic disease, which usually renders the patient inoperable. Periesophageal lymph nodes are usually removed at surgery and their involvement with tumor does not contraindicate esophagectomy. The staging system differs depending on whether the esophageal cancer is located proximally or distally. An important goal is to decrease the numbers of patients undergoing surgical treatment unnecessarily. Positron emission tomography (PET) is the single best method to stage the entire body for metastatic spread of esophageal cancer.

STAGING AND PROGNOSIS

T stage	
TX	Not assessable
T0	No evidence of primary
Tis	*In situ*
T1	Invades lamina propria or submucosa
T2	Invades muscularis propria
T3	Invades adventitia
T4	Invades adjacent structures
N stage	
Nx	Nodes not assessable
N0	No nodes involved
N1	Regional nodes involved
M stage	
M0	No metastases
M1	Metastatic disease

STAGE 5-YEAR SURVIVAL (%)

Stage I	T1 N0 M0	60
Stage II	T2/3 N0 M0	30
Stage III	T3 N1 M0	15
	T4 any N M0	
Stage IV	Any T Any N M1	<5

Treatment response to neoadjuvant therapy is increasingly important to assess as it can predict outcome. Generally patients with the largest declines in tracer uptake are most likely to have the best prognosis. Transient increases in esophageal uptake can be seen with esophagitis from radiation and other causes and these should not be confused with residual cancer.

KEY MANAGEMENT ISSUES

KEY MANAGEMENT ISSUES
Staging of primary
Therapy response (including neoadjuvant response)
Diagnosis of recurrence

The role of PET in esophageal cancer

PET imaging of patients with newly diagnosed esophageal cancer is considered essential so that patients with systemic metastases are not inappropriately exposed to the major risk of esophagectomy.

PET is a very useful tool for staging for the presence/absence of systemic metastases of esophageal carcinoma. PET appears to be the single most accurate noninvasive imaging tool for detection of metastases. Sensitivity for the detection of primary tumors has been over 90 percent in most studies; however, these have not focused on the smallest of tumors. In spite of these figures, PET probably does not have a significant role in the primary diagnosis of esophageal cancer or for screening. Lymph node staging is of importance as patients lacking nodal metastases have a superior prognosis to those with nodal metastases. PET, computed tomography (CT), and endoscopic ultrasound (EUS) are used in periesophageal lymph node staging. Endoscopic ultrasound is probably the most accurate of these methods but all can fail to detect small nodal metastases and indeed, these nodes are usually removed at esophagectomy. Single-center studies have generally shown [^{18}F]2-fluoro-2-deoxy-D-glucose (FDG) PET to be the most accurate method for detecting systemic metastatic disease. In a prospective study of 74 patients, Flamen *et al.* (2000) showed a sensitivity and specificity of 74 percent and 90 percent, respectively, for PET and 41 percent and 83 percent, respectively for CT. Compared with CT, 15 percent of patients were upstaged and 7 percent downstaged using PET. PET and EUS are commonly undertaken to stage esophageal cancer before surgery.

Neoadjuvant chemotherapy is commonly used in patients with esophageal cancer. Rapid declines in FDG uptake with such treatment predict the best response. Weber *et al.* (2001) showed a 54 percent drop in FDG uptake in responders but only a 15 percent drop in FDG uptake in nonresponders at 2 weeks after chemotherapy was initiated. Assessment of response of metastatic disease is also possible with FDG PET. Caution must be used in assessing primary esophageal cancers as they can have confounding patterns of increased FDG uptake in inflammation related to esophagitis.

PET can also be used to detect recurrences of esophageal cancer. Unfortunately, salvage therapies are not too effective, so close monitoring of these patients may not be needed, unless useful salvage treatment is available. Thus, FDG PET plays its greatest role early in the management of patients with esophageal cancer.

EXAMPLES TO ILLUSTRATE KEY ISSUES

CASE 7.1	Diagnosis: Esophageal cancer – staging

Clinical history:

This patient was diagnosed with moderately differentiated adenocarcinoma and staged as T3 N1 M_x on CT and endoscopic ultrasound. There was also bilateral adrenal enlargement on CT. PET/CT was requested for staging.

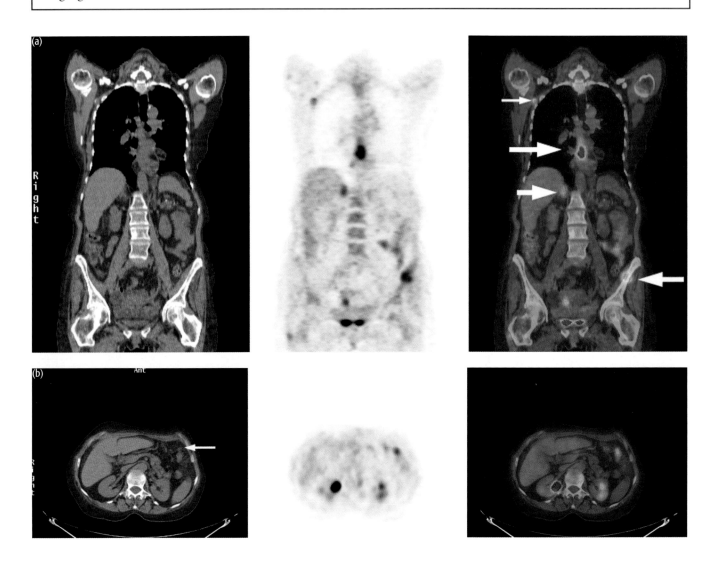

PET/CT findings:

PET showed uptake in the esophageal primary and a periesophageal node. There was also uptake in a right axillary lymph node, in the enlarged right adrenal gland, and in several bone sites including the left iliac bone (a). Increased uptake was also seen within two small peritoneal deposits (b). The patient had metastatic disease and was not suitable for surgery. (Not shown is uptake associated with a metastasis in the left sacrum, probable inflammatory uptake in the uterus and uptake associated with a calcified nodule in the right gluteal muscle.)

Key points:

1 PET/CT is sensitive in the detection of metastatic disease in esophageal cancer.
2 PET/CT did detect local nodal disease in this case, but sometimes it can be difficult to resolve uptake in nodes adjacent to the primary tumor.
3 PET/CT helps to distinguish peritoneal disease from physiologic bowel uptake.

CASE 7.2	Diagnosis: Esophageal cancer – staging

Clinical history:

This patient was referred with adenocarcinoma of the esophagus. The CT scan demonstrated an enlarged right paratracheal lymph node and multiple smaller nodes in the mediastinum. PET/CT was requested for staging.

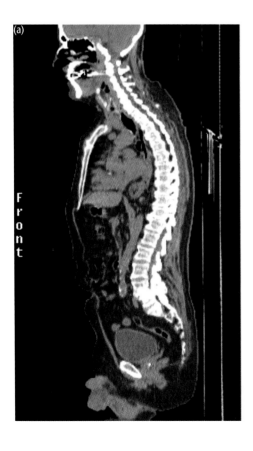
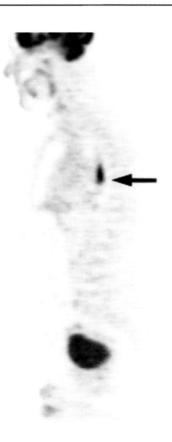
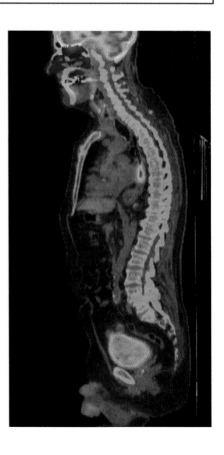

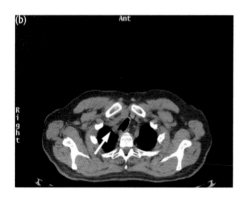

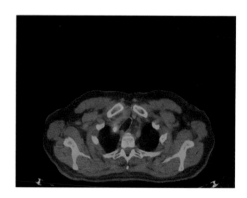

PET/CT findings:

There was increased uptake at the site of the primary cancer (a) and in the enlarged right paratracheal lymph node (b) indicative of a metastasis.

Key point:

PET detects metastatic disease in approximately 15–20 percent of patients with carcinoma of the esophagus who are candidates for surgery on CT.

CASE 7.3 | Diagnosis: Esophageal cancer – staging

Clinical history:

This patient with known esophageal carcinoma had small pulmonary nodules on a staging CT scan. PET/CT was requested to characterize these lesions and to stage the patient's disease.

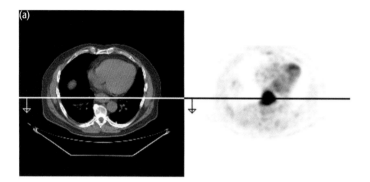

(a)

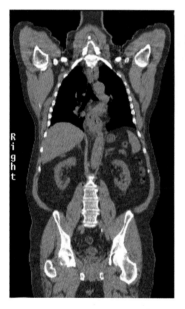
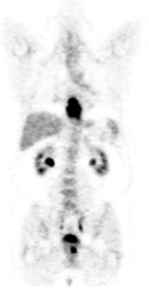
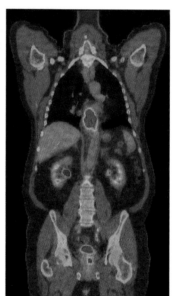

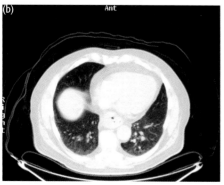
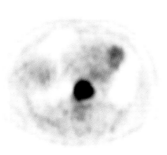
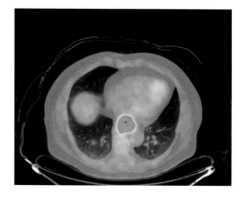

(b)

PET/CT findings:

There was avid uptake in the primary cancer in the distal third of the esophagus (a), but there was no uptake in the pulmonary nodules (b). The patient proceeded to surgery.

Key point:

PET/CT can be used to detect metastatic disease in esophageal cancer although the sensitivity of PET in the lower lobes of the lungs is reduced and cannot always exclude disease in sub-centimeter nodules.

CASE 7.4	Diagnosis: Esophageal cancer – staging

Clinical history:

This patient with adenocarcinoma of the esophagus had an indeterminate liver lesion on CT. PET/CT was requested to characterize the liver lesion and to stage the patient's disease.

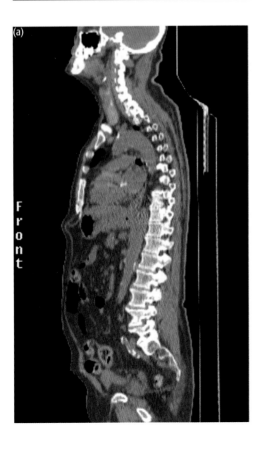
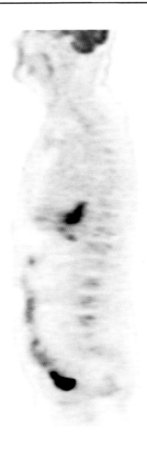
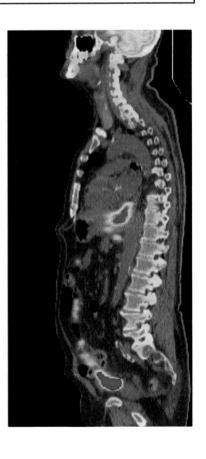

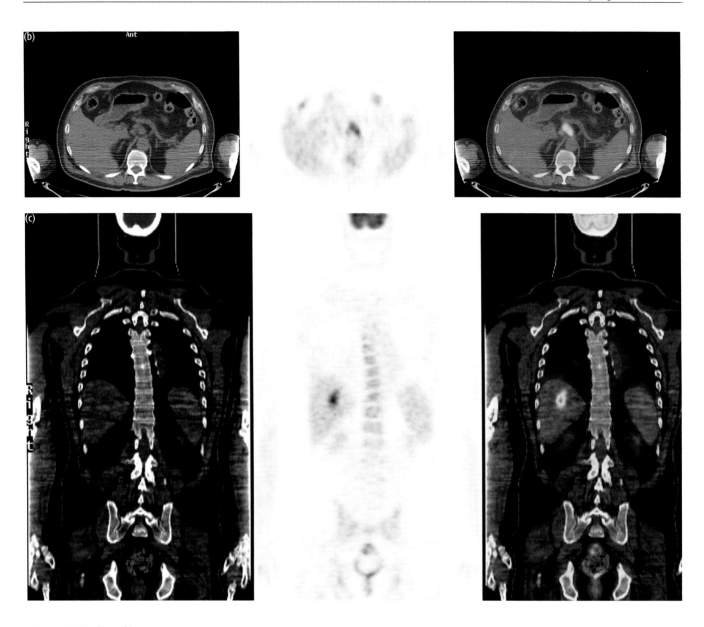

PET/CT findings:

There was uptake in the primary esophageal cancer (a) and metastases in celiac nodes (a, b) and in the liver (c).

Key point:

There was high uptake in this primary adenocarcinoma although uptake can be low grade in some cases of adenocarcinoma of the esophagus. In cases where the primary has low-grade uptake, sensitivity for the detection of metastases is reduced.

CASE 7.5	Diagnosis: Esophageal cancer – therapy response

Clinical history:

This patient with known esophageal adenocarcinoma was treated with neoadjuvant chemotherapy prior to surgery. PET/CT was used to monitor treatment response.

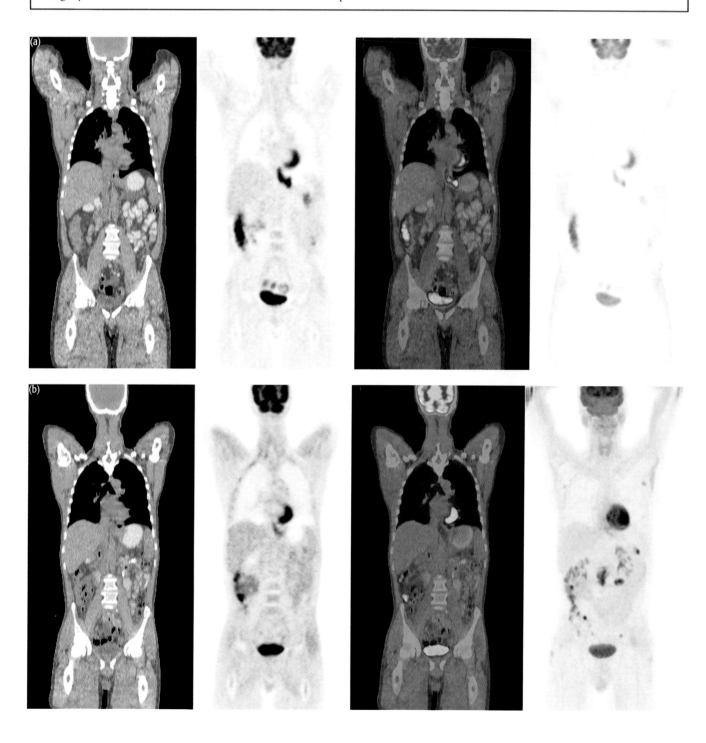

PET/CT findings:

There was high uptake in the primary cancer at the gastroesophageal junction prior to treatment (a) with significant reduction in FDG uptake following chemotherapy (b). Note there is marked physiologic uptake in the cecum in the first scan (a) and physiologic uptake throughout the large bowel in the second scan (b).

Key point:

PET/CT can be used to differentiate responders from nonresponders receiving neoadjuvant chemotherapy for esophageal cancer.

CASE 7.6	Diagnosis: Esophageal cancer recurrence

Clinical history:

This patient had an Ivor Lewis esophagectomy for cancer of the esophagus. He developed vomiting 1 year after surgery and required stenting. CT suggested nodal recurrence. PET/CT was requested to confirm recurrence and restage the patient's disease.

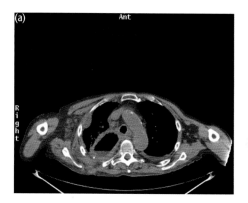

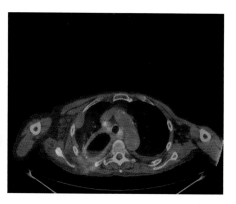
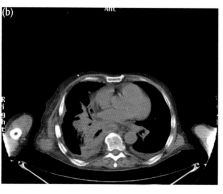

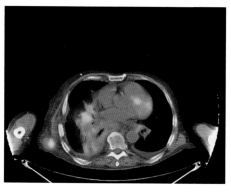

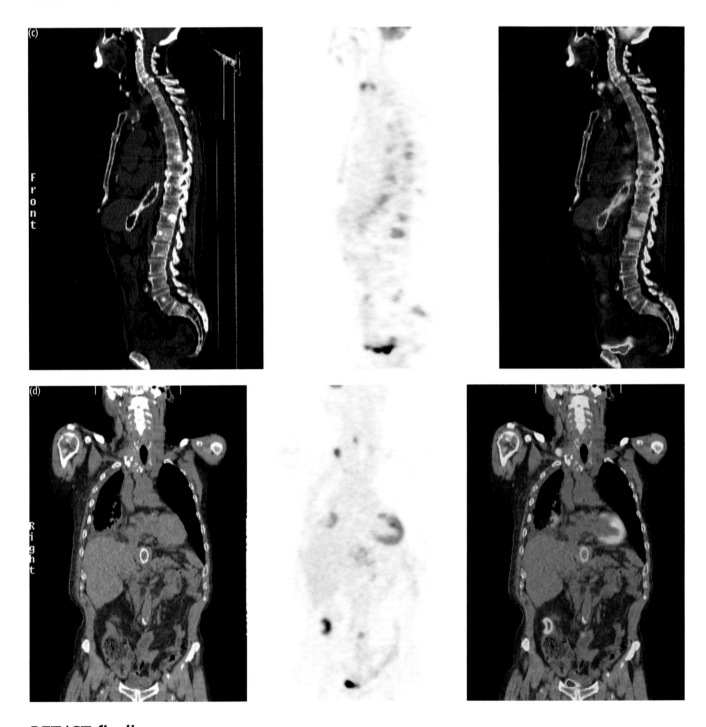

PET/CT findings:

There was extensive recurrent disease. There was nodal disease in the mediastinum (a, b), a deposit in the right latissimus dorsi muscle (b), metastases in the spine (c), and right supraclavicular fossa (d). Further uptake was seen in the ascending colon consistent with a primary colorectal neoplasm (d). Note the presence of the gastric pull-up and stent.

Key points:

1 PET/CT identifies recurrent disease.
2 PET/CT can identify unsuspected colorectal neoplasm.

CASE 7.7 | Diagnosis: Esophageal cancer – recurrence

Clinical history:

This patient with a history of esophageal cancer had been treated with surgery and chemotherapy. Four months postoperatively he developed symptoms suggestive of pneumonia with right upper lobe consolidation on chest radiograph and CT. The changes on CT did not resolve and the patient developed right chest wall pain. PET/CT was requested to determine if there was recurrent cancer.

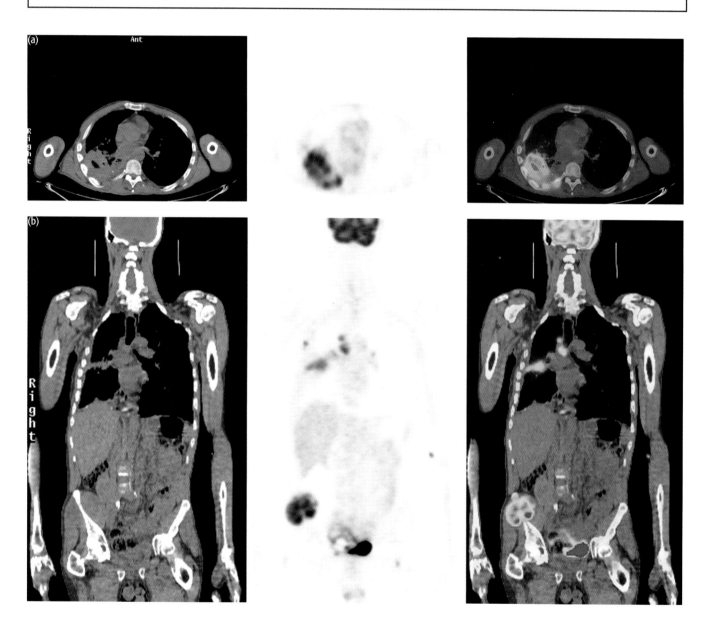

PET/CT findings:

There was massive uptake associated with consolidated lung with uptake extending through the posterior right chest wall indicative of recurrent cancer (a). Uptake was also seen in metastases in right paratracheal and right axillary lymph nodes and in the right iliac bone (b). (Not shown is uptake in bilateral pleural nodules, left supraclavicular and subcarinal nodes, and other bone sites including vertebrae and right sacroiliac joint and multiple sites in subcutaneous tissues in the back.)

Key point:

PET/CT identifies metastatic disease in multiple sites including lung, chest wall, lymph nodes, and bone.

CONCLUSIONS

Figure 7.1 indicates a possible diagnostic pathway.

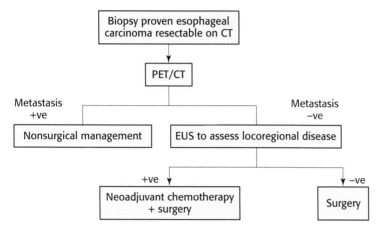

Suggested diagnostic pathway for esophageal carcinomas

REFERENCES AND FURTHER READING

Dehdashti F, Siegel BA (2004) Neoplasms of the esophagus and stomach. *Semin Nucl Med* **34**, 198–208.

Flamen P, Lerut A, Van Cutsem E *et al.* (2000) Utility of positron emission tomography for the staging of patients with potentially operable esophageal carcinoma. *J Clin Oncol* **18**, 3202–10.

Flanagan FL, Dehdashti F, Siegel BA *et al.* (1997) Staging of esophageal cancer with 18F-fluorodeoxyglucose positron emission tomography. *AJR Am J Roentgenol* **168**, 417–24.

Fukunaga T, Enomoto K, Okazumi S *et al.* (1994) Analysis of glucose metabolism in patients with esophageal cancer by PET: estimation of hexokinase activity in the tumor and usefulness for clinical assessment using 18F-fluorodeoxyglucose. *Nippon Geka Gakkai Zasshi* **95**, 317–25.

Rankin SC, Taylor H, Cook GJ, Mason R (1998) Computed tomography and positron emission tomography in the pre-operative staging of oesophageal carcinoma. *Clin Radiol* **53**, 659–65.

Wallace MB, Nietert PJ, Earle C *et al.* (2002) An analysis of multiple staging management strategies for carcinoma of the esophagus: computed tomography, endoscopic ultrasound, positron emission tomography, and thoracoscopy/laparoscopy. *Ann Thorac Surg* **74**, 1026–32.

Weber WA, Ott K, Becker K *et al.* (2001) Prediction of response to preoperative chemotherapy in adenocarcinomas of the esophagogastric junction by metabolic imaging. *J Clin Oncol* **19**, 3058–65.

Yasuda S, Raja S, Hubner KF (1995) Application of whole-body positron emission tomography in the imaging of esophageal cancer: report of a case. *Surg Today* **25**, 261–4.

Yoon YC, Lee KS, Shim YM *et al.* (2003) Metastasis to regional lymph nodes in patients with esophageal squamous cell carcinoma: CT versus FDG PET for presurgical detection prospective study. *Radiology* **227**, 764–70.

CHAPTER 8
HEAD AND NECK CANCER

INTRODUCTION AND BACKGROUND

Cancer of the head and neck is relatively uncommon in Western countries (~3–5 percent of all cancers) but may be extremely common (up to 40 percent of all cancers) in some Asian countries. The vast majority in the industrialized Western countries are squamous cell cancers, which have variable aggressiveness depending on the site and histological type. There is a strong environmental link associating their occurrence with tobacco and alcohol usage together with other factors such as chemicals, fumes and viruses such as the human papilloma virus (HPV). Head and neck tumors in Asia are more commonly adenocarcinomas, often nasopharyngeal carcinomas associated with Epstein–Barr viral (EBV) infections. Good therapeutic outcomes are dependent on patients being treated in specialized centers with experienced multidisciplinary teams that include head and neck surgical oncologists, radiotherapists, imaging specialists, and medical oncologists. Because of the site of the tumor, treatment is directed at maintaining form and function of the head and neck structures as well as eradicating disease. Imaging has an important role in the management of these tumors because of the need to limit surgery and because local nodal spread is the most important prognostic factor aside from the presence or absence of systemic metastases. After treatment, the conventional anatomic imaging procedures are much less useful because of the distortion of anatomy due to treatment. [18F]2-Fluoro-2-deoxy-D-glucose (FDG) positron emission tomography (PET) therefore has a particularly important role in follow-up and for suspected recurrence. FDG PET has also been used in surveillance for tumor recurrence and to monitor early response to therapy.

Approximately 3–5 percent of all malignancies are tumors of the head and neck, and, in the Western world, most are squamous cell in etiology. Head and neck cancers represent nearly half of the tumors in Asian countries such as Hong Kong where EBV-associated nasopharyngeal carcinomas predominate over squamous cell histologies. Men are more likely to develop this cancer than women. The incidence has fallen, particularly in men. In the USA, head and neck squamous cell carcinomas are responsible for about 2 percent of cancer deaths.

Nearly all the tumors are histologically squamous cell in origin with only 1 : 10 other cell types. Nasopharyngeal is most commonly undifferentiated. These tumors may arise from any of the structures in the aerodigestive tract, the most frequent sites being the nasopharynx and oral cavity.

EPIDEMIOLOGY OF HEAD AND NECK CANCERS	
Annual incidence	
Men	19 new cases per 100 000/ 4371 cases UK
	28 new cases per 100 000/ 19 100 cases USA
Women	8 new cases per 100 000/ 1974 cases UK
	13 new cases per 100 000/ 10 270 cases USA
Male/female ratio	~2:1
Peak age	85% >50 years
3–5% all new cancers	
2–3% all cancer deaths	

PATHOLOGY	
Tumor type	Tumor site
Squamous cell (90%)	Maxillary sinus
Adenocarcinoma	Ethmoid sinus
Mucoepidermal	Nasopharynx
Adenoid cystic carcinoma	Nasal cavity
Others	Lip and oral cavity
	Oropharynx
	Hypopharynx
	Larynx
	Salivary glands

Overall there is only a 50 percent 5-year survival rate but this figure conceals a wide variation from small localized, quite curable, tumors of the lip and glottic larynx with survival in excess of 80 percent to highly malignant tumors of the floor of the mouth. The stage at presentation is critical to prognosis – early presentation has a much better prognosis whatever the site. Recurrence rate is very high (50 percent) mostly in first year.

Staging is important to the planning of treatment and prognosis. The single most important prognostic variable is the presence or absence of regional lymph node involvement and this may help determine how radical the surgical nodal dissection should be. Computed tomography (CT) and magnetic resonance imaging (MRI) are currently the cornerstone but with relatively low sensitivity. Over a third of patients with new head and neck cancers have nodal metastases at presentation. One in five patients who are clinically N0 have pathologically involved nodes. Second primary cancers and metastases are not uncommon. About 10 percent of patients harbor distant metastatic disease at the time of initial diagnosis, emphasizing the importance of staging imaging studies.

PROGNOSIS OF SQUAMOUS CELL CANCER

Death rate	5/100 000/ 2999 deaths per year

5-year survival (%)

Overall	50
Early oral	>75
Advanced	35
Cervical esophagus	70
Lip, glottic larynx	>80

STAGING

TNM	Description
Primary tumor (T – Size (oral cavity and oropharynx))*	
Tx	Primary not assessable
T0	No evidence of primary
Tis	*In situ*
T1	<2 cm
T2	2–4 cm
T3	>4 cm
T4a	Local invasion (resectable)
T4b	Local invasion (unresectable)
Lymph nodes (N)	
N0	No nodes
N1	Ipsilateral node <3 cm
N2	
a	Single ipsilateral node 3–6 cm
b	Multiple ipsilateral nodes <6 cm
c	Bilateral or contralateral node <6 cm
N3	Lymph node >6 cm
Metastases (M)	
M1	Distant metastasis

Stage	TNM
Stage I	T1 N0 M0
Stage II	T2 N0 M0
Stage III	T3 N0 M0
	T1 or T2 N1 M0
Stage IV	(T1 T2 T3) N1 M0
	T4 N0 or N1 M0
	Any T N2 or N3 M0

*The T size criteria apply to cancers of the lip, oral cavity, oropharynx, and salivary glands. For the remainder (nasopharynx, hypopharynx, larynx, maxillary sinus, nasal cavity, and ethmoid sinus) the T stage depends on site and local spread.

Not uncommonly in head and neck cancers, lymph node metastasis is the first means by which the cancer presents. In such circumstances, a search is done for the 'unknown' primary lesions, which usually involves anatomic imaging, panendoscopy, and blind biopsies of oral mucosal tissues. PET imaging can help locate some primary lesions not identified by other methods. Chemotherapy and radiotherapy can be very effective in some head and neck cancers. Rapid assessments of treatment response are feasible with PET and can be used to help determine which patients may avoid surgery.

There is an established probability of which nodal groups will be involved from a particular tumor site (Fig. 8.1). This can be helpful in defining the probability of node involvement on PET scans. These tumors usually spread locally initially, but with advanced disease they may spread to lung and elsewhere. Nodal draining regions, 'levels', have been described by Som *et al.* (1999) and are commonly used in characterizing the location of nodal metastases.

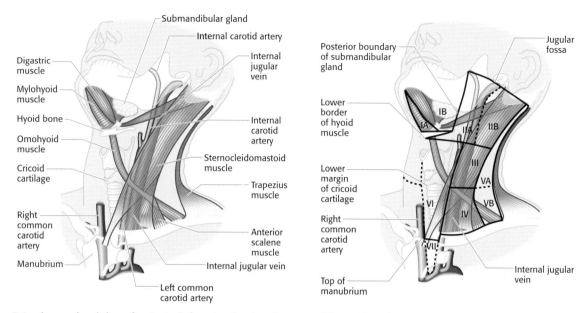

Figure 8.1 *Locoregional sites of metastasis from head and neck cancers. Adapted from Som PM, Curtin HD Mancuso AA (1999) An imaging-based classification for the cervical nodes designed as an adjunct to recent clinically based nodal classifications.* Arch Otolaryngol Head Neck Surg **125**, *388–96.*

KEY MANAGEMENT ISSUES

KEY MANAGEMENT ISSUES
Detection of unknown primary when nodal metastasis present
Extent of primary disease
Nodal and whole-body staging/restaging
Detection of recurrence
Response to therapy

Role of PET in head and neck cancers

Head and neck carcinomas in Western countries are most commonly of squamous cell origin and are generally well imaged with PET using FDG. Although [^{11}C]L-methionine can be used, the majority of clinical studies are performed with FDG. Several studies evaluating FDG PET imaging performance in known primary lesions have shown sensitivity ranging from 88 percent to nearly 100 percent, with some failures in detection in very small lesions. Many studies have shown the highest levels of FDG uptake in primary lesions to be correlated with the least good prognosis. Malignancies of the parotid are not as well imaged as those originating from the squamous mucosa, and sensitivities for parotid cancers have been <70 percent and worse than those reported for MRI. The sensitivity of PET is lower in patients who present with 'unknown' primary lesions, with nodal metastases, and no obvious primary tumor on other tests. In this setting, PET finds about a third of the previously unknown primary tumors. While useful and recommended, this represents a minority of patients and may be related to the small lesions associated with this syndrome.

The accuracy of FDG PET for staging lymph node metastases of primary head and neck carcinoma varies in several reports. In the earliest reports, accuracy for staging was reported to be comparable with that of CT or MRI; however, in a later report (Anzai et al., 1996) PET was significantly more accurate than MRI (p<0.05): 75 percent accuracy for MRI, but >90 percent accuracy for PET. A recent review of the literature showed average PET sensitivities of 87–90 percent, while average specificities were 80–93 percent. Figures are similar in the MRI and CT literature. Thus, PET appears to be at least as good as, and quite possibly better than, standard anatomic imaging for staging primary head and neck carcinoma. MRI does continue to improve, however, and nodal contrast agents may improve MRI performance. Nonetheless, PET commonly detects tumor metastases in normal-sized lymph nodes but can fail to detect small metastases to lymph nodes. Similarly, some lymph nodes may have increased tracer uptake because of an inflammatory reaction, which is glycolytically active. Thus, PET is a useful, but not perfect, tool for staging nodal anatomy of the head and neck.

Systemic staging is very important in patients with head and neck carcinoma as distant metastases can render the patient inoperable. In addition, patients with head and neck cancer not uncommonly have second primary lesions which may be associated with the very same risk factors responsible for their original head and neck cancer, and it is not unusual for 5–10 percent of patients to have second primary lesions.

PET with FDG excels at assessing treatment response and in evaluating the neck postoperatively or after radiation, which is exceedingly difficult to do with standard imaging methods after surgery. Several series have now shown FDG PET to be more accurate than CT or MRI in detecting recurrent head and neck cancer. Indeed, some have proposed that FDG PET should be the first imaging test ordered when evaluating for recurrent head and neck cancer, i.e. before MRI or CT. A caution in the interpretation of FDG PET studies in the head and neck after treatment is that there are some reports of a high false-negative rate at one month following radiotherapy alone, but with better results (and fewer false negatives) when assessments are done at 4 months post radiotherapy. This has not been seen following chemotherapy. In such a situation, waiting until several months after radiation treatment before PET imaging is recommended to assess treatment response.

Detection of recurrent disease after treatment is important for PET because salvage therapy can be quite successful for managing residual/recurrent tumor if identified sufficiently early in the course of the illness. Depending on how the scans are interpreted, false-positive readings can occur. Biopsy should usually be considered to confirm the first recurrence of head and neck cancers. Recently, PET has been shown to be able to detect more recurrences when used in a surveillance mode than was possible with standard physical examination or anatomic imaging. This role of PET is expected to grow.

There is abundant normal FDG uptake in head and neck structures, and the anatomy of the head and neck is complex, especially after surgery. PET/CT imaging is rapidly becoming a favored method in the head and neck as it allows for the precise localization of abnormalities identified on PET and appears to increase diagnostic accuracy compared to PET alone. Certainly, interpretation of PET benefits from anatomic correlative studies and these are well provided for by PET/CT.

Normal uptake of FDG in the head and neck

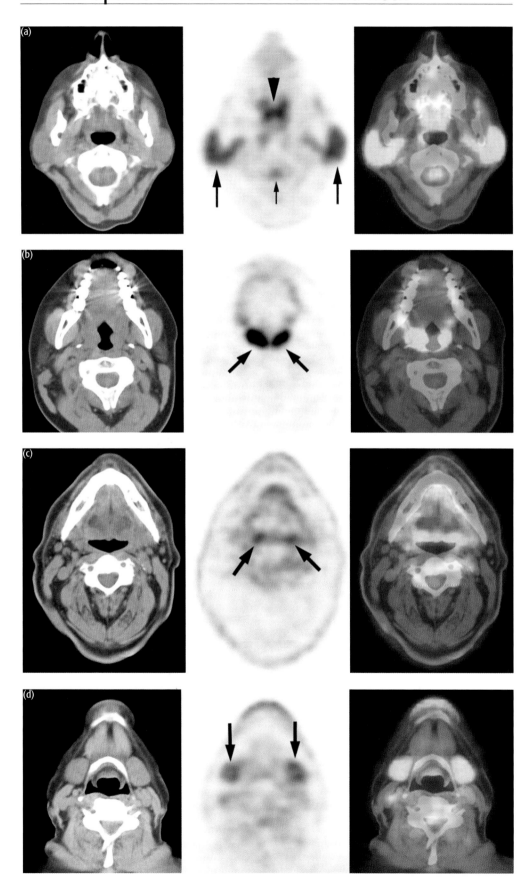

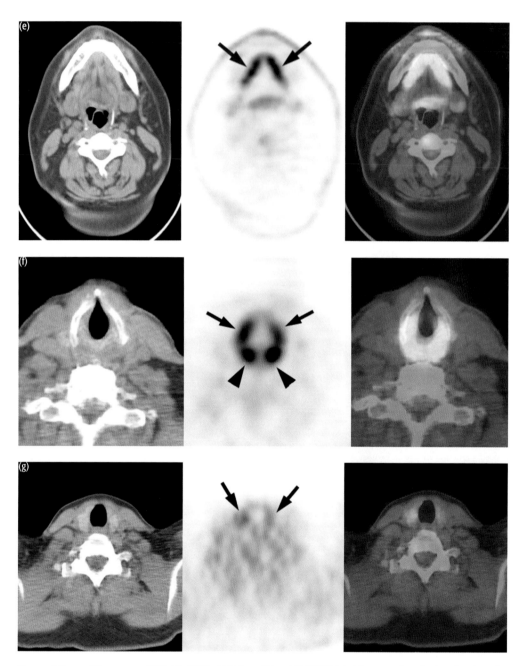

Figure 8.2   a–f Transverse CT (left), PET (middle), and fused PET/CT (right) images of major head and neck structures: (a) parotid glands (large arrows), soft palate (arrowhead), spinal cord (small arrow); (b) palatine tonsils (arrows); (c) lingual tonsils (arrows); (d) submandibular glands (arrows); (e) sublingual glands and possible uptake in mylohyoid muscle (arrows); and (f) vocal cords (arrows) and posterior cricoarytenoid muscles (arrowheads). (g) Although the thyroid gland is usually depicted as a 'cold' area, in this case, mild uptake in the normal thyroid gland (arrows) is observed. Reproduced with kind permission from Nakamoto Y, Tatsumi M, Hammoud D et al. (2005). Normal FDG distribution patterns in the head and neck: PET/CT evaluation. Radiology **234**, 879–85

EXAMPLES TO ILLUSTRATE KEY ISSUES

CASE 8.1	Diagnosis: Head and neck cancer – finding the primary

Clinical history:

This patient presented with neck nodes containing squamous cell cancer. PET/CT was requested to determine the primary site.

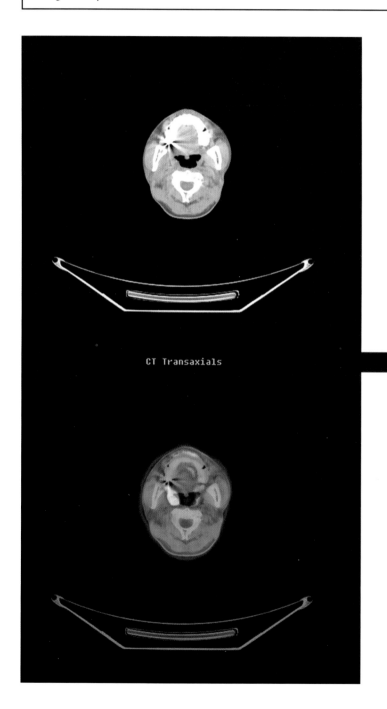
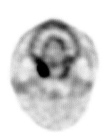
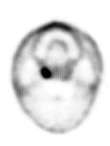

PET/CT findings:

There was avid uptake in the right tonsil which turned out to be the primary cancer.

Key point:

PET/CT can be used to detect the unknown primary in patients presenting with secondaries in the head and neck.

CASE 8.2	Diagnosis: Supraglottic cancer – staging the primary

Clinical history:

This patient was referred with squamous cell supraglottic carcinoma. The patient was staged as T3 N1 Mx on CT scan. There was a nodule in the right lower lobe of the lung, the nature of which was uncertain. PET was requested to stage the patient's disease with a view to surgery.

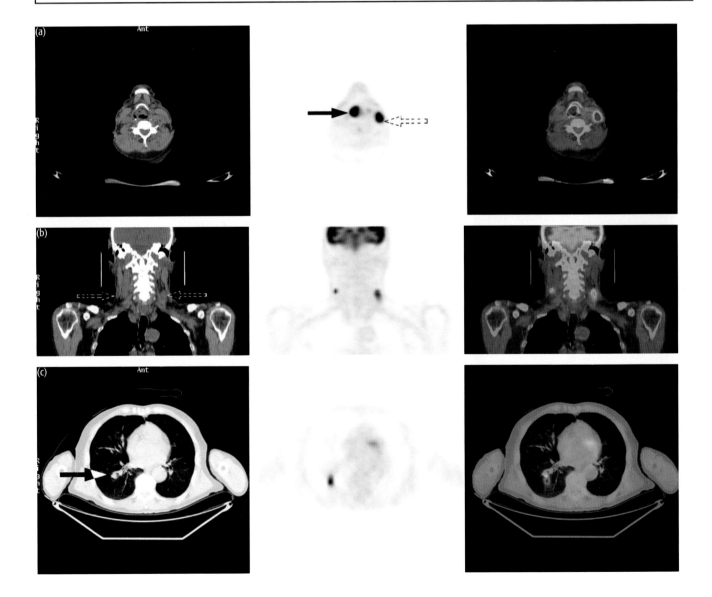

PET/CT findings:

There was uptake in the primary cancer (solid arrow in a) with uptake in cervical lymph nodes bilaterally (broken arrows in a, b) and within the lung nodule (c) indicating systemic metastasis or a new primary lesion.

Key points:

1 PET/CT can be used for staging where there are equivocal findings on other imaging.
2 PET/CT established disease was not localized to the head and neck.

| CASE 8.3 | Diagnosis: Cancer of the tongue – restaging of recurrent disease |

Clinical history:

This patient was referred with previously treated T2 N0 squamous cell carcinoma of the left side of the tongue. A partial glossectomy and selective neck dissection had been performed followed by radiotherapy. The patient then developed induration on the right side of the tongue. Biopsy revealed recurrent squamous cell carcinoma. PET/CT was requested to assist with surgical planning.

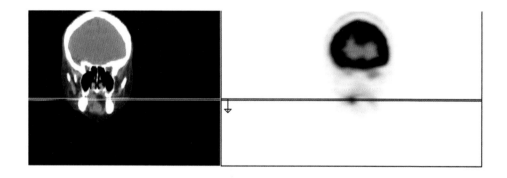

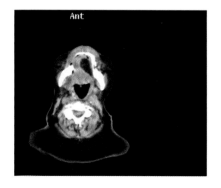

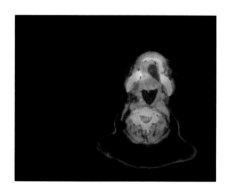

PET/CT findings:

There was intense uptake in the anterior right tongue consistent with the known recurrent tumor. No uptake was seen outside this region indicating local recurrent disease.

Key points:

1 PET/CT can restage in patients with recurrent disease to determine operability.
2 Anatomical imaging is particularly difficult in postoperative patients.

CASE 8.4	Diagnosis: Head and neck cancer – restaging of recurrent disease

Clinical history:

This patient was treated with chemotherapy and radiotherapy for a primary tumor in the right piriform fossa followed by radical neck dissection for local nodal recurrence. He subsequently developed dysphagia. Biopsy during panendoscopy showed recurrence. PET/CT was requested to restage the patient's disease to determine whether the recurrence was operable.

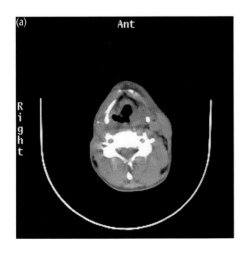

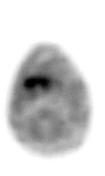

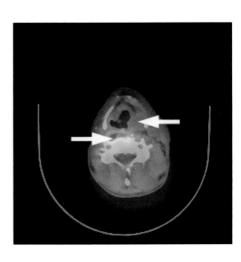

(b)

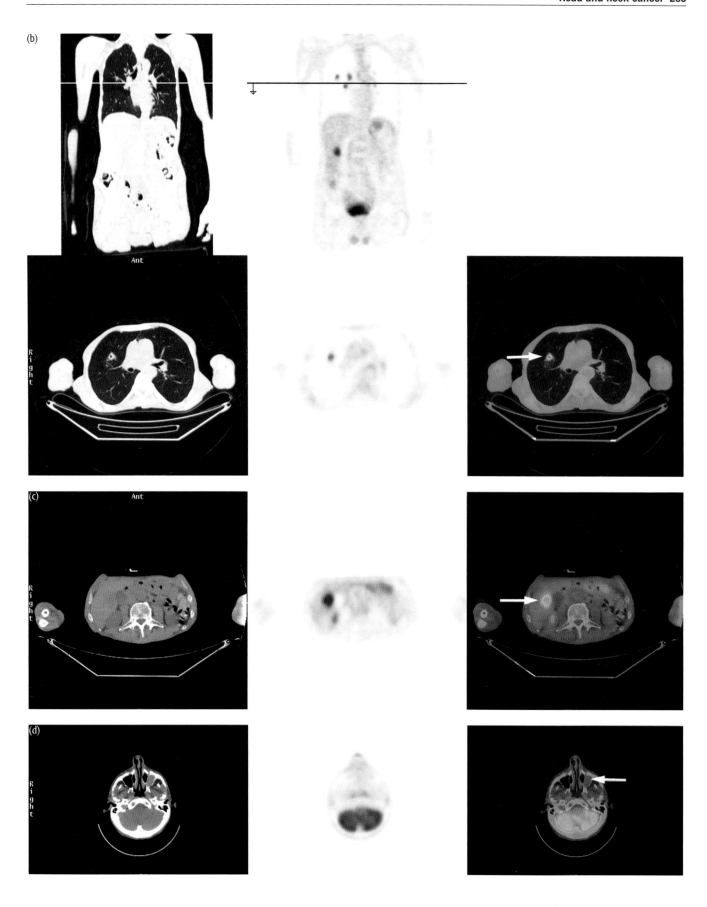

PET/CT findings:

There was FDG uptake in the right piriform fossa extending posteriorly and inferiorly to the esophagus indicating recurrent tumor (a). No FDG uptake was seen associated with abnormal soft tissue in the piriform fossa on the left suggesting this was related to previous treatment rather than new disease (a). Increased uptake was also seen in nodules in the right upper lobe of the lung (b), at the right lung hilum (b), and associated with a low attenuation lesion in the liver (c). There was opacification of the left maxillary sinus on CT which did not take up FDG, consistent with sinusitis (d). (Diagnostic CT performed prior to PET had been reported as showing recurrence on the right side of the neck, new tumor in the left piriform fossa, inflammatory change in the right lung and a possible metastasis in the liver.) Not shown is low grade uptake at the left lung hilum and in the aortopulmonary window which was also suspicious for disease.

Key point:

This case contrasts with Case 8.3. Both cases indicate that FDG PET can differentiate active tumors from the effects of treatment. In the former case there was local recurrence only and the patient was suitable for surgery; however, this case showed extensive metastatic disease.

CASE 8.5	Diagnosis: Head and neck cancer – recurrent disease

Clinical history:

This patient had been treated with radical radiotherapy for posterior cricoid carcinoma. There was a history of neurofibromatosis. She presented with pain in the neck and upper thoracic region. PET/CT was requested to determine if there was disease recurrence.

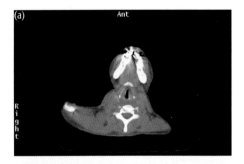

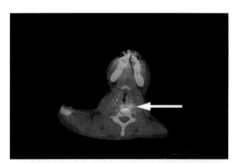
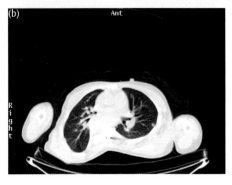

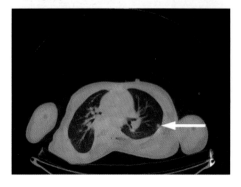

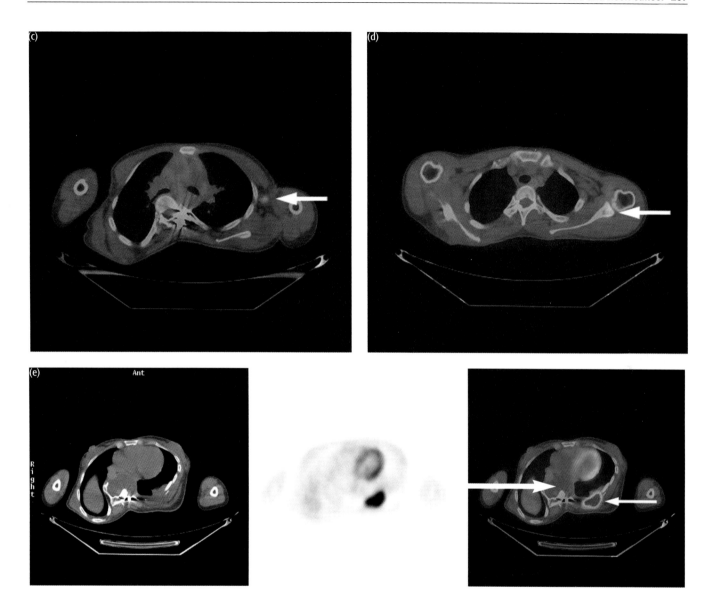

PET/CT findings:

There was recurrent disease in the posterior cricoid space (a) with metastases in lung (b), left axilla (c), and left scapula (d). There was also a large destructive lesion in the posterior chest wall with high FDG uptake (thin arrow in image e), possibly due to metastasis or malignant change within a neurofibroma. On this section a large thoracic meningocele can also be seen due to previous spinal surgery. There is no FDG uptake within it (thick arrow in image e). Note there are multiple subcutaneous neurofibromata seen best on CT.

Key points:

1 PET/CT differentiates active cancer from the effects of treatment.
2 PET can be used to assess malignant transformation within neurofibroma.
3 Note that uptake can be seen in very small lung nodules (b) if they have high metabolic activity.

CASE 8.6	Diagnosis: Head and neck cancer

Clinical history:

This patient was referred with a history of low-grade adenocarcinoma of the right maxilla treated with surgery and radiotherapy 10 years earlier. She complained of headaches. Clinical examination was difficult. MRI revealed a small area of soft tissue in the posterolateral aspect of the right maxillary sinus and soft-tissue changes in the left maxillary sinus – sinusitis? PET/CT was requested to exclude disease recurrence.

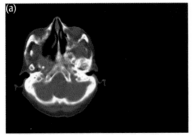
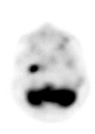
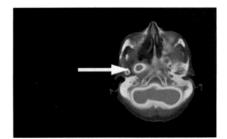
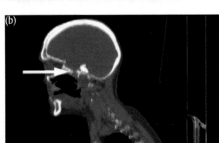
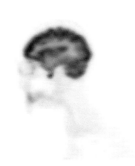
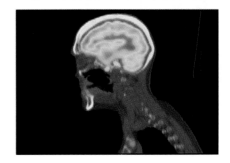

PET/CT findings:

The PET showed high uptake at the site of abnormal soft tissue posterolateral to the surgical cavity (a) consistent with disease recurrence. Note on the sagittal image that the uptake is extending into the base of the skull and is associated with bone destruction (b). Biopsy of the right posterolateral maxillary cavity revealed low-grade adenocarcinoma, confirming recurrence.

Key point:

PET can identify recurrent disease after treatment better than anatomic imaging.

| CASE 8.7 | Diagnosis: Head and neck cancer – response to therapy |

Clinical history:

This patient was diagnosed with right tonsillar squamous cell carcinoma. PET/CT was requested to monitor treatment with chemoradiotherapy.

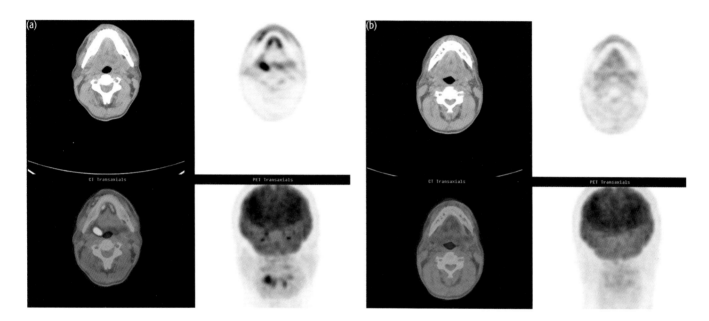

PET/CT findings:

There was avid uptake in the right tonsil prior to treatment with complete resolution of uptake post radiotherapy, indicating complete response.

Key point:

PET/CT can be used to monitor radiotherapy treatment in the head and neck, although inflammatory changes can give false-positive results early after treatment.

CASE 8.8	Diagnosis: Paraganglioma

Clinical history:

This patient was referred with a right glomus vagale tumor. She had previously had a resection of a left glomus vagale tumor. PET was requested to rule out other paragangliomas.

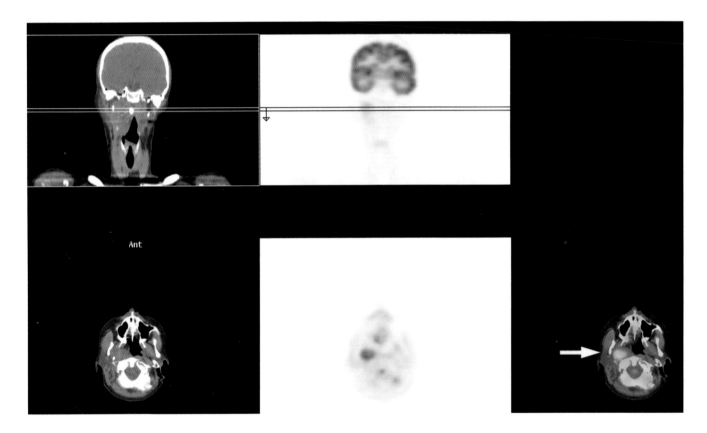

PET/CT findings:

There was a single region of increased uptake seen within the known lesion in the right parapharyngeal space.

Key point:

Glomus tumors are usually benign but may require surgical resection if they cause compression. They may be multiple and PET can be used to identity occult tumors.

CONCLUSIONS

CURRENT CLINICAL INDICATIONS

1 Initial staging of primary, nodal, and systemic disease
2 Investigation of suspected recurrence when anatomic imaging is equivocal
3 Following a negative or equivocal biopsy when the clinical suspicion remains high
4 Staging for surgical planning (especially maxillary sinus)
5 Identifying the primary when presenting with a nodal metastasis
6 Assessment of therapy response
7 Determining if salvage surgery is required
8 Determining if organ-sparing procedures are appropriate

A possible algorithm for the use of FDG PET in evaluating suspected recurrence of head and neck cancers is shown in Figure 8.3.

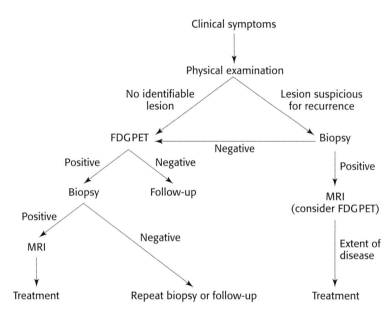

Figure 8.3 *Use of FDG PET for the evaluation of suspected recurrence*

POSSIBLE INDICATIONS

1 Nodal staging to determine if radical surgery should be performed
2 Periodic surveillance in groups at high risk for early recurrence

REFERENCES AND FURTHER READING

Allal AS, Dulguerov P, Allaoua M *et al.* (2002) Standardized uptake value of 2-[(18)F] fluoro-2-deoxy-D-glucose in predicting outcome in head and neck carcinomas treated by radiotherapy with or without chemotherapy. *J Clin Oncol* **20**, 1398–404.

Anzai Y, Carroll WR, Quint DJ *et al.* (1996) Recurrence of head and neck cancer after surgery or irradiation: Prospective comparison of 2-deoxy-2-[F-18] fluoro-D-glucose PET and MR imaging diagnoses. *Radiology* **200**, 135–41.

Anzai Y, Piccoli CW, Outwater EK *et al*; Group (2003) Evaluation of neck and body metastases to nodes with ferumoxtran 10-enhanced MR imaging: phase III safety and efficacy study. *Radiology* **228**, 777–88.

Bailet JW, Abemayor E, Jabour BA *et al.* (1992) Positron emission tomography: A new, precise imaging modality for detection of primary head and neck tumours and assessment of cervical adenopathy. *Laryngoscope* **102**, 281–8.

Greven KM, Williams DW 3rd, Keyes JW Jr *et al.* (1994) Distinguishing tumor recurrence from irradiation sequelae with positron emission tomography in patients treated for larynx cancer. *Int J Radiat Oncol Biol Phys* **29**, 841–5.

Haberkorn U, Strauss LG, Dimitrakopoulou A *et al.* (1991) PET studies of fluorodeoxyglucose metabolism in patients with recurrent colorectal tumors receiving radiotherapy. *J Nucl Med* **32**, 1485–90.

Jabour BA, Choi Y, Hoh CK *et al.* (1993) Extracranial head and neck: PET imaging with 2-[^{18}F] fluoro-2-deoxy-D-glucose and MR imaging correlation. *Radiology* **186**, 27–35.

Lindholm P, Leskinen-Kallio S, Minn H *et al.* (1993) Comparison of fluorine-^{18}fluorodeoxyglucose and carbon-11-methionine in head and neck cancer. *J Nucl Med* **34**, 1711–16.

Lowe VJ, Dunphy FR, Varvares M *et al.* (1997) Evaluation of chemotherapy response in patients with advanced head and neck cancer using [F-18]fluorodeoxyglucose positron emission tomography. *Head Neck* **19**, 666–74.

Lowe VJ, Boyd JH, Dunphy FR *et al.* (2000) Surveillance for recurrent head and neck cancer using positron emission tomography. *J Clin Oncol* **18**, 651–8.

McGuirt WF, Greven KM, Keyes JW *et al.* (1995a) Positron emission tomography in the evaluation of laryngeal carcinoma. *Ann Otol Rhinol Laryngol* **104**, 274–8.

McGuirt WF, Williams D, Keyes JW *et al.* (1995b) A comparative diagnostic study of head and neck nodal metastases using positron emission tomography. *Laryngoscope* **105**, 373–5.

McGuirt WF, Williams D, Keyes JW *et al.* (1995c) Preoperative identification of benign versus malignant parotid masses: A comparative study including positron emission tomography. *Laryngoscope* **105**, 579–84.

Minn H, Joensuu H, Ahonen A, Klemi PI (1988a) Fluorodeoxyglucose imaging: A method to assess the proliferative activity of human cancer in vivo. Comparison with DNA flow cytometry in head and neck tumors. *Cancer* **61**, 1776–81.

Minn H, Paul R, Ahonen A (1988b) Evaluation of treatment response to radiotherapy in head and neck cancer with fluorine-18 fluorodeoxyglucose. *J Nucl Med* **29**, 1521–5.

Mukherji SK, Drane WE, Mancuso AA *et al.* (1996) Occult primary tumors of the head and neck: detection with 2-[F-18] fluoro-2-deoxy-D-glucose SPECT. *Radiology* **199**, 761–6.

Schoder H, Yeung HW (2004) Positron emission imaging of head and neck cancer, including thyroid carcinoma. *Semin Nucl Med* **34**, 180–97.

Schoder H, Yeung HW, Gonen M, Kraus D, Larson SM (2004) Head and neck cancer: clinical usefulness and accuracy of PET/CT image fusion. *Radiology* **231**, 65–72.

Som PM, Curtin HD, Mancuso AA (1999) Imaging-based classification for the cervical nodes designed as an adjunct to recent clinically based nodal classifications. *Arch Otolaryngol Head Neck Surg* **125**, 388–96.

Wong W, Chevretton EB, McGurk M *et al.* (1997) A prospective study of PET-FDG imaging for the assessment of head and neck squamous cell carcinoma. *Clin Otolaryngol* **22**, 209–14.

CHAPTER 9
BREAST CANCER

INTRODUCTION AND BACKGROUND

Breast cancer is the most common visceral cancer in women, and it is the second most frequent cause of death from cancer (after lung cancer) in women overall in the UK and the USA. In the USA, breast cancer is responsible for about 40 000 deaths/year, and it is the most common single cause of death of women in the age group of 35–50 years. Early diagnosis through screening programs and early treatment can be curative but requires a multidisciplinary approach to the overall management. Breast cancer is one of the few cancers in which image-based screening programs have been shown to improve patient survival. Treatment includes surgery, which has become progressively less radical than in previous years, together with chemotherapy. Lumpectomy is now more common for localized cancers than is mastectomy. External beam radiation therapy is often used in treating primary lesions (after surgical excision) and for palliation of metastatic disease. Chemotherapy can be given at several stages of the disease, as part of primary therapy (neoadjuvant therapy), after surgery as adjuvant therapy, or as palliation for recurrent or metastatic disease. Hormonal therapies and radiation therapy are also key parts of the therapeutic regimens. Imaging is an important part of detection, staging, and management of most patients with breast cancer.

Breast cancer incidence is increasing in Western industrialized countries although death rates are falling. However, breast cancer remains infrequent in Japan. Approximately 11 percent of all women will be affected at some point in their lifetime.

EPIDEMIOLOGY	
Annual incidence	
Men	0.8 new cases per 100 000/ 240 cases UK
	1.2 new cases per 100 000/ 1690 cases USA
Women	134 new cases per 100 000/ 40 467cases UK
	135 new cases per 100 000/ 211 240 cases USA
Lifetime risk (female)	1:12
Peak age	At menopause
32% all new cancers in women	
15% all cancer deaths in women	
(Lung cancer now kills more women than breast cancer)	

Most breast cancers are of the infiltrating ductal type with the upper outer quadrant and axillary tail being the most frequent site. This distribution of tumors parallels the distribution of glandular tissue in the breast.

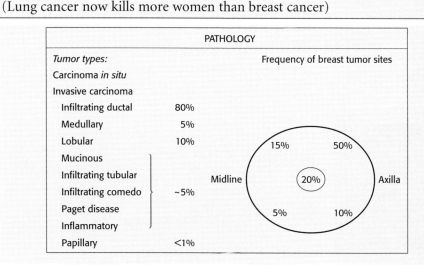

PATHOLOGY		
Tumor types:		Frequency of breast tumor sites
Carcinoma *in situ*		
Invasive carcinoma		
Infiltrating ductal	80%	
Medullary	5%	
Lobular	10%	
Mucinous		
Infiltrating tubular		
Infiltrating comedo	~5%	Midline 20% Axilla
Paget disease		15% 50%
Inflammatory		5% 10%
Papillary	<1%	

The lymph node staging of the axilla has historically been performed by axillary dissection, but is increasingly being replaced by sentinel node sampling, which is less destructive and of excellent accuracy in experienced hands. Although removal of tumor-involved nodes in the axilla decreases the risk of tumor recurrence in the axilla, the major role of surgical assessments of axillary nodal status is to assess patient risk/prognosis for recurrence and to help determine whether and how much systemic therapy is needed.

STAGING

Stage	TNM features
I	Tumor up to 2 cm
	No lymph nodes affected
	No metastatic spread
II	Tumor between 2 cm and 5 cm, and/or
	Lymph nodes in armpit affected
	No metastatic spread
III	Tumor more than 5 cm
	Lymph nodes in armpit affected
	No metastatic spread
IV	Metastatic spread outside breast

Overall 30–40 percent of newly diagnosed breast cancer patients will have axillary lymph node involvement at presentation. Clinical examination has poor accuracy (25 percent false positive, 30 percent false negative). Internal mammary nodes are less frequently involved with metastatic cancer than are axillary nodes but they are much more difficult to identify. Medial breast cancers are three times more likely to involve the internal mammary nodes than outer quadrant tumors. Internal mammary node involvement with tumor has comparably poor prognostic value as axillary tumor involvement. In many practices, the status of the internal mammary nodes is not defined surgically.

LYMPH NODE METASTATIC SITES

Lymph nodes involved	Axillary	40% +ve
	Internal mammary	
	Supraclavicular	
Frequency of axillary nodes related to tumor size	Tumor <2 cm	18% +ve
	Tumor 2–5 cm	35% +ve
	Tumor >5 cm	56% +ve
Internal mammary nodes	Tumor <5 cm	19% +ve
	Tumor >5 cm	37% +ve

DISTANT SITES

Lung
Liver
Bone
Pleura
Adrenals
Skin
Brain

The prognosis in breast cancer is highly dependent on the size of the primary lesion, whether there is involvement of axillary or internal mammary nodes, and the histology of the tumor. Systemic metastatic disease is predictive of an unfavorable outcome.

PROGNOSIS

Stage	10-year survival (%)
I	~80
II	~60
III	~30
IV	<10

KEY MANAGEMENT ISSUES

KEY MANAGEMENT ISSUES

Staging/restaging of high-risk patients:
- nodal disease in bulky medial tumors
- distant metastases

Tumor response

Detection of recurrent disease (including assessment of brachial plexopathy)

Role of PET in breast cancer

Breast cancer can be imaged with positron emission tomography (PET) using several radiopharmaceuticals including [^{18}F]2-fluoro-2-deoxy-D-glucose (FDG), [^{11}C]L-methionine, ^{18}F-labeled estrogen analogs, and fluorothymidine. Breast cancer metastatic to bone can be imaged with ^{18}F-NaF as well as FDG. In practice, virtually all clinical PET imaging studies have been performed using FDG because of the substantially increased glucose metabolism seen in breast cancers. Although early studies showed that essentially all large primary, regionally metastatic, and systemic metastases of breast cancer could be imaged with FDG, and that some breast cancers could be detected by PET but not by standard imaging methods (e.g. in radiodense breasts), the exact role of PET in the management of patients with breast cancer is still in evolution.

As the literature on breast cancer imaging has grown, it is apparent that FDG accumulation in breast cancers may be somewhat lower in intensity on average than seen in lung cancers. Thus, the accuracy of PET using whole-body PET imaging scanners in the detection of primary breast cancers varies depending on the histological type and size of the breast cancer. Tumors of lobular histology, tubular carcinomas, and small *in situ* carcinomas have lower FDG uptake than other types of breast cancer and may not be detectable by PET. In tumors under 1 cm, sensitivity of PET for lesion detection was 57 percent in one study, much lower than the sensitivity of 92 percent seen in lesions over 1 cm in size. Given that smaller breast cancers and some histologic types, including the lobular type, are often falsely negative on PET, PET with standard PET imaging devices designed for the whole body cannot be considered as a substitute for anatomic methods which have superior spatial resolution. Nonetheless, PET can be helpful in some settings, and it has recently been shown to be complementary to magnetic resonance imaging (MRI) in the assessment of breasts at high risk for multifocal disease. There is a growing level of interest in performing PET imaging of breast cancer with dedicated high-resolution instruments designed for breast imaging. PET, if positive, is highly predictive of the presence of breast cancer. At present, there is greater clinical use of MRI with contrast enhancement in primary breast cancer imaging than of FDG PET due to the limitations of the latter.

For detection of regional lymph node metastasis, the literature is varied, with early reports showing high sensitivity, in excess of 90 percent in several series. However, these early series were probably biased as patients with more advanced cancers, and thus larger metastases, were included. The largest trial of PET in axillary nodal staging was performed prospectively and showed FDG PET to be only 61 percent sensitive and 80 percent specific for detection of axillary nodal metastases. The ability to detect tumor is quite dependent on the tumor burden and PET systematically underestimates the total number of tumor-positive lymph nodes. Thus, sensitivity of PET is well below that of axillary dissection and below that of sentinel node sampling and it cannot routinely be recommended as an accurate tool to image patients with newly diagnosed breast cancers. Although PET is not particularly sensitive, when intensely positive, PET can predict with good certainty the presence of axillary nodal metastases. Thus PET may have a role in bulky tumors in patients in whom neoadjuvant chemotherapy is planned or in assessing internal mammary lymph nodes in patients with bulky medial breast primary tumors. High FDG uptake in primary lesions has been associated with a less good prognosis than for those tumors which have lower tracer uptake.

Whole-body PET imaging is increasingly used in an effort to stage the entire body for the presence/location or absence of active tumor. PET can detect some bone metastases not identified by bone scan, especially lytic metastases which may have relatively low FDG uptake. However, some blastic metastases of breast cancer are not FDG avid, but are apparent on bone scan. Thus, at present, FDG cannot be suggested as the only method with which to stage patients for the presence/absence of active breast cancer. Determining the true accuracy of PET versus computed tomography (CT) and versus histologic truth is difficult outside of the setting of the primary lesion or axillary nodes, as there are systematic differences in determining 'truth' as it is not possible to biopsy all locations in the body. However, in general, PET is more sensitive than CT and more predictive of survival. For example, one study showed an 85 percent sensitivity and 79 percent specificity for PET in detection of metastatic disease. Changes in stage and management in over a third of patients has been reported in some studies when the results of PET scanning have been compared with those of conventional imaging.

Chemotherapy treatment monitoring is a strength of PET. Metabolic changes occur before anatomic changes and in general, the greater the decline in FDG uptake, the better the response to treatment and the better the outcome. Generally, responses to breast cancer treatment are assessed by comparing a baseline PET with another one done after one or two cycles of treatment. Bone marrow uptake of FDG can rise following treatment, especially if the patient is receiving colony-stimulating factors which can complicate assessment of the bone marrow for tumor response. Although [^{18}F]-fluoroestradiol has been used to image estrogen receptors, it has not proved to be superior to FDG in practice.

In summary, the role of FDG PET continues to evolve. Its greatest role is likely in staging diseases in high-risk patients, in detecting tumor recurrence, and in being used to predict response to therapy based on early changes in FDG uptake. It is anticipated the use of PET in breast cancer will continue to grow in the coming years as clinicians become more familiar with its capabilities. Appropriate use of PET (or PET/CT) in patients with breast cancer requires a clear understanding of the limitations of the method, especially when imaging low-volume disease.

EXAMPLES TO ILLUSTRATE KEY ISSUES

CASE 9.1	Diagnosis: Breast cancer restaging

Clinical history:

This patient was treated with neoadjuvant chemotherapy and radiotherapy to the breast and right supraclavicular fossa for grade III T3 breast carcinoma. The patient complained of paresthesiae in the arm. MRI showed a lesion at T2. Bone scan was reported as normal. PET/CT was requested to characterize the lesion at T2 and to determine if there were other sites of disease.

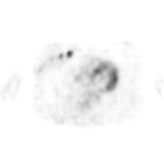
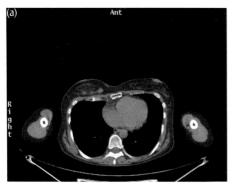
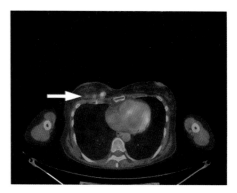

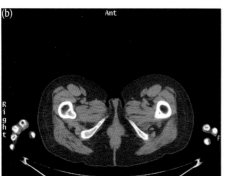
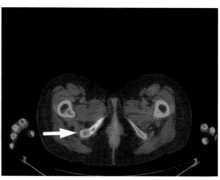

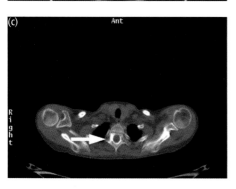
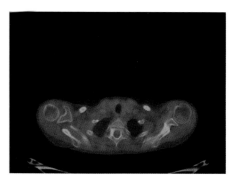

(d)

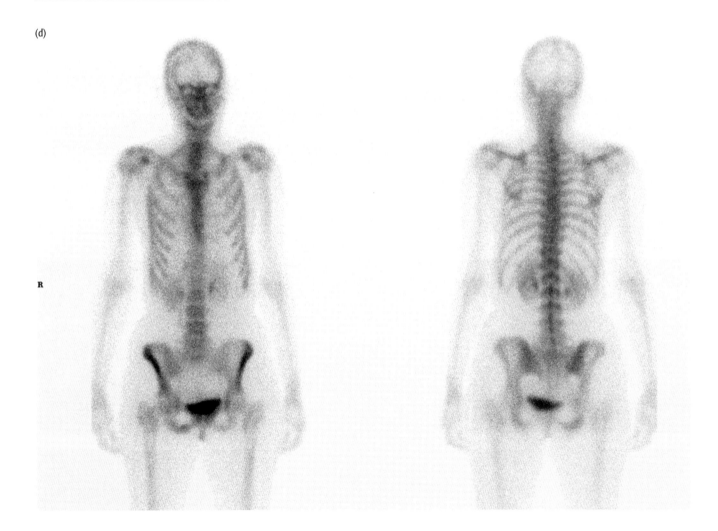

PET/CT findings:

There was increased uptake within two lesions in the right breast consistent with residual disease (a) and in the right inferior pubic bone indicative of metastasis (b) although there was no obvious bone abnormality seen on the CT component of the scan. The sclerotic metastasis at T2 was not FDG avid (c). Review of the bone scan showed low-grade uptake in the right inferior pubic bone at the site of the bone metastasis demonstrated on PET (d).

Key points:

1 Lytic and mixed lesions tend to show increased uptake with FDG, whereas sclerotic bone metastases may not. Bone metastases, which are FDG avid are associated with a poorer prognosis.
2 PET/CT can detect early bone metastases and is more sensitive overall for the detection of bone metastases from breast cancer than is bone scanning.

CASE 9.2 | Diagnosis: Breast cancer – staging

Clinical history:

This patient with previous left breast cancer presented with a new primary in the right breast. PET/CT was requested for staging the patient's disease.

(a)

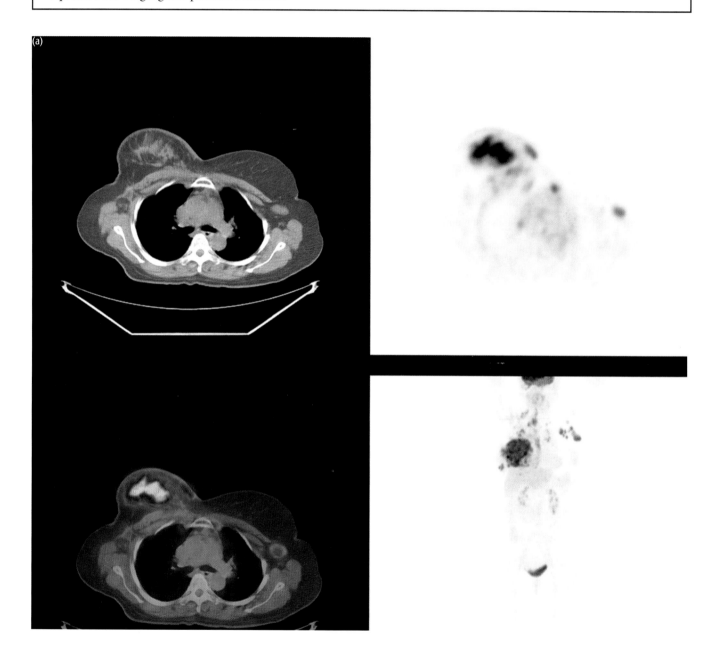

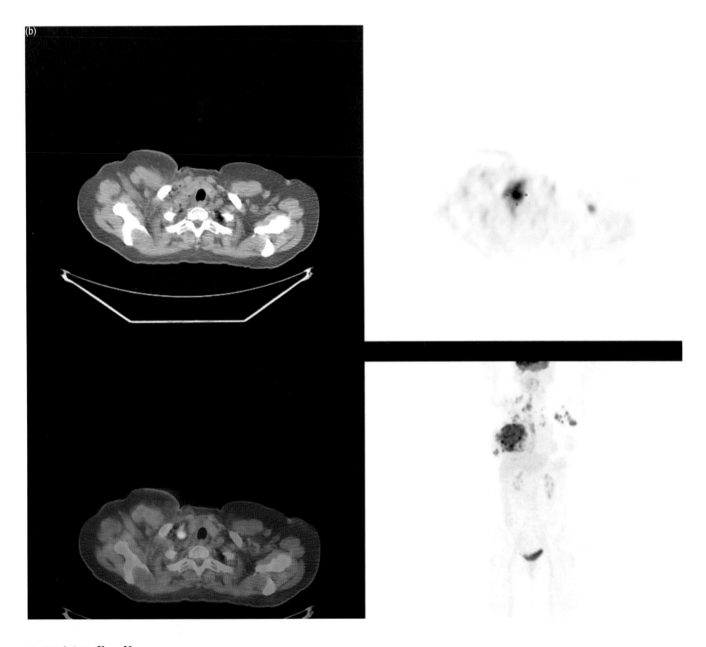

PET/CT findings:

There was high uptake in the primary right breast cancer extending onto the skin (a) and metastatic disease in bilateral axillary (a, b), internal mammary (a) and right supraclavicular lymph nodes (b) consistent with advanced locoregional disease.

Key point:

PET/CT is sensitive for nodal disease in breast cancer and, in particular, can detect disease in the internal mammary chains, although sentinel lymphoscintigraphy is more sensitive in low-volume disease.

CASE 9.3 | Diagnosis: Breast cancer – staging the primary

Clinical history:

This patient with a newly diagnosed breast cancer measuring 4 cm in the left axillary tail was referred for staging.

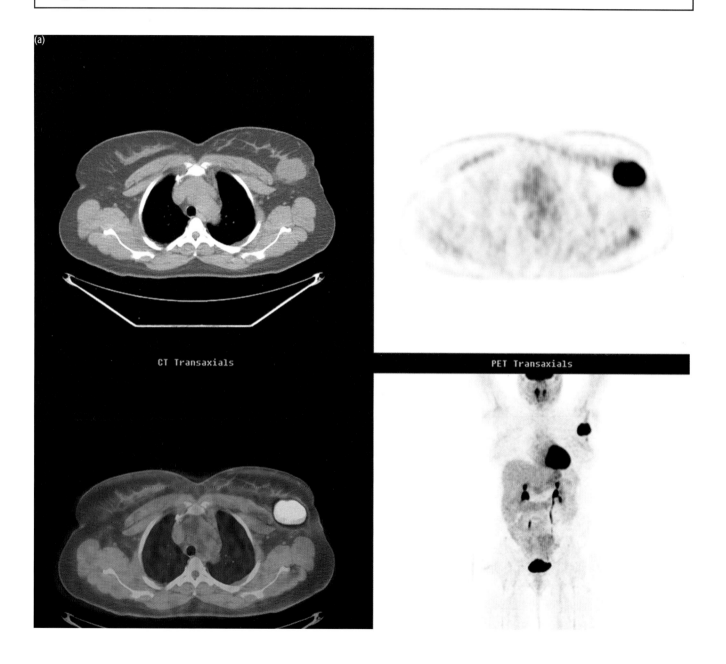

(a)

CT Transaxials

PET Transaxials

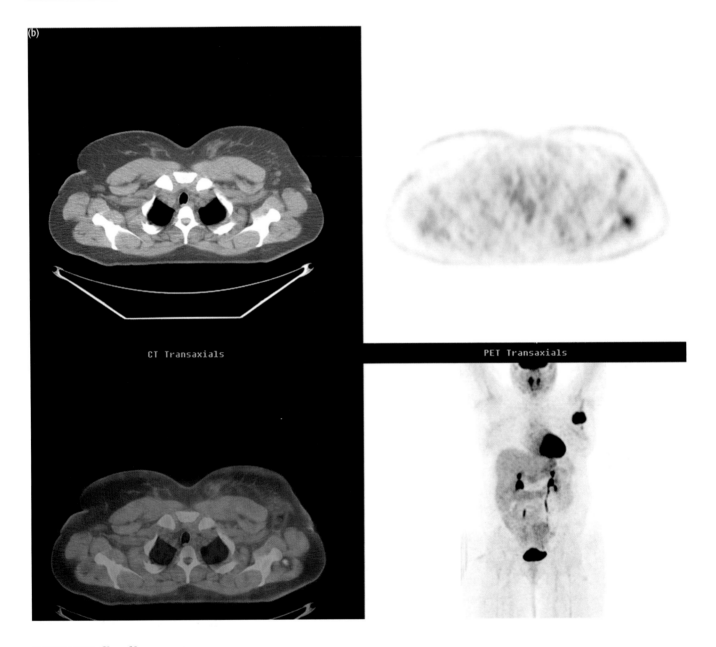

CT Transaxials

PET Transaxials

PET/CT findings:

There was high uptake in the primary cancer (a) with uptake in a left axillary lymph node (b). No uptake was associated with a smaller left axillary lymph node but this may be below the size that can be resolved by PET. In addition, physiologic uptake in muscle is seen posteriorly (b).

Key point:

PET/CT can be used in selected cases for staging breast cancer.

CASE 9.4 | Diagnosis: Breast cancer – tumor response

Clinical history:

This patient with a right breast tumor was scanned before and after chemotherapy. PET/CT was used to monitor the effects of treatment prior to surgery.

(a)

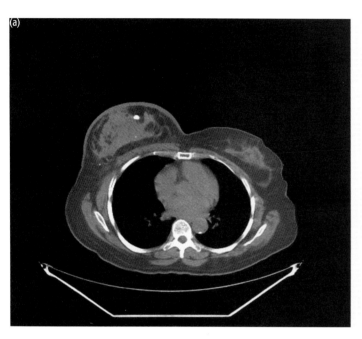

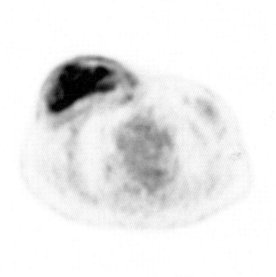

(b)

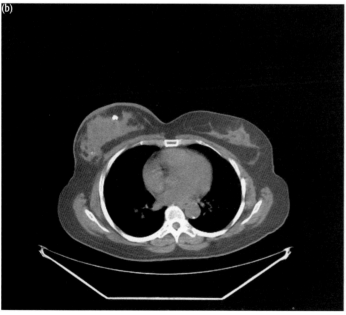

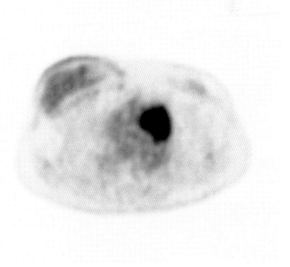

PET/CT findings:

There was reduction of uptake in the tumor but not complete resolution of uptake indicating a partial response.

Key point:

PET/CT gives an early indication of treatment response, which precedes clinical response.

CASE 9.5	Diagnosis: Breast cancer – recurrence

Clinical history:

This lady was referred with a history of breast cancer dating back 20 years. She had received chemotherapy for axillary recurrence and bone metastases 7 years earlier and then remained completely well. She was admitted to hospital with suspected cholecystitis. Investigation with ultrasound showed gallstones and a single lesion in the right lobe of the liver. CT confirmed the presence of a single liver lesion and PET/CT was requested to further characterize the lesion and to restage the patient's disease.

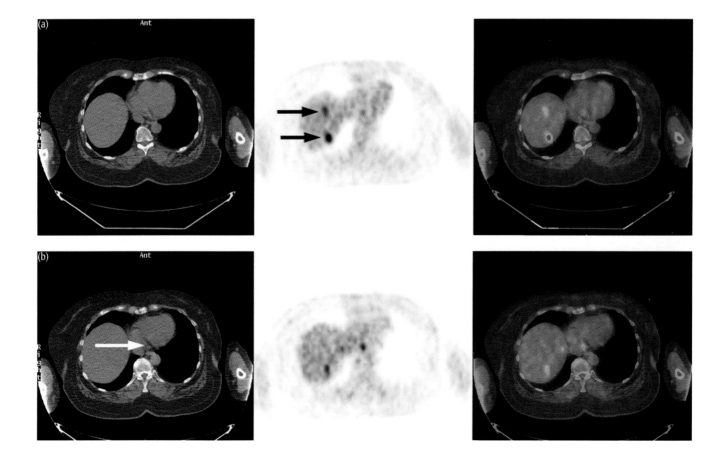

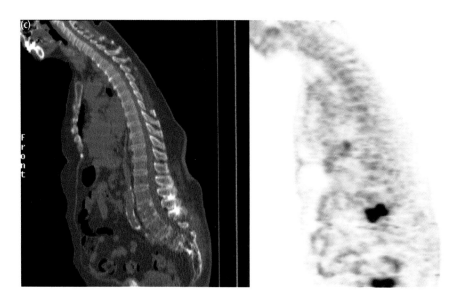
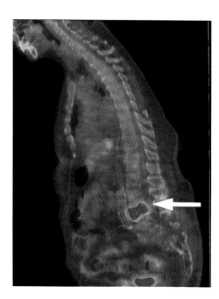

PET/CT findings:

There were two foci of increased uptake in the liver (a) in a celiac lymph node, which was not enlarged (b), and in the L3 vertebra (c). Findings indicated liver, lymph node, and bone metastases. (Not shown is an equivocal area of uptake in the liver in approximately segment VIII, possibly a further low-volume metastasis. There were also metastases in a left para-aortic lymph node at the level of L3 and in the left sacroiliac joint.)

Key points:

1 PET/CT detects breast cancer recurrence.
2 PET/CT is sensitive for the detection of metastatic disease.

CASE 9.6	Diagnosis: Breast cancer – recurrent disease

Clinical history:

This patient with breast cancer and back pain with probable bone metastases was referred for assessment of relapse and restaging.

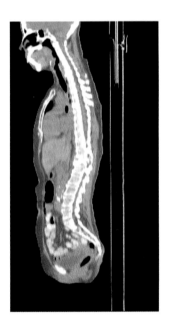 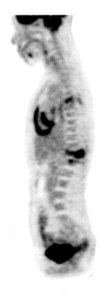 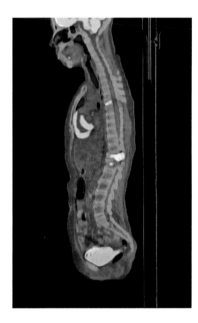 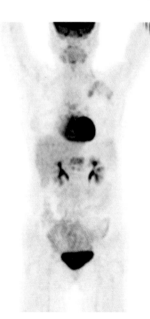

PET/CT findings:

There was high uptake in thoracic vertebrae consistent with metastatic bone disease.

Key point:
PET/CT is sensitive for metastatic bone disease in breast cancer.

CASE 9.7	Diagnosis: Breast cancer

Clinical history:

After finishing breast feeding, this patient complained that her left breast had not returned to normal. Mammography was performed but in view of the high radiographic density within a recently lactating breast, the examination was technically difficult and no tumor was seen. The patient was referred for PET.

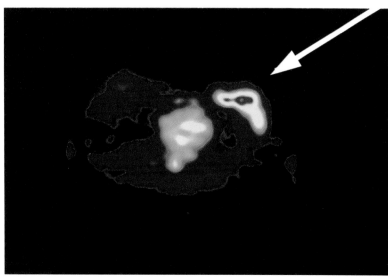

Reproduced with kind permission from Wahl RL, Zasadny KR, Helvie M et al. (1993) Metabolic monitoring of breast cancer chemohormonotherapy using positron emission tomography: initial evaluation. J Clin Oncol 11, 2101–11 (Figure 3b)

PET/CT findings:

Intense uptake of FDG within a large tumor in the left breast is seen in the above transaxial emission image. Biopsy confirmed the diagnosis of breast cancer. Disease was localized to the breast without evidence of nodal or distant spread.

Key point:

PET can sometimes be helpful in the assessment of radiodense breasts which are difficult to image with other methods.

| **CASE 9.8** | **Diagnosis: Breast cancer** |

Clinical history:

This patient with breast prosthesis was assessed for a breast lump. Mammogram of the left breast showed a large prosthesis and adjacent mass (arrowheads in image a). Magnification coned compression displacement view showed a 1.5 cm × 1.0 cm mass (arrows in b) which was moderately well circumscribed and had two microcalcifications.

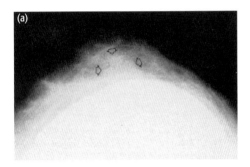

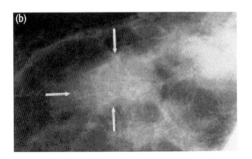

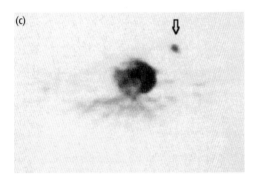

Reprinted by permission of the Society of Nuclear Medicine from: Wahl RL, Helvie MA, Chang AE, Andersson I (1994) Detection of breast cancer in women after augmentation mammoplasty using fluorine-18-fluorodeoxyglucose-PET. J Nucl Med 35, 874 (Figures 2A–C)

PET/CT findings:

Transverse FDG PET scan (c) at the level of the mass demonstrated an FDG-avid nodule in the left breast (arrow) beyond the prosthesis (which did not accumulate FDG) and which was not particularly attenuating of 511 keV photons. Normal myocardial uptake is noted.

Key point:

FDG PET may be used in circumstances where mammography is technically difficult including:
1 dense breasts
2 breast implants
3 lumpy breasts/multifocal disease
4 postoperative/post-biopsy breast.

CONCLUSIONS

CURRENT CLINICAL INDICATIONS
1 Staging/restaging of high-risk patients
2 Brachial plexopathy
3 Recurrent disease equivocal on clinical grounds/other imaging
4 Breast implants – recurrence + conserved breast?
5 Treatment response

FURTHER READING

Adler LP, Crowe JP, al-Kaisi NK, Sunshire JL (1993) Evaluation of breast masses and axillary lymph nodes with [18F] 2-deoxy-2-fluoro-D-glucose PET. *Radiology* **187**, 743–50.

Avril N, Dose J, Janicke DF *et al.* (1996) Metabolic characterization of breast tumors with positron emission tomography using 18F fluorodeoxyglucose. *J Clin Oncol* **14**, 1848–57.

Avril N, Dose J, Janicke F *et al.* (1996) Assessment of axillary lymph node involvement in breast cancer patients with positron emission tomography using radiolabeled 2-(fluorine-18)-fluoro-2-deoxy-D-glucose. *J Natl Cancer Inst* **88**, 1204–9.

Bos R, van Der Hoeven JJ, van Der Wall E *et al.* (2002) Biologic correlates of fluorodeoxyglucose uptake in human breast cancer measured by positron emission tomography. *J Clin Oncol* **20**, 379–87.

Clavo AC, Wahl RL (1996) Effects of hypoxia on the uptake of tritiated thymidine, L-leucine, L-methionine and FDG in cultured cancer cells. *J Nucl Med* **37**, 502–6.

Cook G, Houston S, Maisey M *et al.* (1997) Detection of bone metastases in breast cancer by 18-FDG-PET. Differing metabolic activity in osteoblastic and osteolytic lesions. *J Nucl Med* **5**(S), 127.

Dejdasjti F, Mortimer JE, Siegel BA *et al.* (1995) Positron tomographic assessment of estrogen receptors in breast cancer. Comparison with FDG-PET and in vitro receptor assays. *J Nucl Med* **36**, 1766–74.

Eubank W, Mankoff DA (2004) Current and future uses of positron emisson tomography in breast cancer imaging. *Semin Nucl Med* **34**, 224–40.

Eubank WB, Mankoff D, Bhattacharya M *et al.* (2004) Impact of FDG PET on defining the extent of disease and on the treatment of patients with recurrent or metastatic breast cancer. *AJR Am J Roentgenol* **183**, 479–86.

Jansson T, Westlin JE, Ahlstrom H *et al.* (1995) Positron emission tomography studies in patients with locally advanced and/or metastatic breast cancer: A method for early therapy evaluation? *J Clin Oncol* **13**, 1470–7.

Leskinen-Kallio S, Nagren K, Lehikoinen P *et al.* (1991) Uptake of 11C-methionine in breast cancer studied by PET. An association with the size of S-phase fraction. *Br J Cancer* **64**, 1121–4.

McGuire AH, Dehdashti F, Siegel BA *et al.* (1991) Positron tomographic assessment of 17 alpha-[18F] fluoro-17 beta-estradiol uptake in metastatic breast carcinoma. *J Nucl Med* **32**, 1526–31.

Mortimer JE, Dehdashti F, Siegel BA *et al.* (2001) Metabolic flare: indicator of hormone responsiveness in advanced breast cancer. *J Clin Oncol* **19**, 2797–803.

Oshida M, Uno K, Suzuki M *et al.* (1998) Predicting the prognoses of breast carcinoma patients with positron emission tomography using 2-deoxy-2-fluoro[18F]-D-glucose. *Cancer* **82**, 2227–34.

Scheidhauer K, Scharl A, Pietrzyk U *et al.* (1996) Qualitative [18F]FDG positron emission tomography in primary breast cancer: clinical relevance and practicability. *Eur J Nucl Med* **23**, 618–23.

Schirrmeister H, Guhlmann A, Kotzerke J *et al.* (1999) Early detection and accurate description of extent of metastatic bone disease in breast cancer with fluoride ion and positron emission tomography. *J Clin Oncol* **17**, 2381–9.

Schirrmeister H, Kuhn T, Guhlmann A *et al.* (2001) Fluorine-18 2-deoxy-2-fluoro-D-glucose PET in the preoperative staging of breast cancer: comparison with the standard staging procedures. *Eur J Nucl Med* **28**, 351–8.

Utech CI, Young CS, Winter PF (1996) Prospective evaluation of fluorine-18 fluorodeoxyglucose positron emission tomography in breast cancer for staging of the axilla related to surgery and immunocytochemistry. *Eur J Nucl Med* **23**, 1588–93.

Wahl RL, Cody R, Hutchins GD, Mudgett E (1991) Primary and metastatic breast carcinoma: Initial clinical evaluation with PET with the radiolabeled glucose analog 2-[18F]-fluro-deoxy-2-D-glucose (FDG). *Radiology* **179**, 765–70.

Wahl RL, Zarachy KR, Helvie M *et al.* (1993) Metabolic monitoring of breast cancer chemohormonotherapy using positron emission tomography (PET): Initial evaluation. *J Clin Oncol* **11**, 2101–11.

Wahl RL, Helvie MA, Chang AE, Andersson I (1994) Detection of breast cancer in women after augmentation mammoplasty using positron emission tomography: Initial clinical evaluation. *J Nucl Med* **35**, 872–5.

CHAPTER 10
GYNECOLOGICAL CANCERS

INTRODUCTION AND BACKGROUND

Tumors of the uterus, cervix, and ovaries are newly diagnosed in over 40 000, 10 000, and 20 000 women in the USA per year, respectively. These tumors cause over 7000, 4000, and 14 000 deaths per year in the USA, respectively. Similar population adjusted rates of these cancers are found in the UK. Cervical cancer is associated with risk factors of early sexual activity, multiple sexual partners, and, increasingly clearly, with viral infections such as with the human papilloma virus (HPV). Uterine and ovarian cancers have less clearly defined risk factors, but age at childbirth, hormonal therapy, and mutations such as those in the *BRCA1* and *BRCA2* loci are associated with increased cancer risk. Cervical cancer, when diagnosed in the early stages, is highly curable and hopes exist that vaccines against HPV will help reduce rates of cervical cancer in the future.

Cervical cancer is an excellent example of a disease in which the death rate declined after screening programs were put in place to detect early-stage disease (e.g. Pap smears). Unfortunately not all women are screened and cervical cancer detected at a more advanced stage carries with it a substantial risk of death, commonly due to metastatic disease. Whereas surgery or local radiation treatment may be sufficient for treatment of early-stage cervical cancer, more advanced disease requires more extensive radiation treatment and often chemotherapy. Historically, the initial staging of cervical cancer was largely based on physical examination, however, imaging is increasingly key to major therapeutic decisions. Metastasis commonly occurs via lymphatic spread. The metastases require more aggressive treatment than more limited disease.

Uterine (endometrial) cancers are often diagnosed at a more advanced stage than cervical cancers although some are identified at screening. More commonly, bleeding draws attention to the primary neoplasm. Endometrial cancers are somewhat more likely to metastasize hematogenously than cervical cancers. Although a far more common cancer than the other gynecological cancers, endometrial cancer is associated with a substantially lower death rate relative to incidence compared with the other types of gynecological cancer.

Ovarian cancer is often fairly advanced in its extent at diagnosis with intraperitoneal and often nodal dissemination. Over half of women diagnosed as having ovarian cancer ultimately die of their disease, indicating the major challenges in early detection of the illness. Aggressive surgical excision of ovarian cancers is important to minimize tumor burden, but chemotherapy plays a really important role in attempting to manage the disease. Five-year survival in ovarian cancer is typically under 50 percent and is dependent on stage. No widely applied screening programs are in place, and data are not available to determine whether such programs will reduce mortality in ovarian cancer. There is, however, a great deal of promise in the use of serum markers and possibly anatomic imaging such as ultrasound, in patients with marker elevations to detect ovarian cancer at an earlier, more treatable stage. Serum markers are commonly used to follow the disease during therapy.

Imaging with positron emission tomography (PET) is playing an important and growing role in all these types of cancer.

Cervical, ovarian, and uterine (endometrial) cancers represent approximately 5 percent of all cancers in women. Ovarian cancer often presents late and has a worse prognosis than cervical and uterine cancer.

EPIDEMIOLOGY

Incidence

Cervix	9.9 new cases per 100 000/ 2991 cases UK
	8.6 new cases per 100 000/ 10 370 cases USA
	1% of all cancers
Uterus	19.9 new cases per 100 000/ 6002 cases UK
	25.2 new cases per 100 000/ 40 880 cases USA
	2% of all cancers
Ovary	22.3 new cases per 100 000/ 6734 cases UK
	14.4 new cases per 100 000/ 22 220 cases USA
	2% of all cancers

Despite screening programs, cervical cancer remains a major treatment challenge if it is not locally controlled. Although ovarian cancer is far less frequent than endometrial cancer, ovarian cancer is substantially more lethal, killing over half the women afflicted with the disease.

Histologically, the vast majority of cervical carcinomas are of squamous cell type. Cervical cancer is increasingly being shown to be related to HPV infection. Uterine and ovarian cancers are generally adenocarcinomas of one of several types.

PATHOLOGY

Tumor site	Histology
Cervix	Squamous (~90%)
	Adenocarcinoma (~10%)
	Small cell/lymphoma/sarcoma (<5%)
Uterus	Adeno/squamous carcinoma (>90%)
	Sarcoma (<5%)
Ovary	Epithelial (~90%)
	Stromal (~5%)
	Germ cell (~5%)

Early age of sexual activity, number of sexual partners, and viral infections such as HPV are known risk factors for cervical carcinoma. Ovarian and endometrial cancers are more common in women who have not had children. The BRCA mutations (1 and 2) have been associated with increased risks of breast and ovarian cancer. Some hormonal therapies such as tamoxifen are associated with an increased risk of endometrial cancer.

PREDISPOSING FACTORS

Tumor site	Risk factors
Cervix	HPV
	Early age of sexual activity
	Multiple sexual partners
Uterus	Hormonal treatment, e.g. tamoxifen
	Nulliparity
Ovary	Nulliparity
	Genetic, e.g. *BRAC1*, *BRAC2*

STAGING OF GYNECOLOGICAL CANCERS

FIGO* stage	General stage description
Cervical cancer	
I	Limited to cervix
II	Extends beyond cervix excluding lower third of vagina/pelvic wall
III	Spread to pelvic side wall, lower third of vagina or causing hydronephrosis
IV	Spread beyond true pelvis or involvement of bladder mucosa or rectum
Endometrial/uterine cancer	
I	Limited to corpus
II	Involvement of cervix
III	Spread outside of uterus, confined to pelvis (excluding rectum or bladder)
IV	Spread to bladder, rectum, distant sites
Ovarian cancer	
I	Limited to ovary
II	Involvement of ovary with pelvic extension
III	Tumor in ovary with peritoneal implants outside the pelvis and/or retroperitoneal/inguinal nodes or superficial liver metastasis
IV	Distant metastasis

*FIGO, International Federation of Gynecologists and Obstetricians.

PROGNOSIS

FIGO* stage	5-year survival (%)
Cervical cancer	
I	90–95
II	~ 75
III	~ 50
IV	20–30
Uterine cancer	
I	~ 90
II	~ 80
III	~ 55
IV	~ 15
Ovarian cancer	
I	80–90
II	65–70
III	25–60
IV	~ 15

Primary staging of both ovarian and cervical cancer has mainly been based on physical examination, although computed tomography (CT) scans and ultrasound can be used to detect more extensive disease. CT commonly fails to detect small nodal metastases and peritoneal implants. In all these cancers, the prognosis worsens with increases in tumor stage. PET has recently been shown to be able to provide unique prognostic information at disease presentation in cervical cancer.

Early-stage cervical cancer is nearly 100 percent curable with local therapies. Prognosis declines as the stage of the tumor increases. Spread of the tumor to retroperitoneal lymph nodes indicates a much worsened prognosis whereas organ metastatic disease is essentially incurable. Endometrial cancer is less curable than cervical cancer, and ovarian cancer is even more problematic. Although localized early-stage, histologically nonaggressive, ovarian cancers can be cured, it is much more common for women to present with advanced disease and 5-year survival with stage III or IV disease is 15–60 percent.

Surgery effectively cures early-stage cervical cancer, but it cannot control advanced disease. Although surgery is common for all types of gynecological neoplasm, radiation therapy can also be curative on its own in both cervical and endometrial cancer if the cancer is limited to the irradiated field.

Local recurrence of cervical cancer is sometimes curable. Metastasis to the retroperitoneal lymph nodes is not unusual, with direct involvement of bone, as well as visceral metastasis, as the disease progresses – portending a grim prognosis. Ovarian cancer often spreads throughout the peritoneal cavity and can then spread systemically. Local, nodal, and hematogenous metastases are all seen in recurrent/metastatic endometrial cancer.

In the past, staging of these tumors was essentially based on physical examination only. As imaging tests improve, it is clear that the staging systems will evolve to include imaging as it adds prognostic information beyond that available from physical examination alone. This is most clear at present for cervical cancer, where the PET scan at presentation, as well as after treatment, has unique prognostic information.

KEY MANAGEMENT ISSUES

KEY MANAGEMENT ISSUES
Staging (locoregional and systemic) at presentation for extent of disease
Staging (locoregional and systemic) after treatment has been given
Planning radiation therapy port size
Monitoring for recurrence and for possible debulking surgery (ovary)
Assessment of treatment response

Role of PET in gynecological cancers

CERVICAL CANCER

Cervical cancers are usually detected by cytology, colposcopy, and direct inspection of the cervix, and PET does not have a major role in detection of small primary lesions. More advanced primary cancers are commonly detected by PET, and several studies have shown that over 80 percent of untreated primary cervical cancers can be successfully imaged with [^{18}F]2-fluoro-2-deoxy-D-glucose (FDG). These figures are likely biased toward imaging of larger tumors. Sensitivity of PET has been reported to be between 83 and 97 percent for the detection of nodal metastases of cervical cancer – substantially more sensitive than anatomic methods. Specificity has been reported to be in the same range. PET will fail to detect small-volume disease but can often detect tumor foci which are negative on anatomic imaging. Of particular interest is that the PET findings at presentation of cervical cancer are predictive of disease-free recurrence. Patients with positive PET and CT scans of the retroperitoneal nodes have the worst prognosis. Patients with positive PET and negative CT scans have nearly as poor a prognosis, whereas patients with negative PET scans of these nodes, irrespective of CT findings, have a substantially better prognosis (Figure 10.1). The 3-year survival rate of patients who are PET negative for nodal metastasis at presentation is typically 70–80 percent, whereas in patients with para-aortic metastasis a 30–40 percent rate is seen. Effective therapy of cervical

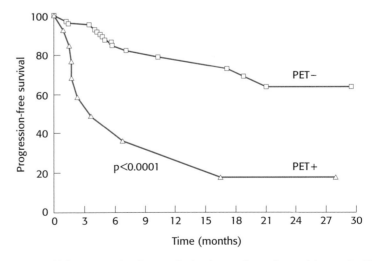

Figure 10.1 *Kaplan–Meier progression-free survival estimates for patients with negative CT scans for para-aortic nodal involvement (n = 94). The graph compares patients with positive PET scans (n = 14) and those with negative PET scans (n = 80), p=0.0001. Redrawn with kind permission from Grigsby PW, Siegel BA, Dehdashti F (2001). Lymph node staging by positron emission tomography in patients with carcinoma of the cervix. J Clin Oncol 19, 3745–9*

cancer reduces tumor FDG uptake quickly and portends a better prognosis than that in patients with persistently positive scans after treatment. FDG PET should strongly be considered in the routine staging and follow-up of patients with cervical cancer; in the USA, Medicare has approved PET for the initial staging of patients with cervical cancer. Similar data on the accuracy of PET have been presented as for the accuracy of PET in recurrent cervical cancer. PET has been shown to change the management of ~20 percent of patients with cervical cancer.

ENDOMETRIAL CANCER

The role of PET in endometrial cancer is less well established than it is in cervical cancer, despite the higher frequency of endometrial cancer. Sensitivity of 80–90 percent and similar specificity has been reported for metastatic disease. PET may also be useful for identifying uterine sarcomas and distinguishing them from myomas. Although it is expected that the role of PET is similar to that in other tumors, there are fewer explicit data on this tumor type. A challenge in uterine uptake of radiotracer is the variability in the intensity of normal uterine uptake during the menstrual period. Modest uptake in the uterus must not be confused with disease.

OVARIAN CANCER

Ovarian cancer often is diagnosed rather late in its course. Unfortunately, whereas a 5-year survival rate of 80–90 percent can be seen in stage I ovarian cancer, survival is only around 15% if the disease is stage IV at presentation, and advanced disease presents more commonly. PET has not proved to be extremely effective in evaluating primary pelvic masses, with a sensitivity for cancer detection of 58% and a specificity of 76%. This may be, in part, due to variable FDG uptake in normal ovary and uptake in ovarian inflammatory processes. Clearly, PET cannot detect small-volume disease. The ability of FDG PET and PET/CT in particular, to detect peritoneal metastases is well described, but is size dependent. Very small peritoneal implants after chemotherapy are often missed by PET. In contrast, lesions >1 cm in diameter are often well detected. PET with FDG has shown very good sensitivity in the setting of the rising CA-125 serum level and can be more sensitive than serum markers. This is because even though recurrence may be diagnosed on the basis of a rising CA-125 level, the lesion(s) cannot be localized by the serum assay. For surgeons who adhere to the philosophy of surgical debulking, PET– and notably PET/CT – has been shown able to identify between 80 and 90 percent of patients who have macroscopic disease amenable to resection, with an approximately 94 percent positive predictive value for macroscopic disease overall.

EXAMPLES TO ILLUSTRATE KEY ISSUES

CASE 10.1	Diagnosis: Cervical cancer

Clinical history:

This patient had a hysterectomy and pelvic lymphadenectomy followed by radiotherapy for squamous cell carcinoma of the cervix. One year later she developed left pelvic wall recurrence and had further surgery and radiotherapy. She then re-presented a further year on with new liver lesions. PET/CT was requested for restaging.

(a)

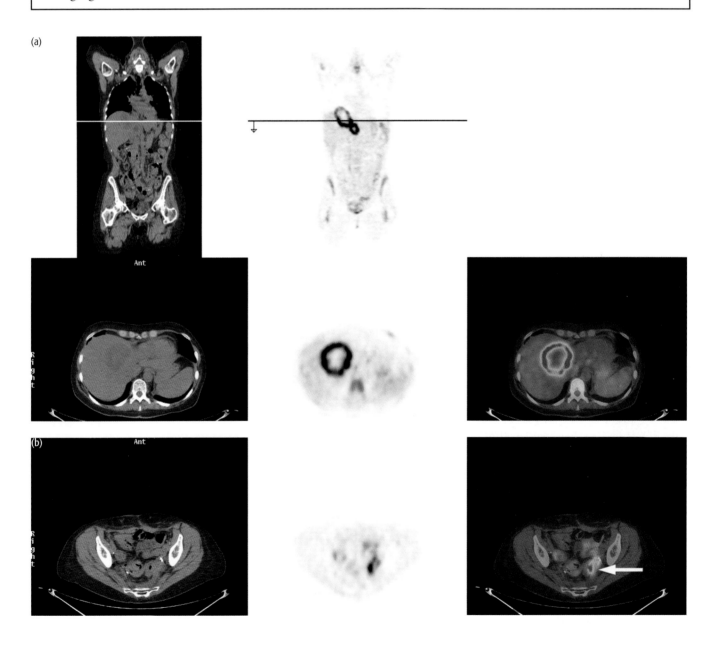

(b)

PET/CT findings:

There was uptake in two liver metastases (a) and intense uptake in the left pelvic side wall posterior to surgical clips (arrowed in b) indicative of tumor recurrence in the left pelvis at the site of previous surgery.

Key point:

PET/CT can differentiate tumor recurrence from treatment effect after surgery and radiotherapy provided sufficient time has elapsed after the treatment to allow resolution of any inflammatory changes associated with therapy.

CASE 10.2	Diagnosis: Cervical cancer

Clinical history:

This patient was treated with surgery followed by radiotherapy 30 years previously. She re-presented with recurrent tumor invading the vaginal vault and extending toward the rectum. Pelvic exenteration was being considered and PET/CT was requested for restaging.

(a)

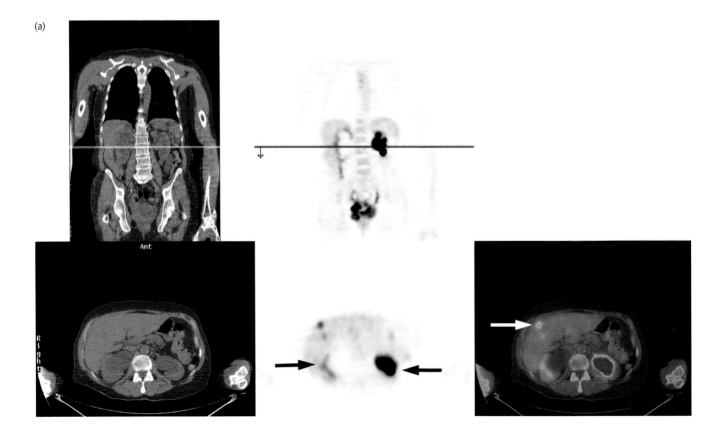

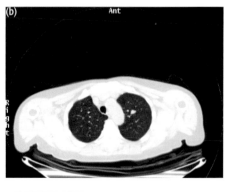

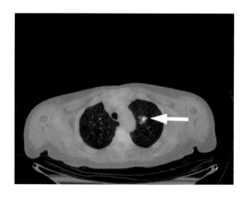
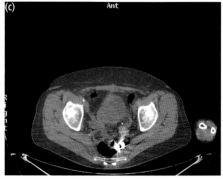

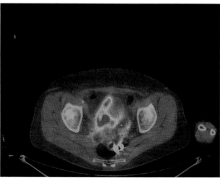

PET/CT findings:

There were metastases in the liver (white arrow in image a) and in the lung (b). There was also avid uptake associated with a pelvic mass involving the vaginal vault and extending over the surface of the bladder toward the anterior abdominal wall (c). There was bilateral hydronephrosis, with uptake only around the rim of the right renal cortex suggesting functional impairment of this kidney (right black arrow in image a). There was marked increased uptake associated with the left renal pelvis indicating likely obstruction on this side (left black arrow in image a).

Key points:

1 PET/CT is sensitive for metastatic disease from cervical cancer.
2 In this case urgent relief of the left renal obstruction was required to prevent renal failure.

CASE 10.3 | Diagnosis: Cervical cancer

Clinical history:

This patient had been treated for carcinoma of the cervix 2 years previously with chemoradiation to the pelvis and para-aortic nodes. She re-presented with acute renal failure and bilateral hydronephrosis due to obstruction in the pelvis. PET/CT was requested to distinguish between recurrent disease and radiation fibrosis as the cause.

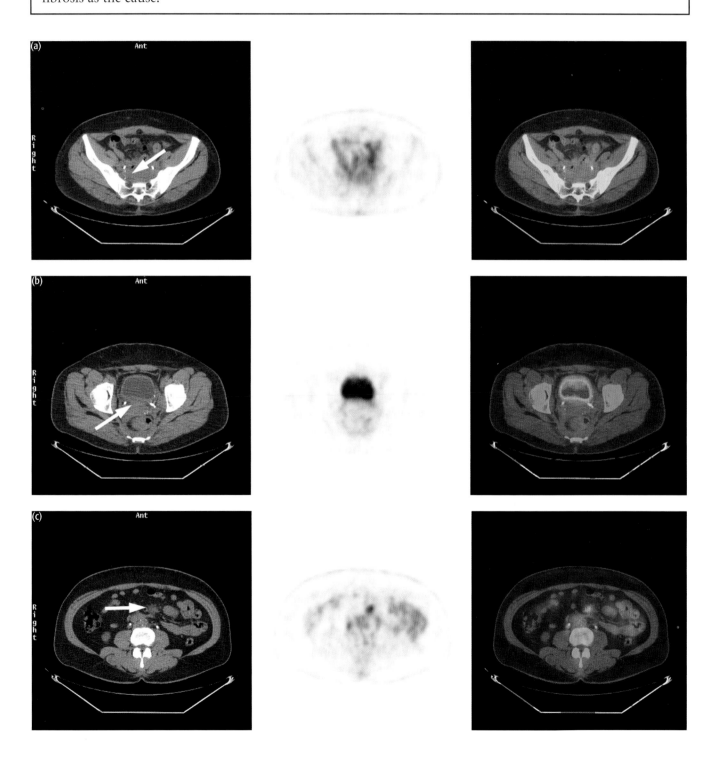

PET/CT findings:

No uptake was associated with the presacral (a) or pelvic soft-tissue masses (b), indicating these were due to radiation fibrosis. However, abnormal uptake was seen in the peritoneum within peritoneal deposits (c).

Key points:

1 PET/CT distinguishes fibrosis from cancer after treatment.
2 In this case the uptake in the peritoneum would have been difficult to differentiate from physiologic uptake in bowel on PET alone. Correlation of the PET with the CT component of the scan is required and PET/CT is superior to PET alone.

CASE 10.4	Diagnosis: Metastatic serous papillary carcinoma

Clinical history:

This patient was referred with a history of right hypochondrial discomfort associated with right pleural effusion. Pleural aspiration, pleural biopsy, bronchoscopy, and CT scanning were not diagnostic. CA-125 (tumor marker) level was marginally elevated. PET/CT was requested to exclude underlying malignancy.

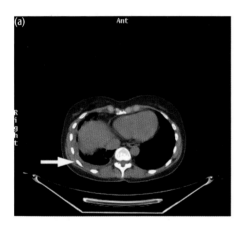 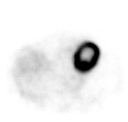 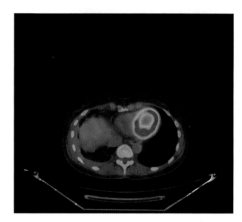

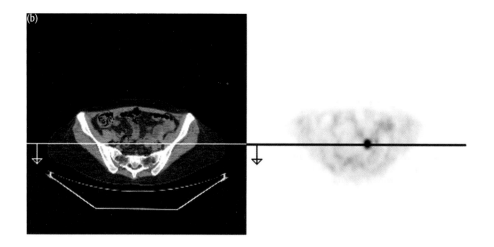

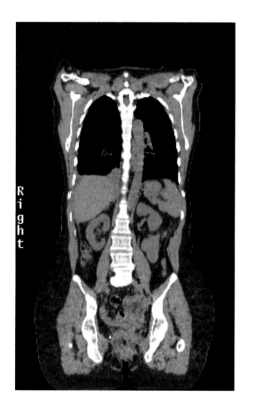

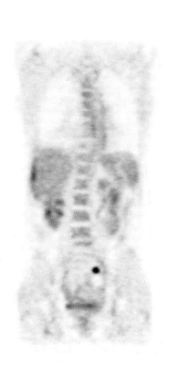

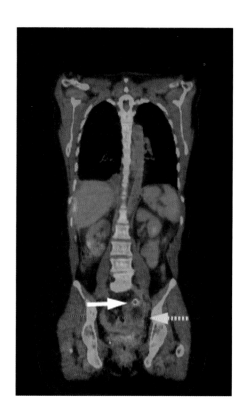

PET/CT findings:

The PET showed no abnormal uptake associated with the pleural effusion (a). There was a small left ovarian cyst with a photopenic centre (broken arrow in b) and intense uptake of FDG in a focus proximal to the cyst (solid arrow in b). Functional uptake can be seen in ovary mid-cycle in premenopausal women but uptake in the region of the ovary in a postmenopausal woman is cause for concern. Transvaginal ultrasound revealed only a simple ovarian cyst, but because of concern over the PET/CT scan findings a laparoscopy was performed. The pelvic cavity including the right ovary was normal on inspection. The left ovary was removed. It contained a benign ovarian cyst, however, a carcinoma was found within the distal left fallopian tube, which accounted for the high uptake on the PET scan. Six weeks after the PET scan, a laparotomy revealed metastatic serous papillary carcinoma in the right ovary, left pelvic side wall, omentum, and posterior aspect of the cervix.

Key points:

1 PET/CT can be helpful in detection of underlying malignancy where there is a high clinical suspicion in difficult cases.
2 In this case metastatic disease may have been 'missed'. It is possible that this was an aggressive tumor that metastasized very quickly, but as the metastatic deposits found were small, it is more likely that micrometastases were already present at the time of the PET/CT scan. The lesions may have been too small to be resolved by PET. The resolution in reconstructed images is typically around 6–8 mm.

| CASE 10.5 | Diagnosis: Ovarian cancer |

Clinical history:

This patient was referred 10 years after treatment for ovarian carcinoma with rising CA-125 (tumor marker) levels. PET/CT was requested to determine the site of probable relapse.

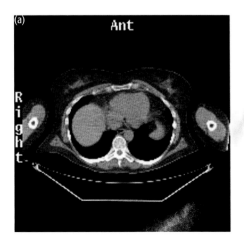
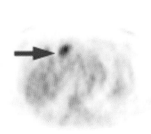
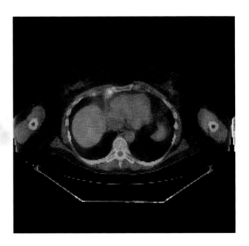

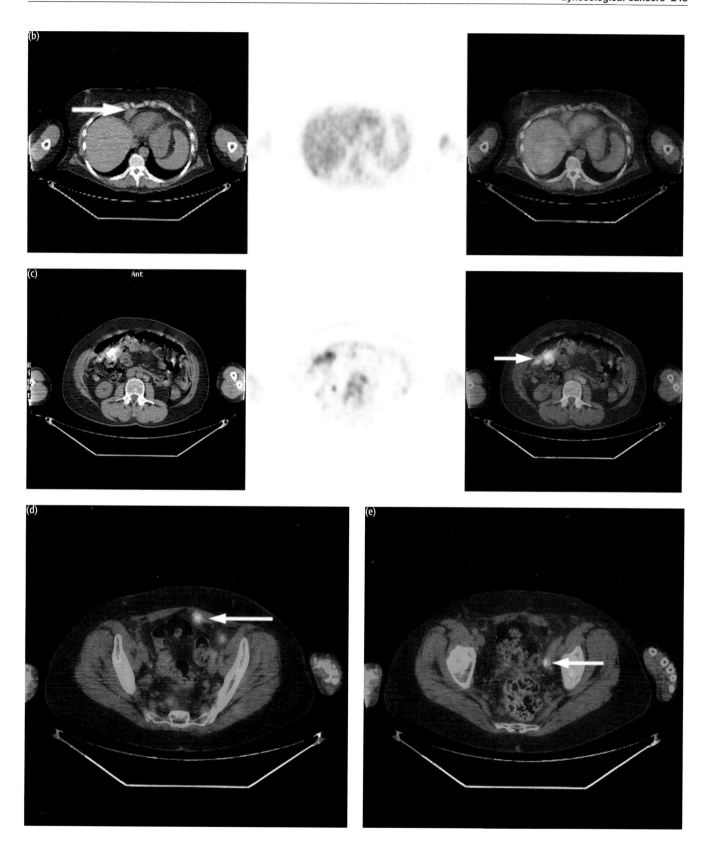

PET/CT findings:

The scan showed multiple metastases: in paracardiac lymph nodes (a,b), calcified peritoneal deposits (c), and several sites in the pelvis, including the left rectus sheath (d) and the left pelvic sidewall (e).

Key point:

Note that there is misregistration between the PET and the CT scans in this patient. The PET uptake seen in one axial section (a) corresponds to the paracardiac lymph node seen in a lower axial section (b) on the CT. Remember that especially around the diaphragm there can be misregistration (typically up to 2–3 mm). It is necessary often 'to scroll up and down' through the images for accurate localization. It may also be necessary to view the nonattenuation-corrected PET images where there is significant breathing artifact.

CONCLUSIONS

CURRENT CLINICAL INDICATIONS

Cervical cancer
1 Staging of primary disease (especially nodal status)
2 Restaging and assessment of recurrence
3 Treatment response

Endometrial cancer
1 Assessment of recurrent disease

Ovarian cancer
1 Assessment of recurrence (especially rising markers)
2 Treatment response

FURTHER READING

Belhocine T, De Barsy C, Hustinx R, Willems-Foidart J (2002) Usefulness of (18)F-FDG PET in the post-therapy surveillance of endometrial carcinoma. *Eur J Nucl Med Mol Imaging* 29, 1132–9. Epub 2002 Jun 19.

Bristow RE, del Carmen MG, Pannu HK *et al.* (2003) Clinically occult recurrent ovarian cancer: patient selection for secondary cytoreductive surgery using combined PET/CT. *Gynecol Oncol* 90, 519–28.

Fenchel S, Grab D, Nuessle K *et al.* (2002) Asymptomatic adnexal masses: correlation of FDG PET and histopathologic findings. *Radiology* 223, 780–8.

Grigsby PW, Siegel BA, Dehdashti F (2001) Lymph node staging by positron emission tomography in patients with carcinoma of the cervix. *J Clin Oncol* 19, 3745–9.

Jadvar H, Conti PS (2004) The reproductive tract. *Semin Nucl Med* 34, 262–73.

Lerman H, Metser U, Grisaru D *et al.* (2004) Normal and abnormal 18F-FDG endometrial and ovarian uptake in pre and post menopausal patients: assessment by PET/CT. *J Nucl Med* 45, 266–71.

Pannu HK, Bristow RE, Cohade C, Fishman EK, Wahl RL (2004) PET-CT in recurrent ovarian cancer: initial observations. *Radiographics* 24, 209–23.

Reinhardt MJ, Ehritt-Braun C, Vogelgesang D *et al.* (2001) Metastatic lymph nodes in patients with cervical cancer: detection with MR imaging and FDG PET. *Radiology* 218, 776–82.

Rieber A, Nussle K, Stohr I *et al.* (2001) Preoperative diagnosis of ovarian tumors with MR imaging: comparison with transvaginal sonography, positron emission tomography, and histologic findings. *AJR Am J Roentgenol* 177, 123–9.

Rose PG, Adler LP, Rodriguez M *et al.* (1999) Positron emission tomography for evaluating para-aortic nodal metastasis in locally advanced cervical cancer before surgical staging: a surgicopathologic study. *J Clin Oncol* 17, 41–5.

Rose PG, Faulhaber P, Miraldi F, Abdul-Karim FW (2001) Positive emission tomography for evaluating a complete clinical response in patients with ovarian or peritoneal carcinoma: correlation with second-look laparotomy. *Gynecol Oncol* 82, 17–21.

Singh AK, Grigsby PW, Dehdashti F, Herzog TJ, Siegel BA (2003) FDG-PET lymph node staging and survival of patients with FIGO stage IIIb cervical carcinoma. *Int J Radiat Oncol Biol Phys* 56, 489–93.

Sugawara Y, Eisbruch A, Kosuda S *et al.* (1999) Evaluation of FDG PET in patients with cervical cancer. *J Nucl Med* 40, 1125–31.

Tatsumi M, Cohade C, Zellars R *et al.* (2003) Initial experience in imaging uterine cervical cancer with FDG PET-CT: direct comparison with PET. *J Nucl Med* 5(Suppl), 394P.

CHAPTER 11
MELANOMA

INTRODUCTION AND BACKGROUND

Malignant melanoma is the most rapidly increasing cancer in Caucasian populations. Its incidence has been increasing at more than 5 percent per year since 1973, with an increasing mortality second only to lung cancer. Malignant melanoma is the most common cancer in young women between the ages of 25 and 29 and contributes to 18 percent of all cancers in young adults between the ages of 15 and 39 years. In the USA, there were about 55 100 cases of melanoma diagnosed in 2004 with nearly 8000 deaths. Risks of melanoma include preexisting skin lesions, but 20–50 percent of malignant melanomas arise *de novo*. Another risk factor is hair color: red-haired individuals have a three times greater risk than average and fair skinned and blond haired individuals have a two times greater risk. The overall increase in risk is thought to be related to strong solar ultraviolet radiation.

Melanoma is one of the most metabolically active tumors in both animal models and patients. Melanoma is curable when diagnosed early (i.e. when thin) and can be completely removed from the skin by surgery. Unfortunately, the thicker melanomas are more likely to metastasize to regional lymph nodes and then systemically. Disseminated melanoma is generally poorly responsive to therapy. The recent approval of recombinant interferon alpha for the treatment of nodal metastasis to regional lymph nodes has increased the importance of early diagnosis of nodal metastases. Similarly, up to 20 percent of patients who present with isolated nodal metastases and no distant metastasis are cured by surgical resection of the tumors. In some series, resection of isolated metastases to brain and to lung has been reported to improve survival. Thus in melanoma, as in many other cancers, detection of both regional lymph node involvement and disseminated metastasis is important. Radical surgical procedures to remove isolated metastases are rational only if disease is truly isolated. PET can play an important role in such decisions.

Malignant melanoma is one of the most rapidly increasing fatal cancers and is now the 14th most common cancer in the UK and 8th most common cancer in the USA.

Lentigo malignant melanoma has better prognosis. Acral lentiginous melanoma has higher incidence in black and Asian populations. The sites of tumor development generally reflect the distribution of skin exposure to sunlight.

EPIDEMIOLOGY	
Incidence	
Men	10.6 new cases per 100 000/ 3028 cases UK
	18.0 new cases per 100 000/ 33 580 cases USA
Women	13.1 new cases per 100 000/ 3939 cases UK
	13.5 new cases per 100 000/ 26 000 cases USA
Proportion of all cancers	3%
Proportion of all skin cancers	10%
Age distribution	18% in 18–39 years age group
Racial distribution	White >> Black/Asian

PATHOLOGY	
Growth pattern	%
Superficial spreading	70
Nodular	15–30
Lentigo maligna	4–10
Acral lentiginous	2–8

The two key prognostic factors are thickness of the primary lesion and lymph node involvement. Extremities have a better prognosis than trunk, and women have a better prognosis than men. Patients presenting with distant metastases have a very poor prognosis.

In-transit means >2 cm from the primary lesion.

STAGING AND PROGNOSIS

TNM	Description	5-year survival (%)
Primary tumor (T)		According to T stage:
T1	≤1 mm	91–95
T2	1–2 mm	77–89
T3	2–4 mm	63–79
T4	>4 mm	45–67
Suffix a/b	b denotes ulceration	
Lymph nodes (N)		
N1	1 node involved	
N2	2–3 nodes/in-transit metastasis/satellite with metastatic nodes	
N2c	In-transit metastasis/satellite without metastatic nodes	
N3	≥4 nodes	
Metastasis (M)		
M1a	Distant skin/subcutaneous/nodal metastasis	
M1b	Lung metastasis	
M1c	Other visceral metastasis/any metastasis with raised lactose dehydrogenase (LDH)	

Stage	TNM	
I	T1a–T2a N0 M0	91–95
II	T2b–T4a N0 M0	45–79
III	Any T N1a–N3 M0	24–67
IV	Any T Any N M1	<10

Among the patients in whom regional nodes are detected clinically, 70–85 percent have distant metastasis (clinical sensitivity about 80 percent). Sentinel lymph node imaging has substantially replaced ELND and is a very good technique for determining if a full axillary dissection is required.

METASTATIC SITES

	Clinical (%)	Autopsy (%)
Skin, subcutaneous and distant nodes	50	60
Lung	30	75
Liver	15	65
Brain	15	45
Bone	15	36
Gastrointestinal tract	5	40
Heart, pancreas, adrenal, thyroid	Rare	35

KEY MANAGEMENT ISSUES

KEY MANAGEMENT ISSUES

Assessment of patients at high risk of metastatic disease
Confirmation of recurrence
Restaging before removal of isolated metastases
Monitoring response

Role of PET in melanoma

Gritters *et al.* (1993) demonstrated in 12 patients that melanoma could be imaged using positron emission tomography (PET) with [^{18}F]2-fluoro-2-deoxy-D-glucose (FDG). In this small study, 15/15 intra-abdominal and lymph node metastases were detected by FDG PET. PET also identified three additional metastatic foci noted only retrospectively on computed tomography (CT). PET correctly identified tumor in 7/7 lymph nodes, including three instances where the nodes were of normal size, and excluded tumor in 6/6 nodal regions for a 100 percent (13/13) accuracy in nodal disease characterization. PET was not as sensitive as CT for small lesions in the lungs. Of particular interest is that small bowel metastases, which are extremely difficult to identify by any method other than autopsy, were detected in several instances in this study.

PET does not currently have an established role in imaging primary melanomas. Once melanoma has been diagnosed, PET can help determine if tumor is present in lymph nodes, but it is sensitive only when tumor volume is adequate for imaging. Microscopic metastatic disease in lymph nodes is commonly missed by FDG PET. In recent publications the sensitivity of PET for the detection of regional lymph node metastases has been ~20 percent. Sentinel lymph node imaging is therefore the preferred method for detecting tumor metastases in lymph nodes. PET is reasonably accurate for characterizing enlarged lymph nodes, i.e. whether they are malignant or benign, but it cannot be recommended for lymph node staging if there are no palpable nodes. In some centers, PET is performed in the assessment of patients with newly diagnosed melanoma after positive lymph nodes have been demonstrated.

Steinert *et al.* (1995) used whole-body PET imaging to survey for melanoma. Using this approach, they showed excellent lesion detection capability, with their failures in detection using the nonattenuation-corrected PET method being only in cases where there were small cutaneous lesions (<3 mm). In their study of 33 patients with known melanoma, the overall sensitivity of PET was 92 percent. Specificity was increased with clinical knowledge of the location of biopsy sites, etc. (77 percent without such clinical information and 100 percent with the clinical information available). Sensitivity of PET for metastatic disease has generally been in the range of 80–100 percent, but for lesions <1 cm, sensitivities are lower than for larger lesions. In a retrospective review of 62 cases in one of our centers, the overall sensitivity for FDG PET was 78 percent and the specificity was 87 percent, however, the sensitivity was only 50 percent in stage I disease and 33 percent in stage II disease. The role of PET in assessing treatment response in melanoma is not as well studied as in other tumors such as lymphoma or breast cancer. Certainly, for assessment of relapse after surgical therapy, PET is an excellent method.

Our current view regarding FDG PET in melanoma is that the method is of greatest value in:

- patients who have a high risk of systemic metastasis based on extensive locoregional tumor
- patients with anatomic findings or symptoms suspicious for distant metastasis
- individuals with known distant tumor metastasis who may benefit from resection
- patients in whom innovative therapies are being assessed.

Small lesions, including lesions in the lungs and the brain, can be missed by PET but detected by anatomic methods. PET/CT may in future be the only method needed to detect recurrent melanoma, but the cost efficacy and benefits in terms of outcomes for such an approach are not yet confirmed.

EXAMPLES TO ILLUSTRATE KEY ISSUES

CASE 11.1	Diagnosis: Melanoma – restaging

Clinical history:

This patient had a primary melanoma on the back followed by local recurrence in the skin and left axillary metastasis treated with surgery 2 years previously. He developed further left axillary lymphadenopathy. PET/CT was requested to restage the patient's disease.

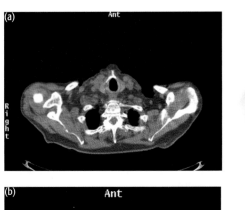

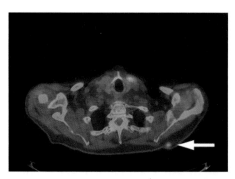

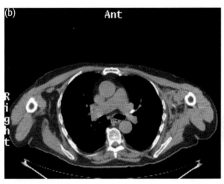
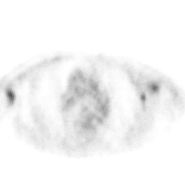
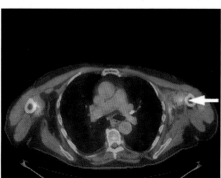

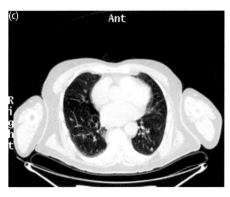
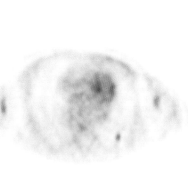
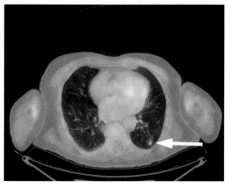

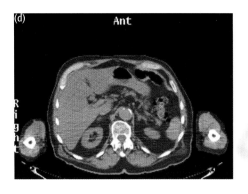 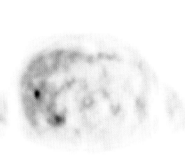 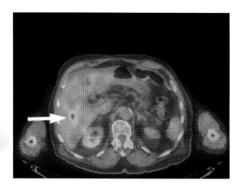

PET/CT findings:

There was metastatic disease in a subcutaneous deposit behind the left scapula (a), in a small left axillary lymph node (b) and in the left lower lobe of the lung (c) and the liver (d). The uptake seen anteriorly in (a) represents physiologic uptake in the left sternocleidomastoid muscle which may be asymmetric. The patient was not suitable for undergoing local resection.

Key points:

1 PET/CT is sensitive in the detection of distant metastases in melanoma.
2 Unnecessary surgery can be avoided where PET/CT detects multiple rather than isolated metastatic disease.

CASE 11.2	Diagnosis: Melanoma – relapse and restaging

Clinical history:

This patient was diagnosed as having melanoma overlying the right shoulder. An incidental mass was found in the left kidney during investigations to stage the melanoma. The mass was excised and found to be renal cell carcinoma. The patient remained disease free for 5 years, when she re-presented with a tender lump in the left axilla/chest wall. Fine needle aspiration revealed adipose tissue and giant cells suggestive only of fat necrosis, however, the clinical suspicion of metastatic disease remained high. PET/CT was requested to determine whether there was relapse.

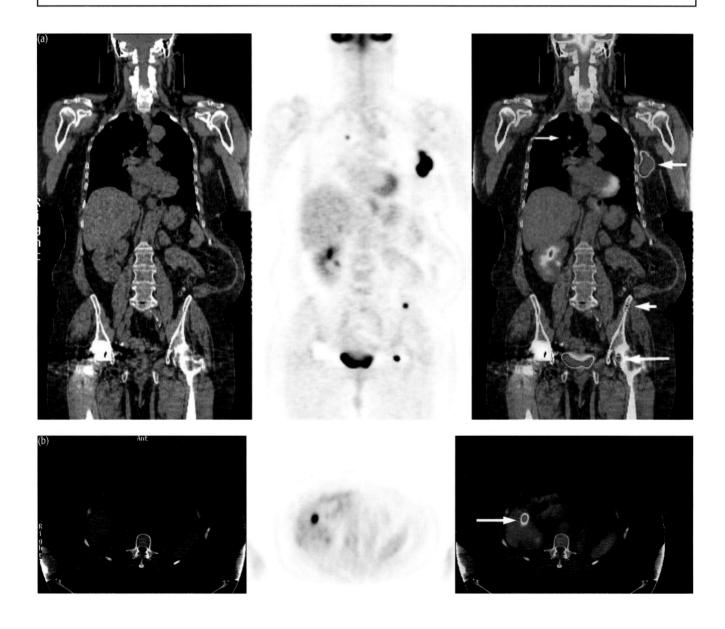

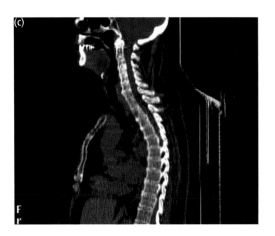 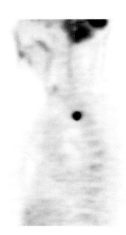 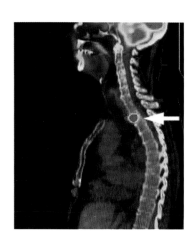

PET/CT findings:

There was extensive uptake in nodes including the left axilla (a), lung (a), liver (b), and bone including the left iliac crest and left femoral head (a) and the thoracic spine (c). Note the lytic lesion on CT at the site of the thoracic spine uptake. Both melanoma and renal cell carcinoma have lytic bone metastases and it was not possible to differentiate the source of metastatic disease from the PET/CT appearances. Excision biopsy of the left axillary lesion revealed metastatic melanoma.

Key points:

1 PET/CT is sensitive for soft tissue, liver, and bone metastases in melanoma.
2 In this patient biopsy was required to determine which tumor was responsible for metastatic disease and decide the most appropriate treatment.

11.3 (three cases)	Diagnosis: Occult metastases (in three patients with no previous evidence of distant disease)

Clinical history:

Patient 1 – This patient was a 42-year-old woman with a history of melanoma on the scalp resected 7 years previously who developed local recurrence in the left parotid.

Patient 2 – This patient was a 52-year-old man with melanoma and a recently diagnosed lung metastasis.

Patient 3 – This patient was a 56-year-old woman with melanoma on the right shoulder and previously resected right maxillary metastases.

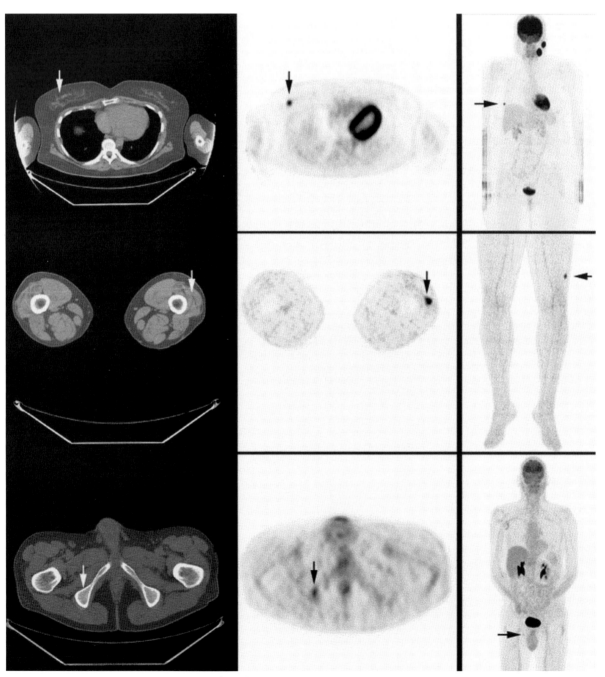

Reproduced with permission from Kent P et al. (2004). Clinical use of positron emission tomography in the management of cutaneous melanoma. Semin Nucl Med **34**, 242–53 © 2004 with permission from Elsevier Inc.

PET/CT findings:

Top row: Patient 1 (a 42-year-old woman). FDG PET demonstrated local recurrence and a distant right breast focus (arrows) that was biopsied and confirmed to be metastatic melanoma.

Middle row: Patient 2 (a 52-year-old man). In addition to lung metastasis, FDG PET demonstrated an occult distant focus in the soft tissues of the left thigh (see arrows). Biopsy confirmed metastatic melanoma.

Lower row: Patient 3 (a 56-year-old woman). In addition to identifying recurrence in the right shoulder, FDG PET demonstrated an occult focus in the right ischium (arrows). Metastatic disease was confirmed by magnetic resonance imaging.

Key point:

PET identified metastatic disease in all three patients with local recurrence of melanoma.

CASE 11.4	Diagnosis: Melanoma – relapse and restaging

Clinical history:

This patient was diagnosed as having melanoma on the surface of the abdomen 8 years previously. Later recurrences of disease in the right groin were treated with surgery, interferon, and radiotherapy. At the time of referral for PET/CT scanning, a surveillance CT examination had shown an enlarged left iliac lymph node. The node had increased marginally in size compared with a CT scan done the previous year. On clinical examination, lymph nodes were also palpable in the left supraclavicular fossa. PET/CT was requested to determine whether the patient had relapsed and to restage the disease with a view to surgery in the left groin.

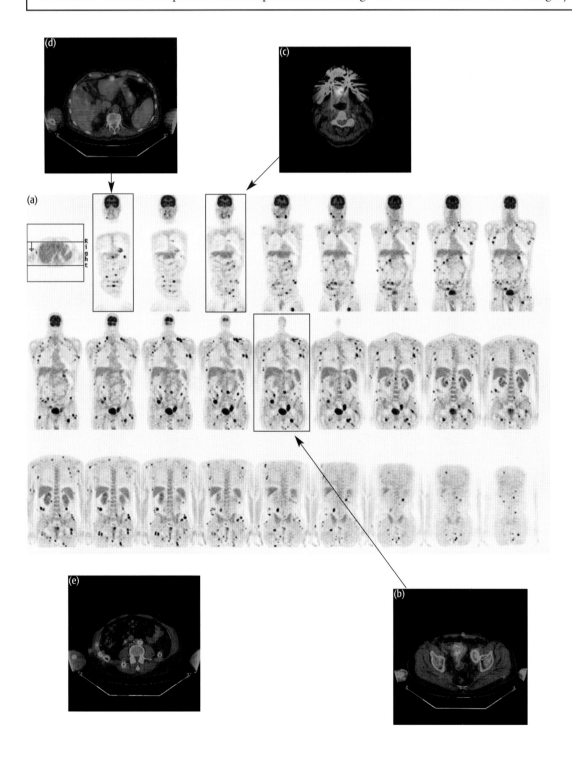

PET/CT findings:

There were multiple areas of increased activity indicative of widespread metastatic disease (a). Axial slices are shown of a peritoneal deposit anterior to the liver (d), a metastasis in the tongue (c), left iliac lymph node involvement (b), and an axial slice through the lower abdomen with left para-aortic disease, and peritoneal, muscle, and subcutaneous deposits (e).

Key point:

In advanced-stage melanoma, PET/CT determines extent of disease, which influences treatment options.

CASE 11.5	Diagnosis: Melanoma staging

Clinical history:

This patient was referred with a primary melanoma on the right foot with palpable lymphadenopathy in the right groin. PET/CT was requested to stage the patient's disease.

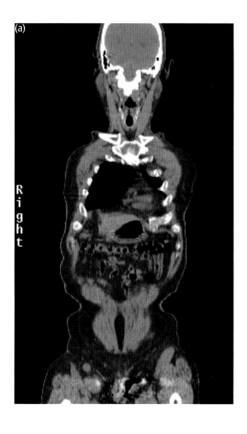

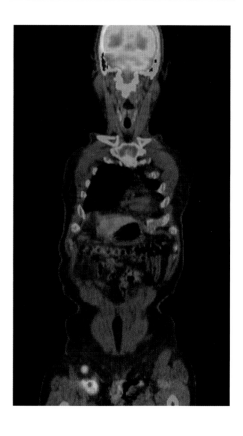

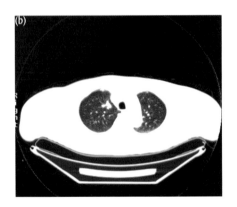

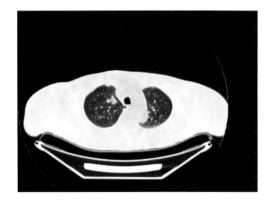

PET/CT findings:

There were metastases in the right inguinal region (a) with low-grade uptake in the right lung, probably representing inflammatory change (b). Bronchoscopic washings revealed no evidence of malignancy. The patient proceeded to right inguinal lymph node dissection. A repeat CT scan of the chest was normal 6 months later confirming that the changes seen in the lungs were due to inflammation and not metastatic disease.

Key point:

PET/CT accurately stages the disease in patients with stage III or IV melanoma.

| CASE 11.6 | Diagnosis: Melanoma – restaging and response assessment |

Clinical history:

Scan 1: This patient was treated for a malignant melanoma overlying the right ear with surgery 4 years previously. She presented with a new lesion on the left upper back. A right axillary lymph node was palpable clinically. Fine needle aspiration of both lesions revealed malignant melanoma. PET/CT was requested to restage the patientís disease.
Scan 2: PET/CT was requested to assess response after two cycles of chemotherapy.

(a)

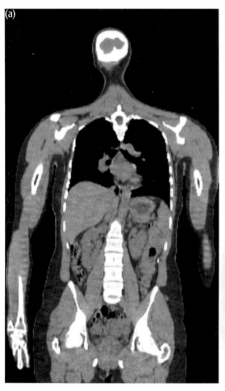
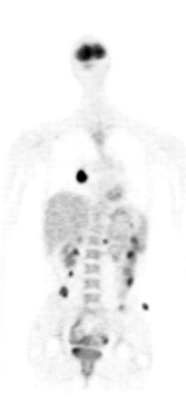
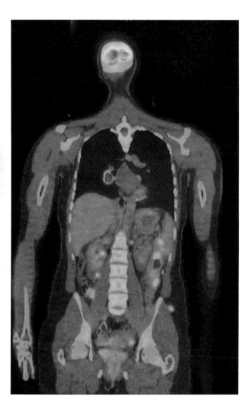

(b)

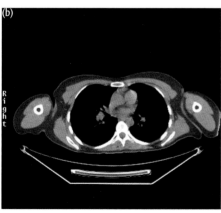

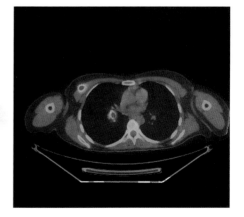

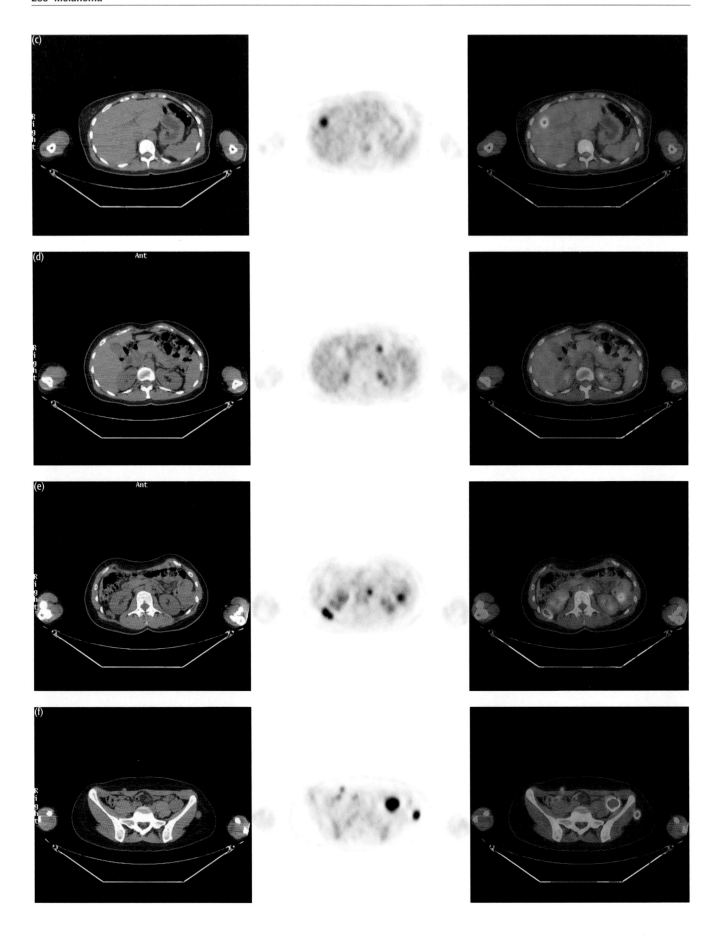

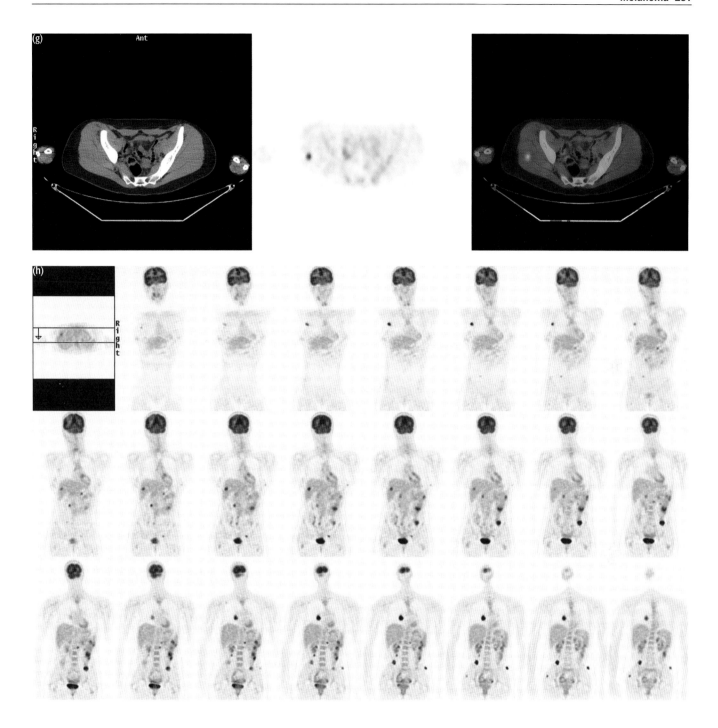

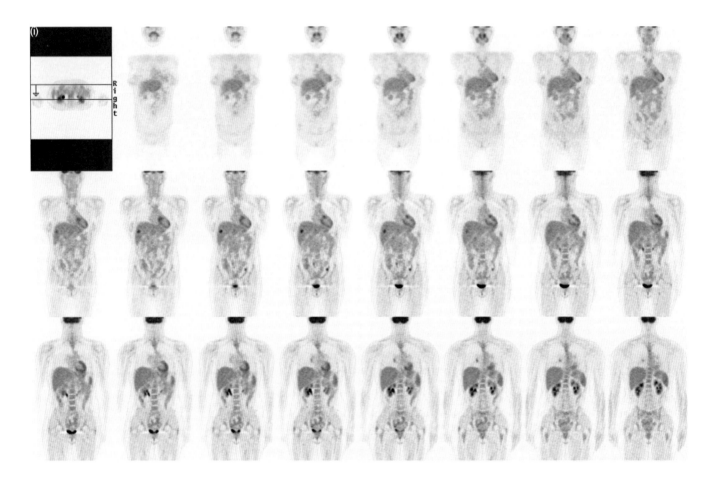

PET/CT findings:

Scan 1: There were multiple metastases (a) including lesions in the right chest and right lung hilum (b), liver (c), mesentery (d), right perirenal and left para-aortic regions (e), right (a) and left (e,f) paracolic gutters, and subcutaneous tissue in the left gluteal region (f) and in the right gluteal muscle (g). A brain metastasis is visible in the coronal whole-body PET images (h).

Scan 2: There was significant response to treatment compared with the original scan (h) with resolution of uptake in many sites, but there was residual disease in the liver, right hilum, and left paracolic gutter (i).

Key points:

1 PET/CT is sensitive for the detection of metastatic disease in malignant melanoma in stage III and stage IV disease.
2 PET/CT can be used to monitor response to treatment.

CASE 11.7 | Diagnosis: Melanoma staging

Clinical history:

This patient had had a melanoma on the anterior abdominal wall excised. Sentinel lymph node biopsy indicated involvement of two axilla nodes. A CT scan with contrast (a) showed a 1.5 cm left para-aortic lymph node, the significance of which was uncertain. PET/CT was requested to stage the patient's disease prior to proceeding with a left axillary lymph node dissection.

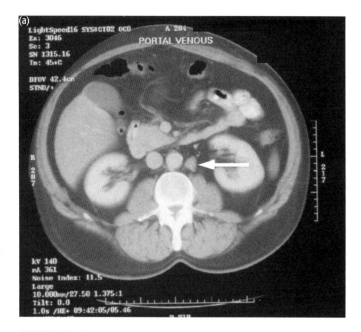

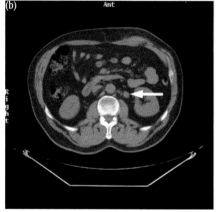
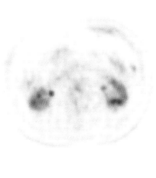
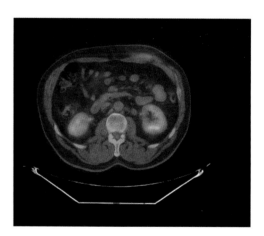

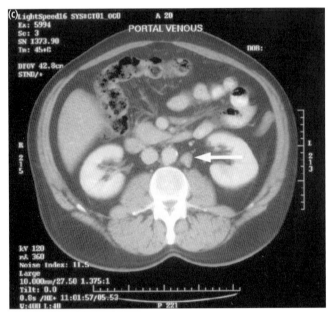

CT images kindly provided by Dr T Sulkin, Radiology Department, Royal Cornwall Hospitals NHS Trust, UK

PET/CT findings:

There was no FDG uptake in the left para-aortic node (b) indicating that it was benign. The patient proceeded to left axillary dissection. Follow-up CT scan 6 months later showed no change in the size of the para-aortic node.

Key point:

PET/CT can exclude melanoma metastases in enlarged lymph nodes.

CONCLUSIONS

CURRENT CLINICAL INDICATIONS
1 Staging in patients with clinical N1–N3 disease at increased risk of metastasis
2 Confirming suspected recurrence or suspected metastasis
3 Response to systemic therapy
4 Determining if 'isolated' metastases for planned resection are indeed solitary
5 Surveillance of high-risk groups

Figure 11.1 shows a possible algorithm for management of metastatic melanoma.

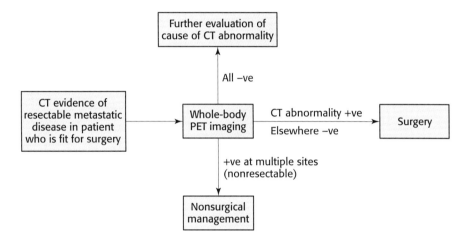

Figure 11.1   *Algorithm for management of metastatic melanoma*

REFERENCES AND FURTHER READING

Acland KM, O'Doherty MJ, Russell-Jones R (2000) The value of positron emission tomography scanning in the detection of subclinical metastatic melanoma. *J Am Acad Dermatol* **42**, 606–11.

Acland KM, Healy C, Calonje E *et al.* (2001) Comparison of positron emission tomography scanning and sentinel node biopsy in the detection of micrometastases of primary cutaneous malignant melanoma. *J Clin Oncol* **19**, 2674–8.

Belhocine T, Pierard G, De Labrassinne M *et al.* (2002) Staging of regional nodes in AJCC stage I and II melanoma 18FDG PET imaging versus sentinel node detection. *Oncologist* **7**, 271–8.

Blessing C, Feine U, Geiger L *et al.* (1995) Positron emission tomography and ultrasonography. *Arch Dermatol* **131**, 1394–8.

Cobben DC, Jager PL, Elsinga PH *et al.* (2003) 3′18F-fluoro-3′-deoxy-L-thymidine a new tracer for staging metastatic melanoma? *J Nucl Med* **44**, 1927–32.

Crippa F, Leutner M, Belli F *et al.* (2000) Which kinds of lymph node metastases can FDG PET detect? A clinical study in melanoma. *J Nucl Med* **41**, 1491–4.

Dalrymple-Hay MJ, Rome PD, Kennedy C (2002) Pulmonary metastatic melanoma – the survival benefit associated with positron emission tomography scanning. *Eur J Cardiothorac Surg* **21**, 611–14; discussion 614–15.

Eigtved A, Andersson AP, Dahlstrom K *et al.* (2000) Use of fluorine-18 fluorodeoxyglucose positron emission tomography in the detection of silent metastases from malignant melanoma. *Eur J Nucl Med* **27**, 70–5.

Fink AM, Holle-Robatsch S, Herzog N *et al.* (2004) Positron emission tomography is not useful in detecting metastasis in the sentinel lymph node in patients with primary malignant melanoma stage I and II. *Melanoma Res* **14**, 141–5.

Gritters LS, Francis IR, Zasadny KR, Wahl RL (1993) Initial assessment of positron emission tomography using 2-fluorine-18–fluoro-2-deoxy-D-glucose in the imaging of malignant melanoma. *J Nucl Med* **34**, 1420–7.

Havenga K, Cobben DC, Oyen WJ *et al.* (2003) Fluorodeoxyglucose-positron emission tomography and sentinel lymph node biopsy in staging primary cutaneous melanoma. *Eur J Surg Oncol* **29**, 662–4.

Holder WD Jr, White RL Jr, Zuger JH (1998) Effectiveness of positron emission tomography for the detection of melanoma metastases. *Ann Surg* **227**, 764–9.

Johnson TM, Smith JW, Nelson BR *et al.* (1995) Current therapy for cutaneous melanoma. *Dermatology* **32**, 689–707.

Krug B, Dietlein M, Groth W *et al.* (2000) Fluor-18-fluorodeoxyglucose positron emission tomography (FDG-PET) in malignant melanoma. Diagnostic comparison with conventional imaging methods. *Acta Radiol* **41**, 446–52.

Lindholm P, Leskinen S, Nagren K *et al.* (1995) Carbon-11-methionine PET imaging of malignant melanoma. *J Nucl Med* **36**, 1806–10.

Longo MI, Lazaro P, Bueno C *et al.* (2003) Fluorodeoxyglucose-positron emission tomography imaging versus sentinel node biopsy in the primary staging of melanoma patients. *Dermatol Surg* **29**, 245–8.

Lucignani G, Paganelli G, Modorati *et al.* (1992) MRI, antibody-guided scintigraphy, and glucose metabolism in uveal melanoma. *J Comp Assist Tomogr* **16**, 77–83.

Macfarlane DJ, Sondak V, Wahl RL (1995) Initial prospective evaluation of FDG-PET in staging regional lymph nodes in patients with cutaneous malignant melanoma (CMM.) *J Nucl Med* **36**, 116.

Macfarlane DJ, Sondak V, Johnson T *et al.* (1998) Prospective evaluation of 2-[18F]-2-deoxy-D-glucose positron emission tomography in staging of regional lymph nodes in patients with cutaneous malignant melanoma. *J Clin Oncol* **16**, 1770–6.

Mercier GA, Alavi A, Fraker DL (2001) FDG positron emission tomography in isolated limb perfusion therapy in patients with locally advanced melanoma Preliminary results. *Clin Nucl Med* **26**, 832–36.

Mijnhout GS, Hoekstra OS, van Tulder MW *et al.* (2001) Systematic review of the diagnostic accuracy of F-fluorodeoxyglucose positron emission tomography in melanoma patients. *Cancer* **91**, 1530–42.

Prichard RS, Hill AD, Skehan SJ *et al.* (2002) Positron emission tomography for staging and management of malignant melanoma. *Br J Surg* **89**, 389–96.

Rinne D, Baum RP, Hor G *et al.* (1998) Primary staging and follow-up of high risk melanoma patients with whole-body 18F-fluorodeoxyglucose positron emission tomography results of a prospective study of 100 patients. *Cancer* **82**, 1664–71.

Rivers JK (1996) Melanoma. *Lancet* **347**, 803–7.

Stas M, Stroobants S, Dupont P *et al.* (2002) 18-FDG PET scan in the staging of recurrent melanoma additional value and therapeutic impact. *Melanoma Res* **12**, 479–90.

Steinert HC, Huch Boni RA, Buck A *et al.* (1995) Malignant melanoma: staging with whole-body positron emission tomography and 2-[18F]-fluoro-2-deoxy-D-glucose. *Radiology* **195**, 705–9.

Swetter SM, Carroll LA, Johnson DL *et al.* (2002) Positron emission tomography is superior to computed tomography for metastatic detection in melanoma patients. *Ann Surg Oncol* **9**, 646–53.

Tyler DS, Onaitis M, Kherani A *et al.* (2000) Positron emission tomography scanning in malignant melanoma. *Cancer* **89**, 1019–25.

Wagner JD, Schauwecker D, Hutchins G *et al.* (1997) Initial assessment of positron emission tomography for detection of nonpalpable regional lymphatic metastases in melanoma. *J Surg Oncol* **64**, 181–9.

Wagner JD, Schauwecker D, Davidson D *et al.* (1999) Prospective study of fluorodeoxyglucose-positron emission tomography imaging of lymph node basins in melanoma patients undergoing sentinel node biopsy. *J Clin Oncol* **17**, 1508–15.

Wagner JD, Schauwecker DS, Davidson D *et al.* (2001) FDG-PET sensitivity for melanoma lymph node metastases is dependent on tumor volume. *J Surg Oncol* **77**, 237–42.

Yang M, Martin DR, Karabulut N *et al.* (2003) Comparison of MR and PET imaging for the evaluation of liver metastases. *J Magn Reson Imaging* **17**, 343–9.

CHAPTER 12
ENDOCRINE TUMORS

INTRODUCTION AND BACKGROUND

Malignant tumors of the endocrine glands are relatively uncommon, but benign tumors are not infrequent. The most common of the endocrine tumors are those affecting the thyroid, adrenal, pituitary, and parathyroid glands. Malignant disease is more common as primary disease in the thyroid, whereas metastatic tumors to the adrenal glands are more common than primary tumors. Tumors in the parathyroid and pituitary glands are more commonly benign. Often benign endocrine tumors present with symptoms related to oversecretion of key hormones and the tumors can thus present at a relatively early stage and small size.

Thyroid cancers can occur at all ages but are relatively common in younger women, a group not typically at high risk for cancers. Most are sporadic cases and no clear etiologic factor is associated with most thyroid cancers. The notable risk factor that has been identified for thyroid cancer is radiation exposure at a young age. Data from the Chernobyl nuclear accident, atomic bomb survivors, and patients who have received therapeutic radiation to the head and neck indicate that radiation exposure is a strong risk factor for thyroid cancer. Familial medullary cancers associated with multiple endocrine neoplasia (MEN) syndromes can also can present at a relatively young age.

EPIDEMIOLOGY		
Incidence (per 100 000 population)	Male	Female
Thyroid cancer*	1.3 (UK)	3.3 (UK)
	3.7 (USA)	11.2 (USA)
Parathyroid cancer	<1 (UK/USA)	<1 (UK/USA)
Adrenocortical cancer	<1 (UK/USA)	<1 (UK/USA)

*Predisposing factors for thyroid cancer include previous radiation exposure, and for medullary cancers the familial MEN syndromes.

Ninety percent of thyroid cancers are papillary or follicular tumors. Medullary and anaplastic cancers make up the remainder. Parathyroid tumors are usually benign; malignant tumors are almost exclusively adenocarcinoma. Adrenal metastases are almost 30 times more common than adrenal primary malignancies, many of which are secretory tumors.

PATHOLOGY	PERCENT
Thyroid cancer	
Papillary/follicular	90
Anaplastic	~5
Medullary	~5
Parathyroid cancer	
Adenocarcinoma	100
Adrenocortical cancer	
Differentiated	20
Anaplastic	20
Hormonal	60

STAGING OF THYROID CANCER

TNM	Description
*Primary tumor (T)**	
T0	No evidence of primary tumor, artery or mediastinal vessels
T1	≤2 cm confined to thyroid
T2	>2–4 cm confined to thyroid
T3	>4 cm limited to thyroid or minimal extrathyroid extension
T4a	Invasion of subcutaneous soft tissues, larynx, trachea, esophagus or recurrent laryngeal nerve
T4b	Invasion of prevertebral fascia or encases carotid
Lymph nodes (N)	
N0	No involved lymph nodes
N1a	Metastasis to level VI (pretracheal, paratracheal, and prelaryngeal/Delphian lymph nodes)
N1b	Metastasis to unilateral or bilateral cervical or superior mediastinal lymph nodes
Metastasis (M)	
M0	No metastasis
M1	Distant metastasis
Subtypes and stage	**TNM**
Papillary/follicular (<45 years)	
I	T1–4 N1–2 M0
II	T1–4 N1–2 M1
Papillary/follicular (>45 years) and medullary	
I	T1 N0 M0
II	T2 N0 M0
III	T1–3 M0
	T3 N0 M0
IVa	T1–3 N1b M0
	T4a N0–1b M0
IVb	T4b N0–N1b M0
IVc	T1–4b N0–N1b M1
Anaplastic	
IVa	T4a N0–1b M0
IVb	T4b N0–N1b M0
IVc	T1–4b N0–N1b M1

*All anaplastic carcinomas are considered as T4.

STAGING OF PARATHYROID CANCER

Stage	Description
Localized	Parathyroid +/− invasion of local tissues
Metastatic	Spread beyond local tissues

STAGING OF ADRENOCORTICAL CANCER

TNM	Description
Primary tumor (T)	
T0	No evidence of primary tumor
T1	≤ 5cm with no invasion
T2	>5cm with no invasion
T3	Invasion in adrenal fat
T4	Invasion of adjacent organs
Lymph nodes (N)	
N0	No involved lymph nodes
N1	Involved lymph nodes
Metastasis (M)	
M0	No metastasis
M1	Distant metastasis
StageTNM	
I	T1 N0 M0
II	T2 N0 M0
III	T1–2 N1 M0
	T3 N0 M0
IV	T3–4 N1 M0
	T1–4 N0–1 M1

Primary staging of thyroid cancer is generally determined by physical examination and surgery/pathologic examination. Iodine scanning following surgery is commonly done to look for residual normal thyroid or residual tumor tissue. PET is not typically used in initial staging of thyroid cancer or other endocrine tumors, except for rare malignant tumors of the adrenal or in pheochromocytomas. However, the single photon emission computed tomography (SPECT) tracer, MIBG is often preferred to FDG in the initial work up of pheochromocytoma.

PROGNOSIS

Thyroid cancer	
Papillary/follicular	Majority are curable
Medullary	5-year OS ~80%
Anaplastic	3-year OS ~30%
Parathyroid cancer	Potentially curable. Indolent if metastatic
Adrenocortical cancer	5-year OS ~30%

Early-stage thyroid cancer is nearly 100 percent curable with local therapies. Prognosis declines only minimally with nodal involvement at presentation. Distal organ involvement is associated with a much worse prognosis.

OS, overall survival.

KEY MANAGEMENT ISSUES

KEY MANAGEMENT ISSUES

Detection of recurrence with rising markers and no iodine uptake in differentiated thyroid cancer (DTC)

Assessment of recurrence in medullary thyroid cancer

Localization of parathyroid tumors where other imaging negative

Role of PET in thyroid disease

[^{18}F]2-Fluoro-2-deoxy-D-glucose (FDG) positron emission tomography (PET) is not reliable in the characterization of primary thyroid masses as benign or malignant. However, if increased FDG uptake is noted in a thyroid nodule as part of whole-body studies for cancer imaging, there is a moderately high risk (approximately 50 percent) that such a nodule is malignant. In Graves disease and thyroiditis there can be diffuse FDG uptake.

No role has been established for PET in the management of primary thyroid disease. FDG PET has its greatest role in determining if thyroid cancer has recurred, and the precise location, in the setting of iodine-negative thyroid cancers that are producing thyroglobulin. Surgery effectively cures most thyroid cancer, but it cannot control advanced disease, which is systemic. Radioiodine therapy is useful in iodine-avid tumors, however it has limited or no value in noniodine-avid disease. When tumors become noniodine avid, they may be detectable with FDG PET which can then guide surgical resection. Whereas surgery is commonly used for all endocrine neoplasms, radiation therapy with external beam has a much lesser role in these than in many other types of cancer.

In a multicenter study of unselected thyroid cancer patients (n=222), Grunwald *et al.* (1999) found that the sensitivity of FDG PET for localizing metastatic disease in patients with differentiated thyroid cancer (DTC) was 75 percent, and for the group with a negative whole-body scan (n=166) it was 85 percent. Feine *et al.* (1996) noticed that there were tumors that accumulated only FDG, others that accumulated only ^{131}I, and some that accumulated both FDG and iodine. He named this alternating pattern of either ^{131}I or FDG uptake in thyroid cancer metastases as the 'flip flop' phenomenon. Thyroid cancer cells that lose their ability to concentrate radioactive iodine may exhibit increased metabolic activity, which results in enhanced glucose uptake. Some studies have reported that increased thyroid stimulating hormone (TSH) levels stimulate FDG uptake by thyroid cancer cells. Sissonet *et al.* (1993) in a case report demonstrated that there was higher FDG uptake in a thyroid cancer metastasis imaged after withdrawal from thyroid hormone therapy compared with when the same cancer was imaged during hormone therapy.

Use of recombinant human thyrotropin (rhTSH) has recently been proposed to increase the sensitivity of FDG PET in the diagnosis of recurrent and metastatic cancer compared with the unstimulated setting. We have found this to be useful for increasing both the number of lesions detected and the intensity of tracer uptake in the lesions.

Hürthle cell cancer is an infrequent histologic subtype of thyroid cancer that is clinically more aggressive and has little or no iodine uptake but which is typically FDG avid. Medullary thyroid cancer is a calcitonin-secreting tumor originating from the parafollicular C cells which is also generally FDG avid. Detection of these tumors is generally volume dependent and most, but not all, nodal metastases will be detected by this approach. We have often identified metastatic systemic disease with this method.

Role of PET in adrenal tumors

The role of PET in identifying adrenal metastases is covered in other chapters, notably Chapter 4 (Lung cancer). PET is quite robust at separating malignant from benign disease such as adrenal adenomas. The benign adenomas are most commonly non-FDG avid, while metastases are typically intensely FDG avid. There can be modest overlap, however. Adrenal primary cancers are rare and there is little literature on the use of PET in these cancers. If pheochromocytoma is suspected, MIBG scanning is generally preferable to FDG PET. Shulkin *et al.* (1993) have reported on non-MIBG but FDG-avid malignant pheochromocytomas.

Role of PET in parathyroid tumors

FDG-avid parathyroid adenomas have been reported, but they appear to be the exception rather than the rule. In contrast, [11C]-methionine appears to accumulate in many parathyroid adenomas. Although this latter approach has not been extensively evaluated, it appears to be at least as accurate as ^{99m}Tc sestamibi scanning. Nonetheless, SPECT would be the typical initial approach in the diagnosis of parathyroid adenomas in most centers, including our own.

Role of PET in pituitary tumors

FDG PET can detect increased uptake in many macroadenomas, but it is not sensitive in microadenomas. Magnetic resonance imaging is more commonly used in pituitary gland assessments. FDG PET has been shown to detect metastatic disease to the pituitary gland.

EXAMPLES TO ILLUSTRATE KEY ISSUES

CASE 12.1	Diagnosis: Thyroid follicular adenoma

Clinical history:

This patient had a previous left thyroid lobectomy for malignant disease 12 months earlier. She re-presented with difficulty swallowing and a firm nodule in the right lobe of the thyroid gland. PET/CT was requested to determine if there was recurrent disease.

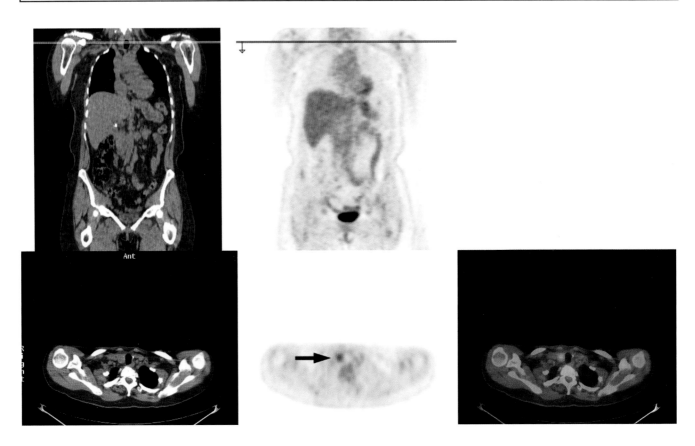

PET/CT findings:

Increased uptake was associated with a nodule in the lower pole of the right lobe of the thyroid gland. Note the surgical clips on the left from previous surgery. The nodule was removed and turned out to be follicular adenoma.

Key points:

1 Benign and malignant thyroid neoplasms may take up FDG but focal uptake in the thyroid gland should be investigated. Reports suggest that ~27–47 percent of focal lesions in the thyroid gland that accumulate FDG turn out to be cancer.
2 Diffuse increased uptake in the thyroid gland may be seen as a normal variant especially in young women or can be seen in association with thyroiditis.

CASE 12.2 | **Diagnosis: Papillary thyroid cancer – recurrence**

Clinical history:

This patient had undergone surgery and radioiodine therapy in the past for papillary thyroid cancer. Thyroglobulin levels were rising but iodine scanning off hormone replacement therapy was negative. PET/CT was requested to determine the site of relapse.

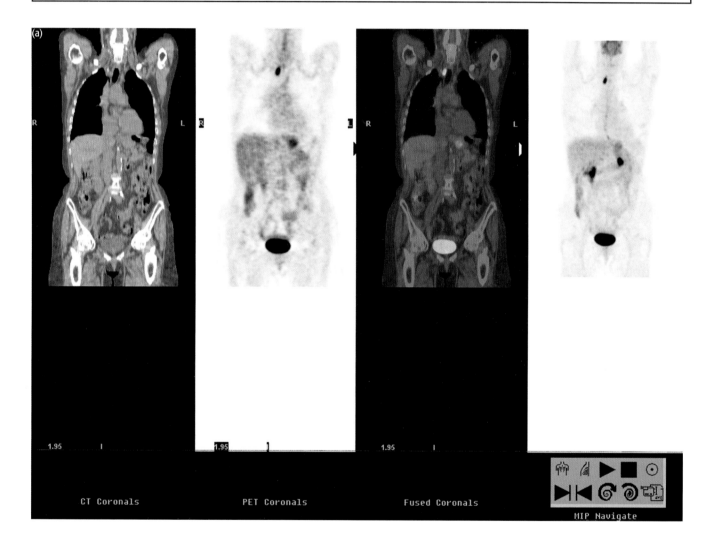

(a)

CT Coronals   PET Coronals   Fused Coronals

MIP Navigate

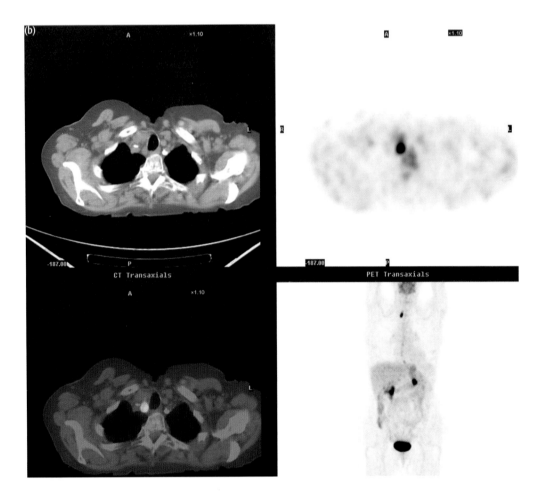

PET/CT findings:

There was increased uptake in the right thyroid bed (a, b) indicative of a single site of recurrent cancer. The patient proceeded to surgery.

Key point:

Local recurrence of thyroid cancer is treatable by surgery (or radioiodine in tumors that are FDG avid) and less often by radiotherapy.

CASE 12.3	Diagnosis: Papillary thyroid cancer

Clinical history:

This patient with a history of papillary thyroid carcinoma was treated with surgery. She then had radiotherapy for recurrence in the right neck. She re-presented with rising thyroglobulin levels. MRI and whole-body radioiodine scans were reported as normal.

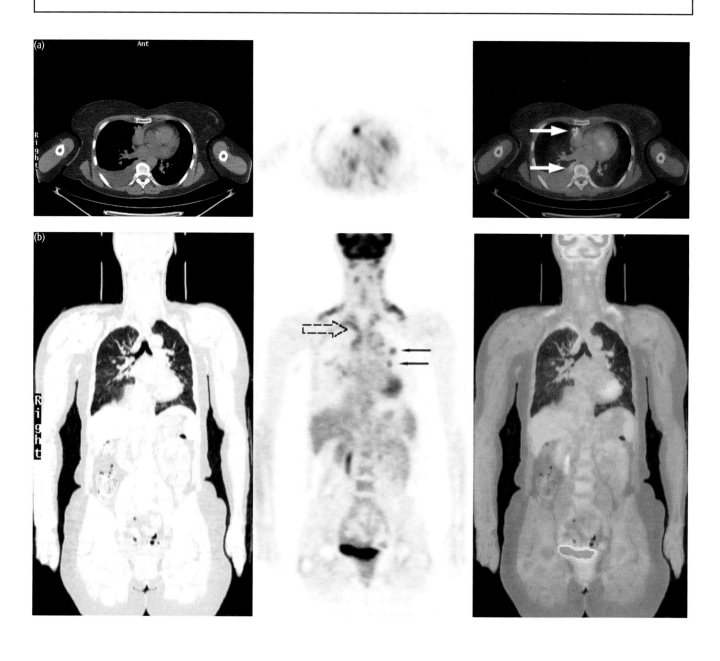

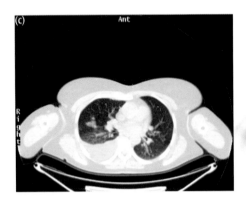

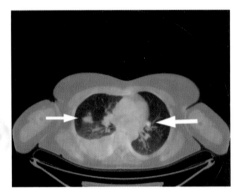

PET/CT findings:

Increased uptake within multiple small lung nodules was associated with a right pleural effusion (a–c) indicative of metastatic disease from thyroid cancer. Increased uptake in the right lung apical margins was ascribed to previous radiotherapy (broken arrow in b). Note also the marked physiologic uptake in brown fat in the neck (b).

Key point:

FDG PET can identify sites of tumor recurrence in papillary thyroid cancer. It may be especially useful in cases where the tumor de-differentiates and no longer takes up iodine.

CASE 12.4	Diagnosis: Medullary thyroid cancer – recurrence

Clinical history:

This patient with a history of medullary thyroid cancer under surveillance developed a rising calcitonin level. PET/CT was requested to confirm relapse and determine the site of tumor recurrence.

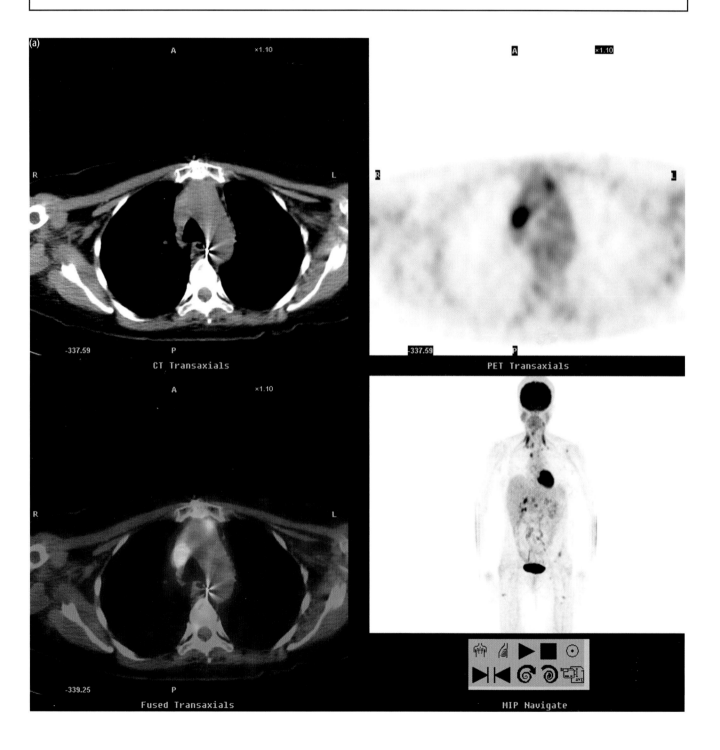

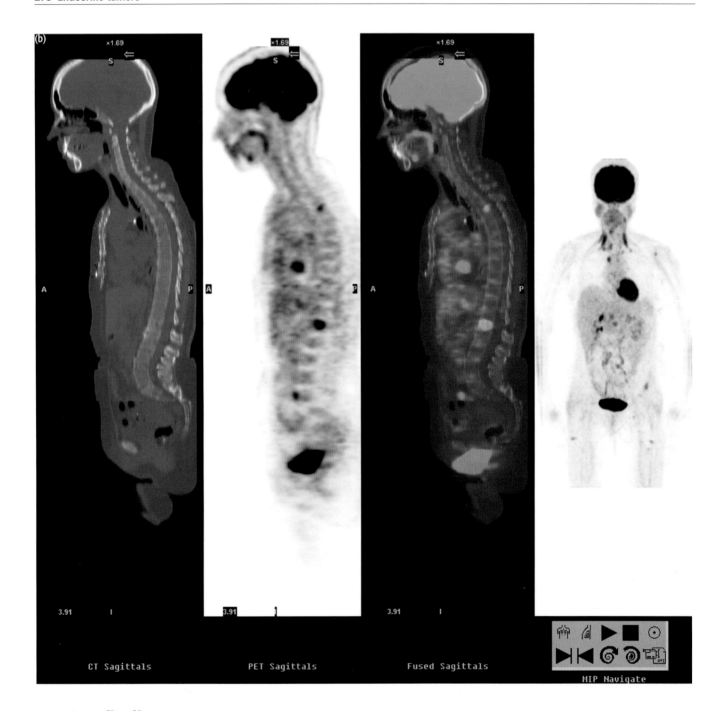

PET/CT findings:

There was metastasis in a right paratracheal lymph node (a), in the anterior mediastinum (a), and in the thoracic and lumbar spine (b) indicative of disseminated disease.

Key point:

PET/CT can detect disease recurrence in patients with functioning medullary thyroid cancer.

| CASE 12.5 | Diagnosis: Thyroid cancer |

Clinical history:

This elderly patient presented with a large mass in the right side of the neck extending into the mediastinum with probable lung metastasis on CT. Fine needle aspiration of the mass confirmed thyroid cancer but the degree of differentiation of the tumor was not clear in the sample obtained. PET/CT was requested to characterize the lesion and guide further management.

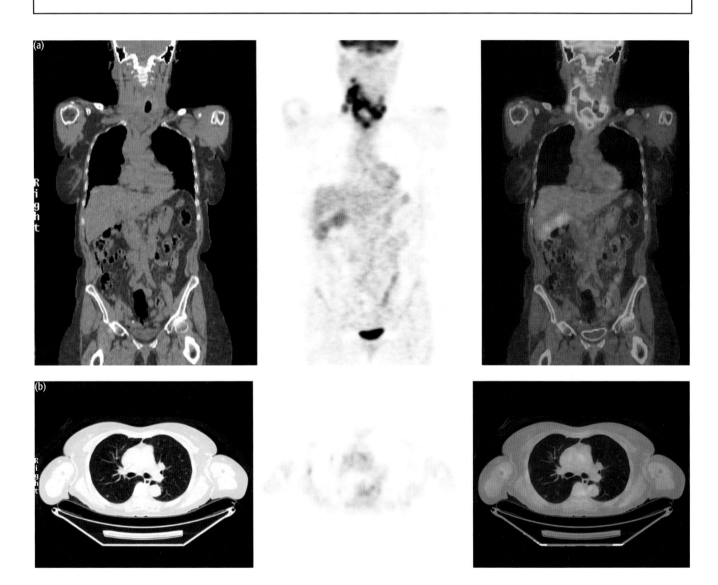

PET/CT findings:

There was intense FDG uptake in the thyroid tumor with uptake in lymph nodes in the neck bilaterally (a) consistent with an aggressive thyroid cancer, probably anaplastic. There were multiple small lung nodules on CT, many of which appeared FDG 'negative' because they were too small to be resolved on PET (b).

Key points:

1 FDG is taken up in aggressive thyroid cancers, which often do not trap iodine.
2 CT is more sensitive for small lung metastases.

CASE 12.6	Diagnosis: Thyroid lymphoma

Clinical history:

Scan 1: This patient presented with a mass in the right neck and a multinodular thyroid goitre. She had been treated with chemotherapy for thyroid lymphoma 10 years previously. Excision biopsy of the right neck node revealed recurrent diffuse large B cell lymphoma of the thyroid gland. PET was requested for staging.

Scan 2: The patient was treated with two cycles of chemotherapy. PET/CT was requested to assess interim treatment response.

Scan 3: The patient completed six cycles of chemotherapy. PET/CT was requested to assess end-of-treatment response.

(a)

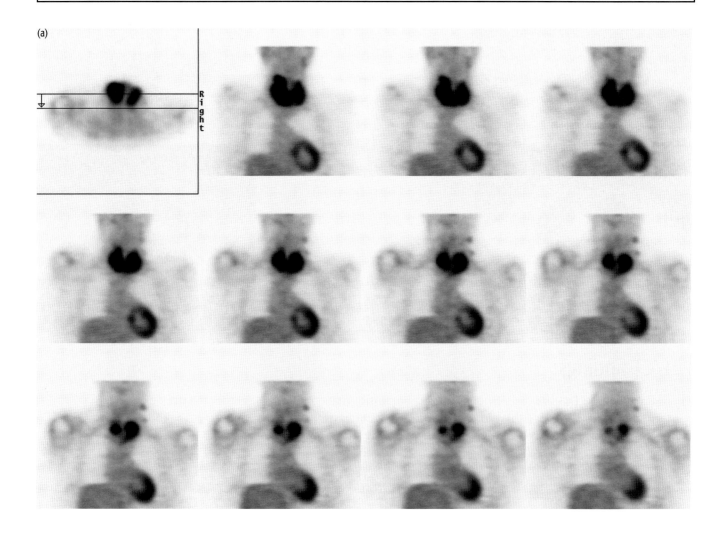

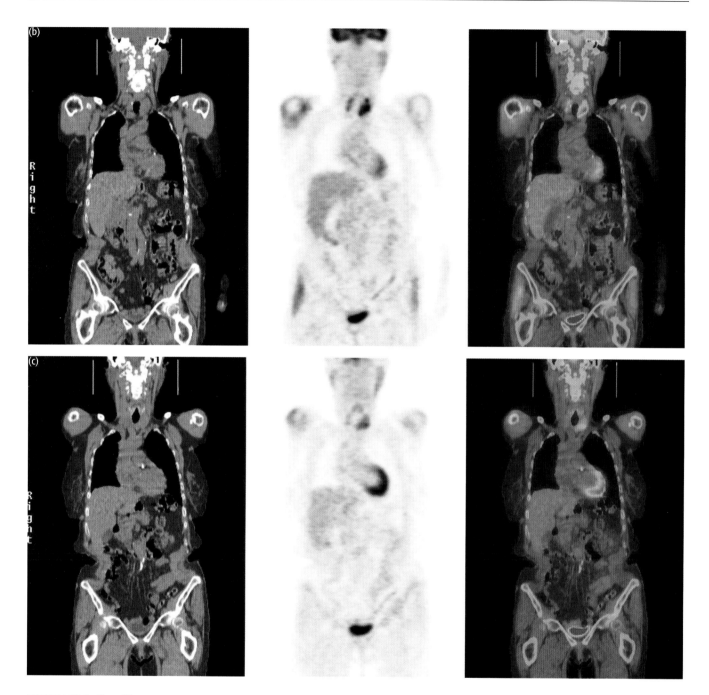

PET/CT findings:

Scan 1 (a): PET-only scan showed uptake in the thyroid consistent with the diagnosis of recurrent lymphoma and uptake at two nodal sites in the left neck.

Scan 2 (b): Following treatment the PET/CT scan showed that the nodal disease had resolved (as indicated by no uptake in the lymph nodes on the scan) but there was residual active disease in the thyroid gland.

Scan 3 (c): There had been partial response to chemotherapy but residual active lymphoma remained in the gland and the patient proceeded to radiotherapy.

Key point:

PET/CT can be used to monitor disease response in thyroid lymphoma as with non-Hodgkin lymphoma in other sites.

CASE 12.7	Diagnosis: Parathyroid adenoma

Clinical history:

This patient with primary hyperparathyroidism was referred after a failed cervical exploration. ^{99m}Tc sestamibi scanning with an iodine subtraction SPECT scan had suggested a functioning parathyroid gland in the posterior mediastinum. PET/CT was requested to confirm the presence of an ectopic gland.

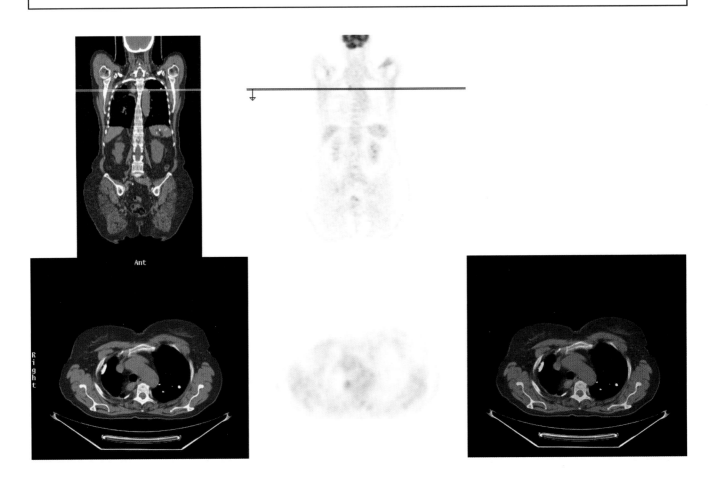

PET/CT findings:

FDG uptake within a soft tissue mass adjacent to the T3 vertebra in the posterior mediastinum was indicative of an ectopic parathyroid gland which was used to direct surgery.

Key point:

There can be FDG uptake in functioning parathyroid adenomas, however, there are variable reports in the literature regarding its sensitivity. In selected cases it may be of value but [^{11}C]methionine is probably more sensitive.

CASE 12.8 | Diagnosis: Parathyroid adenoma

Clinical history:

This patient had previous surgery on the thyroid gland for benign thyroid disease. She presented with symptoms due to hypercalcemia. Biochemistry confirmed primary hyperparathyroidism. PET/CT was requested because of persistent hypercalcemia after a failed surgical exploration.

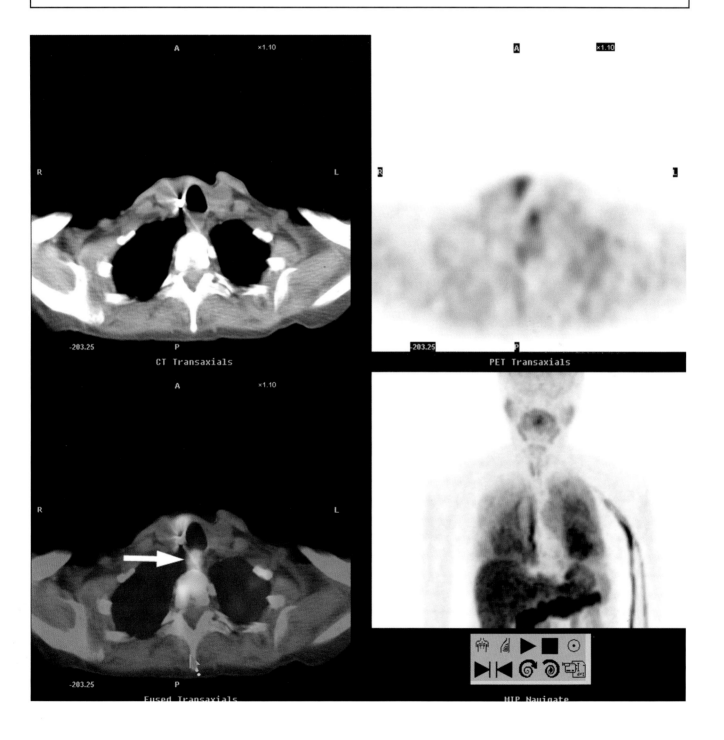

PET/CT findings:

There was high uptake of [^{11}C]methionine in a functioning gland in the right retrotracheal region (arrowed). Note also there is uptake of methionine in normal thyroid remnant on the right.

Key point:

1 [^{11}C]methionine is more sensitive than FDG for the detection of 'ectopic' parathyroid glands.
2 There is physiologic uptake of [^{11}C]methionine in the normal thyroid gland.

CASE 12.9	Diagnosis: Pituitary adenoma and lung cancer

Clinical history:

This patient was referred with a mass in the right upper lobe of the lung. PET/CT was requested to characterize the lesion.

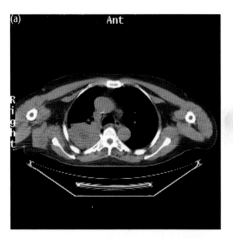

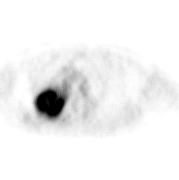

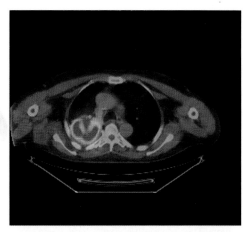

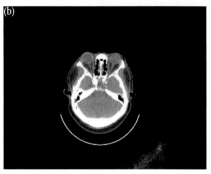

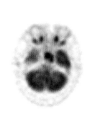

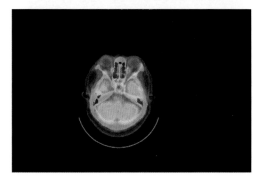

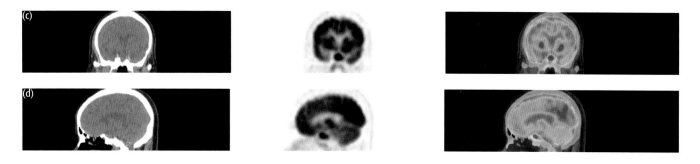

(c)

(d)

PET/CT findings:

Uptake was associated with the right upper lobe mass consistent with a primary lung cancer (a). Uptake was also seen in the pituitary gland (b–d). Trans-sphenoidal resection of the pituitary lesion revealed a gonadotrophin-secreting adenoma.

Key point:

Pituitary macroadenomas may have high FDG uptake, as well as metastasis, to the pituitary gland.

CASE 12.10	Diagnosis: Mixed papillary and follicular thyroid cancer

Clinical history:

This patient was treated with surgery followed by radioiodine ablation for mixed papillary and follicular thyroid cancer. His thyroglobulin levels began to rise and measured 226 micrograms/L off thyroxine and he was re-treated with radioiodine. The post-therapy scan showed no abnormal iodine uptake (a). PET/CT was requested to determine if there was recurrent cancer.

(a)

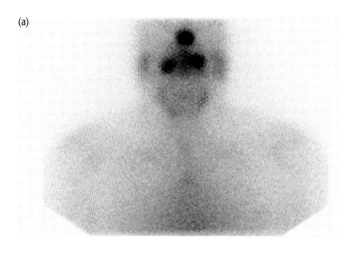

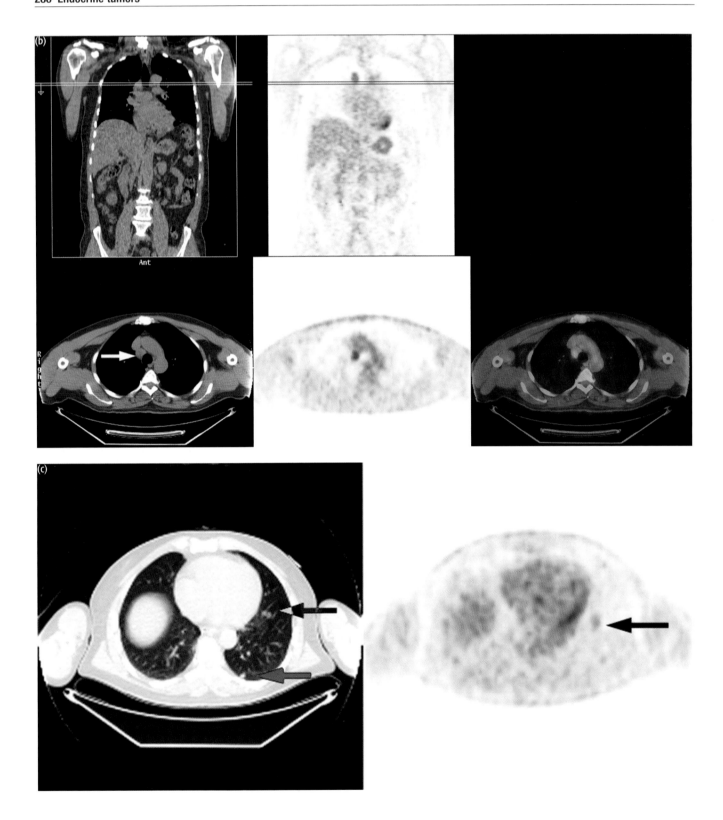

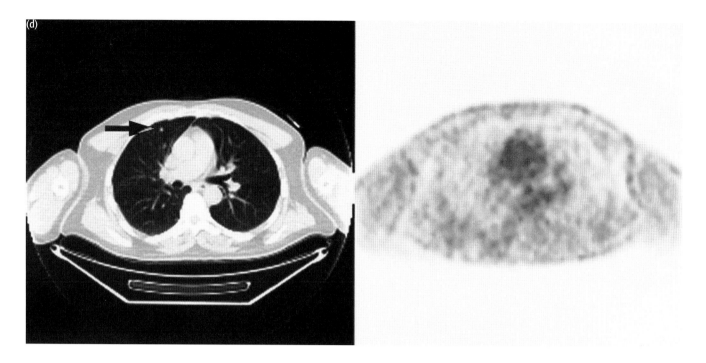

(d)

PET/CT findings:

There was uptake in a right paratracheal node (b) and multiple small lung nodules consistent with metastases. Some of the lung nodules accumulated FDG (black arrow in c), others did not (red arrow in c, black arrow in d) and were probably too small to be resolved using PET.

Key point:

PET/CT is especially useful in patients with rising thyroglobulin and negative iodine scans.

CONCLUSIONS

CURRENT INDICATIONS

Thyroid cancer
1 Restaging with rising thyroglobulin and negative iodine scan
2 Assessment of recurrence in medullary thyroid cancer with rising calcitonin levels and normal/equivocal imaging

Parathyroid tumors
1 Localization where sestamibi scan negative preoperatively using [^{11}C]-L-methionine

Adrenal masses
1 Separation of malignant from benign lesions
2 Assessment of non-MIBG-avid malignant pheochromocytomas for metastatic disease

POSSIBLE INDICATIONS

Thyroid cancer
^{124}I imaging for dosimetry

Parathyroid disease
Assessment for systemic metastases of rare malignant tumors

REFERENCES AND FURTHER READING

Chin BB, Patel P, Cohade C *et al.* (2004) Recombinant human thyrotropin stimulation of fluoro-D-glucose positron emission tomography uptake in well-differentiated thyroid carcinoma. *J Clin Endocrinol Metab* **89**, 91–5.

Cohen MS, Arslan N, Dehdashti F *et al.* (2001) Risk of malignancy in thyroid incidentalomas identified by fluorodeoxyglucose-positron emission tomography. *Surgery* **130**, 941–6.

Cook GJ, Wong JC, Smellie WJ *et al.* (1998) [11C]Methionine positron emission tomography for patients with persistent or recurrent hyperparathyroidism after surgery. *Eur J Endocrinol* **139**, 195–7.

Diehl M, Risse JH, Brandt-Mainz K *et al.* (2001) Fluorine-18 fluorodeoxyglucose positron emission tomography in medullary thyroid cancer: Results of a multicentre study. *Eur J Nucl Med* **28**, 1671–6.

Feine U, Lietzenmayer R, Hanke JP *et al.* (1996) Fluorine-18-FDG and iodine-131-iodide uptake in thyroid cancer. *J Nucl Med* **37**, 1468–72.

Grunwald F, Kalicke T, Feine U *et al.* (1999) Fluorine-18-fluorodeoxyglucose positron emission tomography in thyroid cancer: Results of a multicentre study. *Eur J Nucl Med* **26**, 1547–52.

Kang KW, Kim S-K, Kang H-S *et al.* (2003) Prevalence and risk of cancer of focal thyroid incidentaloma identified by 18F-fluorodeoxyglucose positron emission tomography for metastasis evaluation and cancer screening in healthy subjects. *J Clin Endocrinol Metab* **88**, 4100–4.

Kresnik E, Gallowitsch HJ, Mikosch P *et al.* (2003) Fluorine-18-fluorodeoxyglycose positron emission tomography in the preoperative assessment of thyroid nodules in an endemic goiter area. *Surgery* **133**, 294–9.

Kumar R, Xiu Y, Yu JQ *et al.* (2004) 18F-FDG PET in evaluation of adrenal lesions in patients with lung cancer. *J Nucl Med* **45**, 2058–62.

Lowe VJ, Mullan BP, Hay ID, McIver B, Kasperbauer JL (2003) F-18-FDG-PET of patients with Hurthle cell carcinoma. *J Nucl Med* **44**, 1402–6.

Petrich T, Borner AR, Otto D, *et al.* (2002) Influence of rhTSH on [(18)F]fluorodeoxyglucose uptake by differentiated thyroid carcinoma. *Eur J Nucl Med Mol Imaging* **29**, 641–7.

Schluter B, Bohuslavizki KH, Beyer W *et al.* (2001) Impact of FDG-PET on patients with differentiated thyroid cancer who present with elevated thyroglobulin and negative 131 I scan. *J Nucl Med* **42**, 71–6.

Shulkin BL, Koeppe RA, Francis IR *et al.* (1993) Pheochromocytomas that do not accumulate metaiodobenzylguanidine: localization with PET and administration of FDG. *Radiology* **186**, 711–15.

Sisson JC, Ackermann RJ, Meyer MA, Wahl RL (1993) Uptake of 18-fluoro-2-deoxy-D-glucose by thyroid cancer: implications for diagnosis and therapy. *J Clin Endocrinol Metab* 77, 1090–4.

Wang WP, Macapinlac H, Larson SM *et al.* (1999) F-18-2-fluoro-2-deoxy-D-glucose positron emission tomography localizes residual thyroid cancer in patients with negative diagnostic I-131 whole body scans and elevated serum thyroglobulin levels. *J Clin Endocrinol Metab* 84, 2291–302.

Yasuda S, Shohtsu A, Ide M, Takagi S *et al.* (1997) Diffuse F-18 FDG uptake in chronic thyroiditis. *Clin Nucl Med* 22, 341.

CHAPTER 13
UROLOGIC CANCERS

INTRODUCTION AND BACKGROUND

Approximately 342 000 new cases of cancers affecting the genitourinary system are diagnosed each year in the USA with about 56 000 deaths, based on year 2005 statistics. Cancers of the prostate are most common, with 232 000 new cases per year and 30 000 deaths. Cancers of the bladder are newly diagnosed in 63 000 patients per year and result in 13 000 deaths per year. Renal cancer afflicts 36 000 patients per year and kills 13 000. Testicular cancer is rare; it affects about 8000 patients per year and kills about 400.

The incidence and mortality associated with genitourinary cancers have a great impact on society. The role of FDG PET is limited in prostate cancer but is established in renal and urinary tract cancers and in testicular cancer.

EPIDEMIOLOGY

Incidence of renal and urinary tract cancers

Men	41 new cases per 100 000/ 11 707 cases UK
	48 new cases per 100 000/ 71 090 cases USA
Women	18.5 new cases per 100 000/ 5573 cases UK
	21 new cases per 100 000/ 30 790 cases USA

Incidence of testicular cancers
    7.0 new cases per 100 000/ 2005 cases UK
    5.4 new cases per 100 000/ 8010 cases USA

The majority of renal cell cancers are adenocarcinomas whereas most urinary tract cancers are transitional cell cancers. Testicular cancers are divided into seminomatous and nonseminomatous germ cell tumors (NSGCT) and are rare.

PATHOLOGY	PERCENT
Renal cell cancer	
Adenocarcinoma (clear cell/granular cell)	85
Transitional cell	15
Bladder cancer	
Transitional cell	>90
Squamous cell	6–8
Adenocarcinoma	2
Ureteric cancer	
Transitional cell	85
Squamous cell	15
Testicular cancer	
Seminoma	*
Nonseminoma	
Teratoma	
Choriocarcinoma	
Yolk sac	
Embryonal	

*Less than 50 percent have single cell type. Most have a combination of cell types.

Staging of renal cancers depends on disease extent – size of tumor, nodal status, and the presence or absence of metastatic disease.

STAGING OF RENAL CELL CANCER

TNM	Description
Primary tumor (T)	
T0	No evidence of primary tumor
T1	≤7 cm confined to kidney
T2	> 7 cm confined to kidney
T3	Extends into major veins/invades adrenal gland or perinephric tissues. Not beyond Gerota's fascia
T4	Extends beyond Gerota's fascia
Lymph nodes (N)	
N0	No involved lymph nodes
N1	Single lymph node
N2	>1 lymph node
Metastases (M)	
M0	No metastasis
M1	Distant metastasis
Stage	**TNM**
I	T1 N0 M0
II	T2 N0 M0
III	T1–2 N1 M0
	T3 N0–1 M0
IV	T4 N0–1 M0 T1–4 N2 M0
	T1–4 N0–2 M1

STAGING OF BLADDER CANCER

TNM	Description
Primary tumor (T)	
T0	No evidence of primary tumor
T1	Invades subepithelial connective tissue
T2	Invades muscle
T3	Invades perivesical tissue
T4	Invades prostate, uterus, vagina, pelvic wall, or abdominal wall
Lymph nodes (N)	
N0	No involved lymph nodes
N1	Single lymph node ≤2 cm
N2	Single lymph node 2–5 cm
	Multiple lymph nodes ≤5 cm
N3	Metastases in lymph node > 5 cm
Metastasis (M)	
M0	No metastasis
M1	Distant metastasis
Stage	**TNM**
I	T1 N0 M0
II	T2 N0 M0
III	T3 N0 M0
	T4a* N0 M0
IV	T4b† N0 M0
	T1–4 N1–3 M0
	T1–4 N0–3 M1

*T4a: Tumor invades prostate, uterus, or vagina †T4b: Tumor invades pelvic wall or abdominal wall.

STAGING OF URETERIC CANCER

TNM	Description
Primary tumor (T)	
T0	No evidence of primary tumor
T1	Invades subepithelial connective tissue
T2	Invades muscularis
T3	Invades peripelvic fat, renal parenchyma or periureteric fat
T4	Invades adjacent organs or through the kidney into perinephric fat
Lymph nodes (N)	
N0	No involved lymph nodes
N1	Single lymph node ≤2 cm
N2	Single lymph node 2–5 cm
	Multiple lymph nodes ≤5 cm
N3	Metastases in lymph node >5 cm
Metastasis (M)	
M0	No metastasis
M1	Distant metastasis
Stage	**TNM**
I	T1 N0 M0
II	T2 N0 M0
III	T3 N0 M0
IV	T4 N0 M0
	T1–4 N1–3 M0

The T staging of urinary tract cancers also depends on the depth of the tumor invasion into the wall of the bladder/ureter.

STAGING OF TESTICULAR CANCER (BASED ON EXTENT OF DISEASE AND MARKERS)

TNM	Description
Primary tumor (T)	
Tx	Not assessable
T0	No primary identified
Tis	*In situ*
T1	Confined to testis
T2	As T1 plus vascular and/or lymphatic invasion
T3	Invasion of spermatic cord
T4	Invasion of scrotum
Lymph nodes (N)	
Nx	Nodes not assessable
N0	No nodes
N1	Lymph node/s <2 cm
N2	Lymph node/s 2–5 cm
N3	Lymph node/s >5 cm
Metastasis (M)	
M0	No distant metastasis
M1	Distant metastasis
Stage	**TNM**
I	T1–4 N0 M0
II	Any T N1–3
III	Any T Any N M1
	Each stage will have stage with and stage without positive serum markers

The staging of testicular cancers relies on whether the disease expresses markers as well as on disease extent.

Prognosis of testicular cancers is good, however, cancers of the urinary tract have a poor overall prognosis when there is metastatic disease present and many present at an advanced stage.

DISEASE STAGE PROGNOSIS

Renal cell cancer	
Localized disease	Potentially curable
Metastatic disease	Median 1 year OS variable (10–75%)
Bladder cancer	
Localized disease	Potentially curable but limited data
Metastatic disease	Median OS ~ 1 year
Ureteric cancer	
Localized disease	Potentially curable but limited data
Metastatic disease	Median OS ~1 year
Testicular	
All stages	5-year OS 98%

OS, overall survival.

The role of PET and PET/CT in these tumors is discussed by disease type in the following sections.

KEY MANAGEMENT ISSUES

As in any cancer, tasks for imaging include detection, locoregional and systemic staging, and assessment of the disease after therapy in an effort to monitor treatment. After therapy, or if serum markers are altered, restaging can also be done. In each of these cancers, unique diagnostic problems occur which are not adequately addressed by standard anatomic imaging techniques. For example, detection of nodal metastases is often difficult, as they are often small and appear normal anatomically. Similarly, challenges exist when determining if lesions have fully regressed after treatment. These challenges are major and can be substantially, but not totally, addressed with PET imaging.

KEY MANAGEMENT ISSUES

Staging/restaging of disease especially with raised tumor markers
Assessment of disease activity in residual masses
Monitoring therapy

Role of PET in prostate cancer

Prostate cancer currently represents a disease in which imaging has not been fully successful in the detection of either primary cancer or metastatic disease. Although [18F]2-fluoro-2-deoxy-D-glucose (FDG) positron emission tomography (PET) can detect primary and metastatic prostate cancers in some instances, a variety of reports have shown low avidity of FDG for many prostate cancers. The literature is somewhat confusing, but probably no more than half of active prostate cancers which are metastatic are FDG avid. It does seem clear, however, that the most aggressive, and perhaps those tumors with the highest tumor burden and growth rates, are typically more FDG avid. At present, FDG is not a routine test for imaging prostate cancer metastasis or primary disease in many medical centers, but it is being recognized as having a role in selected patients who appear to have more aggressive disease. The precise role of this test is likely very limited in primary prostate cancer but there may be a greater role in prostate cancer which has progressed or recurred and is associated with rising level of prostate-specific antigen in the blood. In this setting, perhaps 30 percent of patients may have an abnormal FDG scan. Although not extensively evaluated in prostate cancer, sodium fluoride (NaF) PET can provide excellent images of prostate cancer metastatic to bone.

Tracers of other aspects of prostate metabolism include [11C]choline, which is capable of imaging a substantial number of prostate cancers, as well as [18F]fluorocholine, which can image some prostate cancers that are negative on FDG PET. It is believed that this imaging is achieved by active transport of choline through the choline transporters with phosphorylation by choline kinase. Another tracer which is used in the imaging of many prostate cancers is [11C]acetate. This agent accumulates in prostate cancer cells likely through accumulation into cellular lipid pools, although the precise mechanism of tracer uptake is unclear. These tracers are not widely available, however, they are likely to provide imaging superior to that available with FDG alone.

IMAGING OF PROSTATE CANCER – EMERGING TRACERS
[^{11}C]Choline
[^{18}F]Fluorocholine
[^{11}C]Acetate

FDG PET is not a reliable method for detecting prostate cancer located within the prostate gland. A negative FDG PET scan in a patient suspected of having prostate cancer DOES NOT exclude active prostate cancer.

Role of PET in bladder cancer

It is difficult to image primary bladder cancers with FDG because of the substantial excretion of FDG through the kidneys and into the bladder. Although bladder lavage is possible, in general it is not practical to image bladder cancer in the bladder with FDG. It is, however, possible to image locoregional and systemic metastases of bladder cancer with PET. Usually these tumors are histologically transitional cell tumors and typically have high glycolytic activity. At present, only small studies of the accuracy of PET with FDG for staging nodal metastases of bladder cancer have been performed, but they have been encouraging. Obviously, nodal metastases located immediately adjacent to the bladder are difficult to see due to intense activity of the surrounding FDG excreted in the bladder. Delayed imaging, post-void images of the pelvis, and catheterization can help reduce these challenges in diagnosis. Since some of the most common lymph nodes for metastasis parallel the course of the normal ureters, PET/computed tomography (CT) is useful to distinguish the normal ureters from FDG-avid nodes along the course of the ureter. Although most bladder cancers are highly FDG avid, our experience is that only a minority of bladder cancers are currently staged or followed with PET or PET/CT. As bladder cancers respond well to chemotherapy and reasonably well to irradiation, it is important to remember that FDG PET is a good tool for evaluating these tumors.

Role of PET in renal cancer

Renal cancers kill about 40 percent of the individuals who are diagnosed as having these tumors. Since the kidneys cannot easily be palpated, renal cancers presenting due to clinical symptoms are often quite late and advanced in their natural history. However, given that medical imaging including CT scanning is being done with increasing frequency for a variety of ailments, including for screening, renal masses as an incidental finding are being diagnosed more commonly than ever before. A key diagnostic question is how to determine whether a renal mass needs biopsy or removal. Although there are a variety of helpful anatomic characteristics, not all solid renal masses are cancer, whereas some cystic renal masses are indeed malignant. It had been hoped that FDG PET would be able to reliably separate malignant from benign masses noninvasively. Initial data were promising, especially for larger primary cancers, but more recent data suggest that 40–50 percent of renal cancers presenting as solitary renal masses on PET are not detected as foci of increased tracer uptake on FDG PET. Part of the challenge may be that these cancers are located near intense excreted FDG activity in the renal collecting system, although this is only part of the reason as many renal cancers only have modest

FDG uptake. The precise value of FDG PET/CT has not been explored fully in primary renal cancers. Alternative tracers, such as [^{11}C]acetate, may hold more promise but to date have only been explored to a modest extent.

Metastatic renal cancers are imaged much better than the primary lesions and typically 90 percent or more of the metastatic lesions are detected with FDG PET. Thus, FDG PET has a much greater role in assessing metastatic than primary renal cancers.

Role of PET in testicular cancer

Testicular cancers are of several histologic types, but essentially all of them are FDG avid in their untreated state. Thus, seminomas and nonseminomatous germ cell tumors are typically quite easily detected by PET. Because these tumors are rare, the use of PET has not been explored to any substantial extent for the imaging of primary testicular cancers, especially in the screening setting. PET has, however, been evaluated for lymph node staging and for monitoring treatment response. Both of these detection tasks are challenging for anatomic imaging. For initial staging, there has been a historical desire to histologically verify nodal status in the retroperitoneum. Unfortunately, obtaining of specimens for histologic examination can result in significant morbidity, such as impotence, as the specimens are obtained by retroperitoneal lymph node dissection. PET with FDG has been explored as an alternative to this aggressive approach. Although PET cannot detect all metastatic foci as some are too small to be imaged, it can be used to monitor patients for the development of nodal metastasis, thus potentially sparing them the need for the retroperitoneal lymph node dissection.

Often testicular carcinomas present as large masses, and whereas the masses sometimes disappear after treatment, not infrequently residual masses remain which can be difficult to distinguish from viable tumor. In germ cell cancers, it is possible to have residual viable tumor, scarring, or transformation of the malignant tumor to a less malignant form such as benign teratoma. PET may have a role in this setting. While low FDG uptake is seen in both scar and mature teratomas, active tumor typically has high level FDG uptake. Kinetic modeling has been used in this setting. Since the number of patients with testicular carcinoma is rather low, large series of patients with testicular cancer have not been included in studies, so the literature is somewhat less developed than in more common cancers such as lung or breast cancer. Nonetheless, FDG PET appears to have several possible roles in imaging testicular cancer, both in the earliest stages and during and after treatment has been delivered. Other tracers are not routinely used in testicular cancer imaging.

EXAMPLES TO ILLUSTRATE KEY ISSUES

Renal cancer

CASE 13.1	Diagnosis: Renal cancer – negative FDG uptake

Clinical history:

This patient had previously undergone renal transplantation for Alport syndrome and was referred for staging of a known renal cell carcinoma in the transplanted kidney.

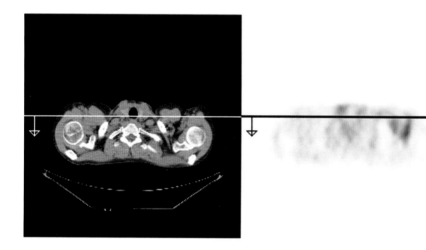

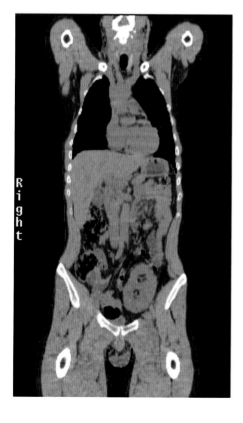
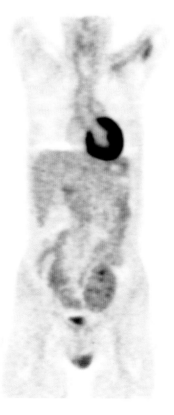
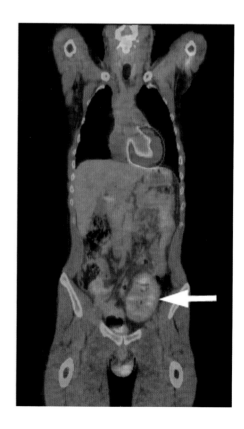

PET/CT findings:

PET/CT showed physiologic uptake only in the transplanted kidney (arrow) with no evidence of cancer.

Key points:

1 Lack of or low FDG uptake in a renal mass does not exclude the possibility of renal cancer.
2 Approximately 40–50 percent of renal cell carcinomas do not take up FDG and in this case PET could not help with tumor staging.

CASE 13.2	Diagnosis: Renal cancer – solitary lung metastasis?

Clinical history:

This patient with renal cancer had a wedge resection of an FDG-avid metastasis in the left lower lobe of the lung 2 years earlier. He was referred because of an apparently solitary enlarging nodule in the left upper lobe on CT. No other sites of disease were reported on CT. PET/CT was requested to characterize the lesion prior to surgery.

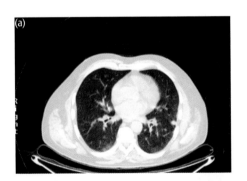

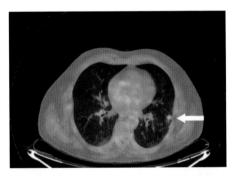
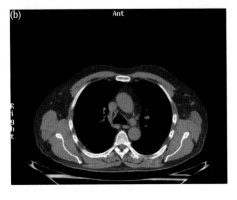

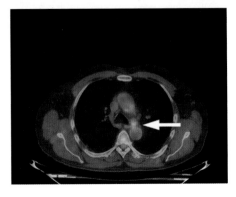

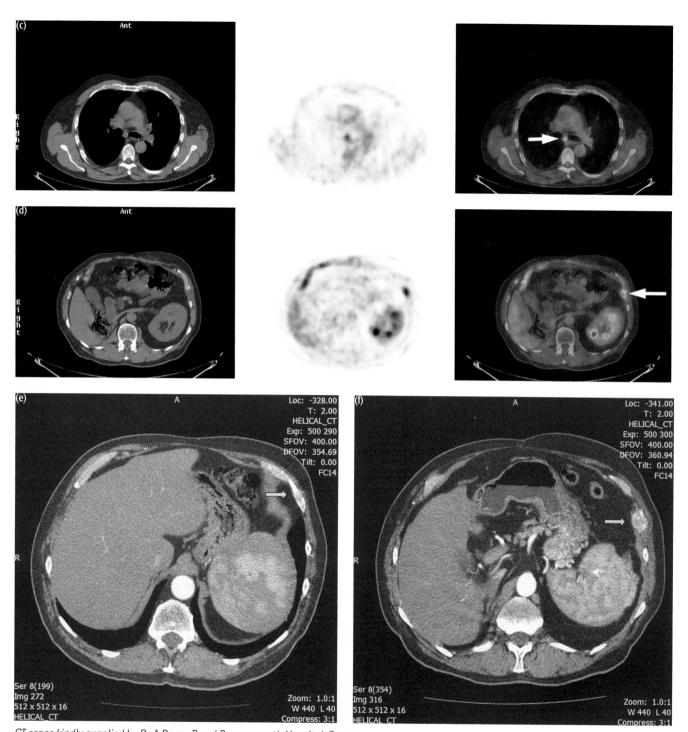

CT scans kindly supplied by Dr A Drury, Royal Bournemouth Hospital, Sussex

PET/CT findings:

FDG uptake was increased in the lung nodule (a) and also in aortopulmonary (b) and subcarinal (c) lymph nodes as well as within the left eighth rib (d), suggestive of additional metastases. Review of the diagnostic CT scan showed that there was an abnormality in the eighth rib (e). The patient was treated with interferon. A successive CT scan 2 months after the PET/CT showed enlargement of the rib deposit (f).

Key points:

1 Detection of metastatic renal cancer is typically quite effective with FDG PET.
2 PET/CT directed treatment away from 'local' surgery to systemic treatment – in this case by detection of unsuspected metastatic disease.

| CASE 13.3 | Diagnosis: Renal cancer and metastasis |

Clinical history:

This patient was referred with a history of renal cell carcinoma T1 N0 M0 treated with right nephrectomy. He subsequently developed a soft-tissue mass anterior to the right scapula which was thought to be a solitary metastasis. A magnetic resonance imaging (MRI) scan showed a further lesion at L3, which was thought to be a hemangioma. PET/CT was requested to determine if the patient should undergo metastasectomy of the lesion.

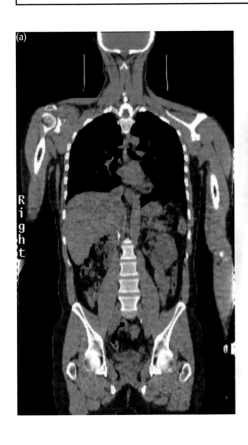 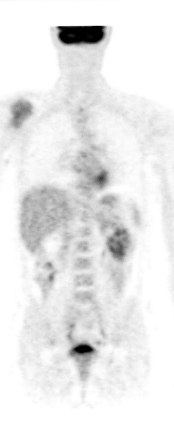 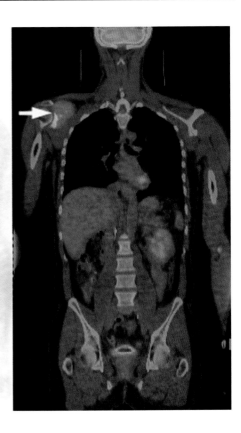

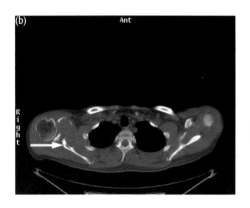

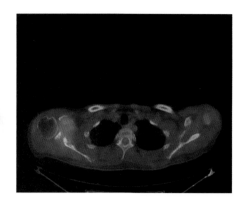

PET/CT findings:

PET showed uptake in a soft-tissue mass anterior to the right scapula (a), with erosion of the scapula posteriorly (b). The mass was excised and confirmed to be a metastasis.

Key point:

Compare with Case 13.2 where disease was disseminated and therefore inoperable.

CASE 13.4	Diagnosis: Renal cancer – residual mass

Clinical history:

This patient was referred with a history of clear cell renal carcinoma with extensive vascular invasion by tumor and thrombosis in the venous channels. He underwent a left nephrectomy and evacuation of thrombus in the inferior vena cava (IVC) into which a filter was inserted. After completion of interferon therapy a soft-tissue mass remained around the IVC. PET/CT was requested to determine if this represented healing thrombus or tumor.

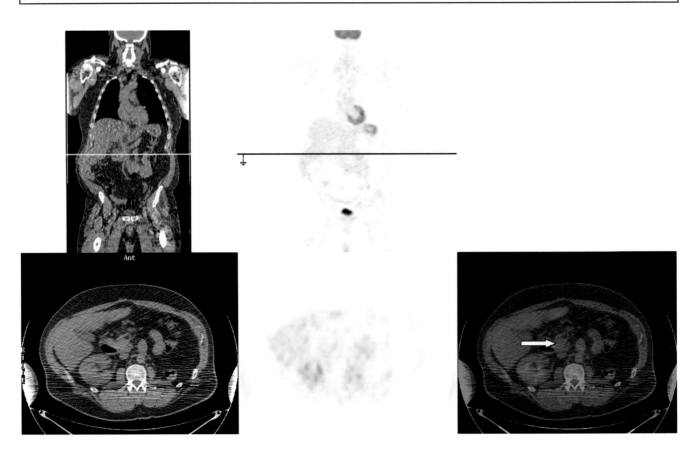

PET/CT findings:

Note a left nephrectomy and a soft-tissue mass adjacent to the IVC but no increased FDG uptake to support residual active cancer. The patient remained well with no changes in appearances on CT 6 months after the PET scan.

Key point:

Metastatic renal cancers are imaged better than the primary lesions. Typically 90 percent or more of the metastatic lesions are detected with FDG PET. Thus, FDG PET has a much greater role in assessing metastatic than primary renal cancers.

| CASE 13.5 | Diagnosis: Renal cancer |

Clinical history:

This patient had previously undergone right nephrectomy and right adrenalectomy with stenting of the inferior vena cava for extensive renal cell carcinoma. There was a left adrenal mass, which was followed up on CT and appeared to be enlarging slowly in size. Laparoscopic biopsy of the mass with a view to adrenalectomy was attempted but was unsuccessful due to extensive peritoneal scarring following postoperative radiotherapy. Radiofrequency ablation was being considered but was also likely to be technically difficult. PET/CT was requested to further characterize the adrenal mass.

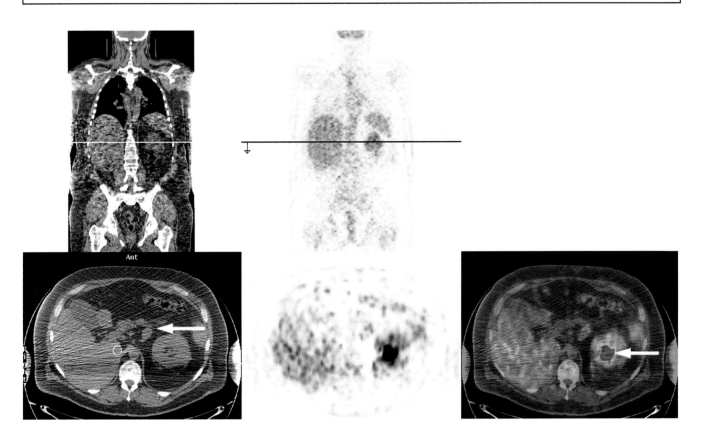

PET/CT findings:

Uptake in the solitary left kidney was associated with a soft-tissue mass with gas within it and a small perisplenic collection (not shown) suggestive of postoperative infection. There was, however, no uptake in the left adrenal mass. The perisplenic collection was drained and revealed infection with *Escherichia coli*. Three months after treatment with antibiotics the collection had resolved and the left adrenal mass had not enlarged further.

Key points:

1 This was a difficult case where correlation with clinical information and CT scanning was crucial for the correct diagnosis.
2 Interpretation with PET/CT of the uptake in the left kidney is easier than using PET alone. Without CT the uptake in the infected kidney could easily have been mistaken for physiologic uptake in the renal pelvis.
3 As this patient had not undergone scanning previously, the 'negative' uptake in the adrenal mass does not definitely exclude malignancy, but in the present difficult circumstances it helped inform clinicians and the patient who decided to adopt a conservative approach.

Bladder cancer

| CASE 13.6 | Diagnosis: Bladder cancer – metastatic disease |

Clinical history:

This patient had bladder cancer treated with cystectomy. PET/CT was requested to characterize small para-aortic lymph nodes seen on CT.

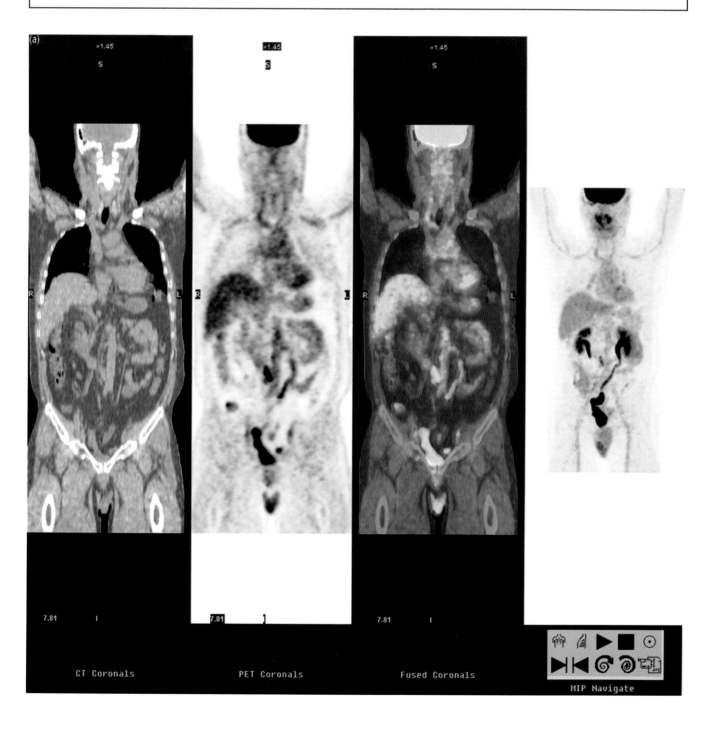

(a)

CT Coronals   PET Coronals   Fused Coronals

MIP Navigate

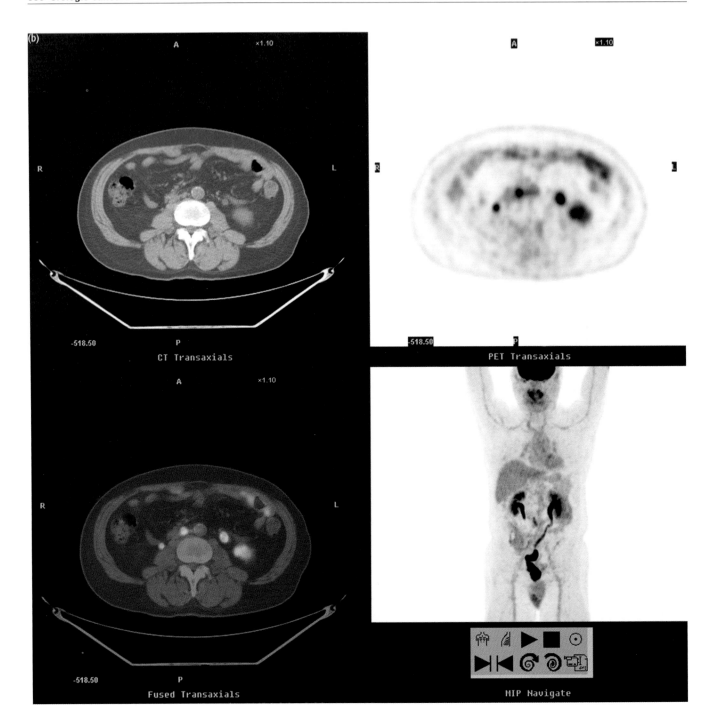

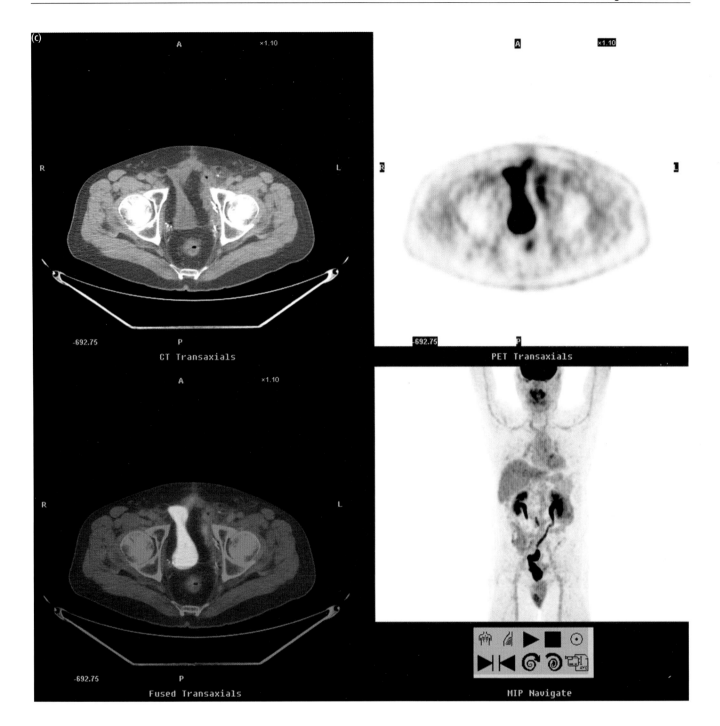

PET/CT findings:

There were metastases in para-aortic lymph nodes (a). Note on the axial images at the level of the lower pole of the left kidney (b) that there is physiologic uptake in the left kidney and both ureters which is the same intensity as the uptake in the metastasis in the right para-aortic lymph node. High uptake of FDG is also seen in urine in neobladder fashioned from ileum and in adjacent bowel, which is best appreciated on axial images (c).

Key points:

1 FDG in the normal genitourinary tissues is a major challenge for evaluating patients with suspected bladder cancers.
2 FDG uptake can be minimized by having the patient void immediately before obtaining the PET images. Catheterization, diuresis, and delayed imaging may also be useful.
3 PET/CT can provide clear separation of the ureters from lymph nodes located along the ureters.

Testicular cancer

CASE 13.7	Diagnosis: Germ cell tumor

Clinical history:

This patient had a history of NSGCT treated with chemotherapy and nodal dissection of left para-aortic disease, with intraoperative damage to the left kidney. Residual masses in the left retroperitoneal region and posterior mediastinum were monitored on CT; enlargement of the mass in the left retroperitoneal region was noted on serial scanning. PET/CT was requested to characterize the masses and plan surgery.

(a)

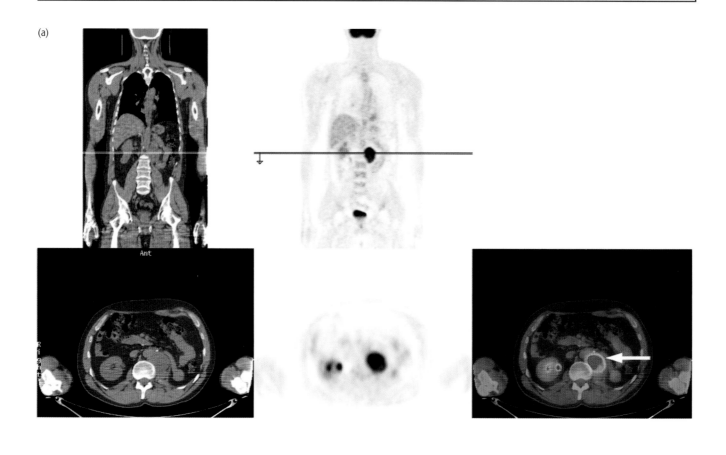

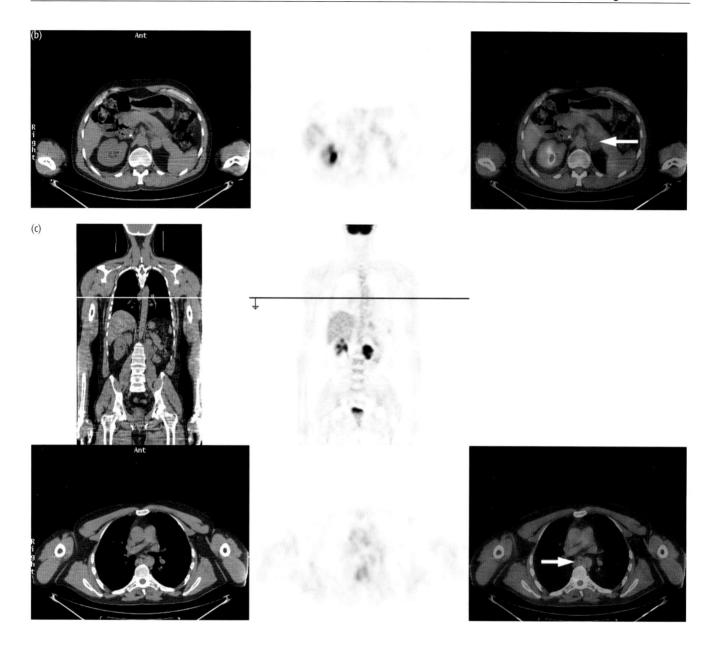

PET/CT findings:

Intense uptake in the left retroperitoneal mass was consistent with active germ cell tumor (a). The small soft-tissue mass immediately above the mass represented the atrophic left kidney (b). No uptake was seen in the posterior mediastinal mass, consistent with fibrosis. At surgery the mass in the retroperitoneal region containing aggressive yolk sac tumor was removed together with the nonfunctioning atrophic left kidney.

Key points:

1 Residual masses are common after treatment in patients with testicular cancer. High FDG avidity suggests cancer, but scar and sometimes mature teratomas have no uptake. A growing non-FDG-avid mass following treatment for germ cell cancer is likely to be due to teratoma.
2 Sometimes PET/CT may be used to stage teratoma as opposed to a retroperitoneal nodal dissection. If this is done, close follow-up scans are likely to be needed as microscopic disease will be missed.

CASE 13.8	Diagnosis: Teratoma

Clinical history:

This patient with teratoma of the left testis with vascular invasion was treated with surgery and chemotherapy. One year after treatment CT showed two cystic masses in the para-aortic region, most likely mature teratoma. Surgery was planned to remove these masses as, although mature teratoma is a benign condition, there is a significant likelihood that mature teratoma will undergo malignant change. PET/CT was requested to determine if there was disease elsewhere which would influence the plan to resect the two para-aortic masses.

(a)

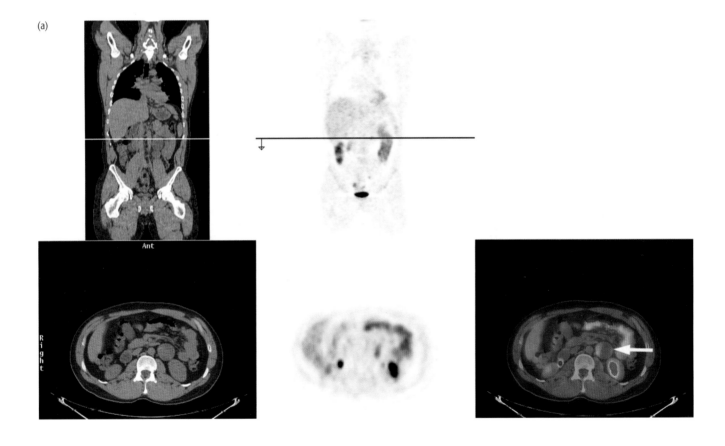

(b)

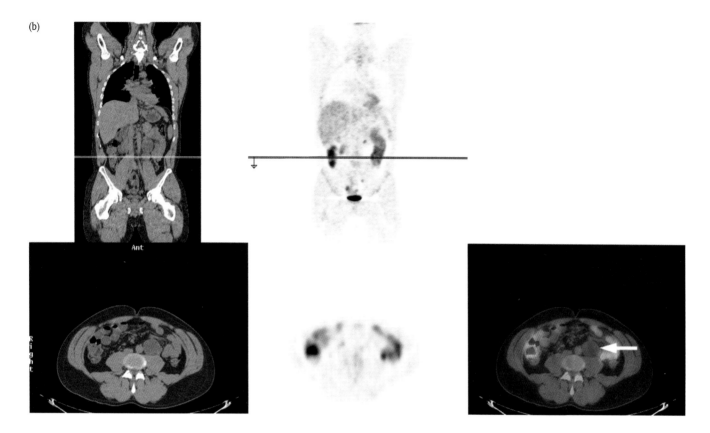

PET/CT findings:

There were two masses in the left para-aortic region. The superior mass had a small area of low-grade activity at its medial rim (a). The inferior mass had no FDG uptake associated with it (b). (Physiologic uptake is seen in bowel and ureters.) The masses were removed; they consisted of mature teratoma.

Key points:

1 PET/CT can differentiate fibrosis and mature teratoma (teratoma differentiated) from undifferentiated teratoma. Mature teratoma has either low-grade or no associated uptake of FDG. However it is not possible to differentiate between mature teratoma and fibrosis.
2 Residual masses after treatment of teratoma are often removed because of the possibility of de-differentiation of mature teratoma.

Prostate cancer

CASE 13.9	Diagnosis: Prostate cancer

Clinical history:

This patient with suspected metastatic disease from cancer of the prostate was referred for PET scanning with [^{11}C]choline for staging.

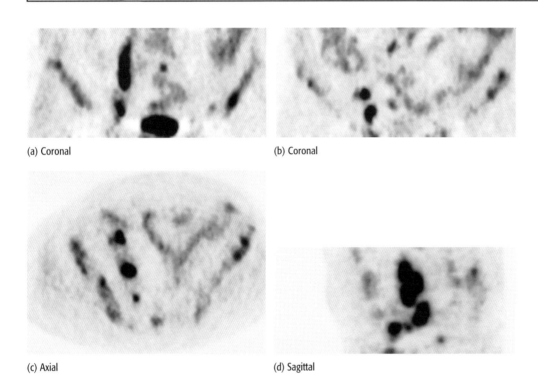

(a) Coronal

(b) Coronal

(c) Axial

(d) Sagittal

PET findings:

There was uptake in para-aortic and iliac lymph nodes (a–c) and in multiple sites in the pelvic bones (a–c) representing metastases. Primary disease in the prostate is well shown on the sagittal image with exophytic tumor arising from the gland (d). Some physiologic uptake is also seen in the bladder (a, d).

Key points:

1 There is high uptake of [^{11}C]choline in prostate cancers and metastases, however, it is not exclusive for cancer. Uptake can be seen in benign prostatic hypertrophy, but in this setting it is usually lower than with cancer and higher than in the normal prostate gland.

2 Physiologic uptake occurs in salivary glands, lungs, liver, kidneys, adrenal glands, and bowel. Generally the uptake in the bladder is lower with [^{11}C] choline than with the fluorinated choline compounds.

CONCLUSIONS

CURRENT INDICATIONS

Renal and urinary tract cancer
1 Assessment of recurrent disease with equivocal imaging

Testicular cancer
1 Detection of recurrence with rising markers or symptoms
2 Assessment of residual masses
3 Prior to metastasectomy
4 Monitoring response to treatment

POSSIBLE INDICATIONS
1 Staging the primary in selected cases (with suspicion of metastatic disease)

FURTHER READING

Dehdashti F, Picus J, Michalski JM *et al.* (2005) Positron tomographic assessment of androgen receptors in prostatic carcinoma. *Eur J Nucl Med Mol Imaging* **32**, 344–50. Epub 2005 Feb 22.

Hain SF, Maisey MN (2003) Positron emission tomography for urological tumours. *BJU Int* **92**, 159–64.

Harney JV, Wahl RL, Liebert M *et al.* (1991) Uptake of 2-deoxy, 2-(18F) fluoro-D-glucose in bladder cancer: animal localization and initial patient positron emission tomography. *J Urol* **145**, 279–83.

Jadvar H, Conti PS (2004) The reproductive tract. *Semin Nucl Med* **34**, 262–73.

Kumar R, Zhuang H, Alavi A (2004) PET in the management of urologic malignancies. *Radiol Clin North Am* **42**, 1141–53.

Kwee SA, Coel MN, Lim J, Ko JP. (2005) Prostate cancer localization with 18fluorine fluorocholine positron emission tomography. *J Urol* **173**, 252–5.

Morris MJ, Akhurst T, Larson SM *et al.* (2005) Fluorodeoxyglucose positron emission tomography as an outcome measure for castrate metastatic prostate cancer treated with antimicrotubule chemotherapy. *Clin Cancer Res* **11**, 3210–16.

Schmid DT, John H, Zweifel R *et al.* (2005) Fluorocholine PET/CT in patients with prostate cancer: initial experience. *Radiology* **235**, 623–8.

Schoder H, Larson SM (2004) Positron emission tomography for prostate, bladder, and renal cancer. *Semin Nucl Med* **34**, 274–92.

Yoshida S, Nakagomi K, Goto S, Futatsubashi M, Torizuka T (2005) ^{11}C-choline positron emission tomography in prostate cancer: primary staging and recurrent site staging. *Urol Int* **74**, 214–20.

CHAPTER 14
MUSCULOSKELETAL CANCER

INTRODUCTION AND BACKGROUND

EPIDEMIOLOGY

Incidence

Men	1 new case per 100 000/ 298 cases UK (bone)
	2.7 new case per 100 000/ 778 cases UK (soft tissue)
	1 new case per 100 000/ 1480 cases USA (bone)
	3.1 new cases per 100 000/ 5530 cases USA (soft tissue)
Women	0.8 new cases per 100 000/ 227 cases UK (bone)
	2.0 new cases per 100 000/ 624 cases UK (soft tissue)
	0.8 new cases per 100 000/ 1090 cases USA (bone)
	2.5 new cases per 100 000/ 3890 cases USA (soft tissue)

Primary malignant bone tumors include osteosarcoma, Ewing sarcoma, chondrosarcoma, lymphoma, and myeloma. Osteosarcoma is the most common primary bone malignancy in children and the second most common in adults after multiple myeloma. Osteosarcomas usually present in the long bones in childhood. Involvement of the axial skeleton is seen more often in adults. The treatment is usually surgical with or without local radiotherapy. Adjuvant chemotherapy can be used to reduce the extent of surgery for limb salvage. Chemotherapy is also used to delay and to control metastatic disease with variable results. Chondrosarcomas occur mostly in young adults and in the fifth and sixth decades. They often present late and have poor prognosis with a 55 percent 5-year survival rate reported even for patients without metastatic disease at presentation. Management is similar to that for osteosarcoma.

Soft-tissue sarcomas represent solid neoplasms arising from nonepithelial extraskeletal tissue (excluding glial cells) with a wide range of tumor types and behavior.

PATHOLOGY

Histologic subtypes

Adipocytic tumors

Fibroblastic/myofibroblastic tumors

Fibrohistiocytic tumor

Smooth muscle tumors

Skeletal muscle tumors

Vascular tumors

Chondro-osseous tumors

Tumors of uncertain differentiation

STAGING

TNM	Description
Primary tumor (T)	
Tx	Primary tumor not assessable
T0	No evidence of primary tumor
T1	Tumor <5 cm diameter
T1a	Superficial
T1b	Deep
T2	Tumor >5 cm
T2a	Superficial
T2b	Deep
Lymph nodes (N)	
Nx	Nodes not assessable
N0	No regional nodes
N1	Regional nodes involved
Metastasis (M)	
M0	No distant metastasis
M1	Distant metastasis
Stage	**TNM**
Stage I	T1 or T2 N0 M0 Low grade
Stage II	T1 or T2a N0 M0 High grade
Stage III	T2b N0 M0 High grade
Stage IV	Any T N1 M0 Any grade
	Any T N0 M1 Any grade

> *The behavior of soft tissue tumors is related to the histologic subtype, and correct classification with a representative biopsy is important in deciding management and predicting prognosis.*

GENERAL CLINICAL BEHAVIOR

Propensity for local recurrence
Clinical aggressiveness correlates with histologic grade
Lungs are most common site for metastatic spread

The treatment of soft-tissue sarcoma is primarily surgical although local radiotherapy may be used if a wide enough surgical excision margin cannot be achieved because of proximity to bone or major nerves. There is a high rate of local recurrence and of late distant metastasis.

KEY MANAGEMENT ISSUES

KEY MANAGEMENT ISSUES

Determining the optimal site of biopsy
Staging at diagnosis
Restaging with recurrence

Role of PET in primary bone malignancy

Plain radiography and magnetic resonance imaging (MRI) are used to assess primary disease. [^{18}F]2-Fluoro-2-deoxy-D-glucose (FDG) positron emission tomography (PET) cannot reliably distinguish benign from malignant disease in the primary lesion but can be used to direct biopsy to the area that is most likely to contain the most aggressive area of tumor – which is crucial for tumor grading. PET may be able to predict prognosis, with one study demonstrating that rates of overall and event-free survival were significantly better in patients with low FDG uptake in tumor compared with patients with high FDG uptake. Metastatic disease occurs commonly in lung and bone and is usually visualized in computed tomography (CT) scans of the chest and bone scintigraphy (although chondrosarcomas tend to have lower uptake on bone scanning than osteosarcoma and Ewing sarcoma). FDG PET has been shown to detect metastatic disease in small numbers of cases, but may be less sensitive than bone scintigraphy in osteosarcoma but more sensitive in Ewing sarcoma.

FDG PET has also been used to monitor chemotherapy response preoperatively. In 33 children with osteosarcoma or Ewing sarcoma a decline in standardized uptake value (SUV) of 30–40 percent was able to correctly predict histologic response at surgery, defined as ≥90 percent necrosis (Hawkins *et al.*, 2002). In another study in adults, tumor to background ratio of FDG uptake was measured before and after chemotherapy (Schulte *et al.*, 1999). Using a cut-off ratio of 0.6, PET identified all responders and 8/10 nonresponders. Thus PET may have a role in the initial biopsy, staging, detection of metastases, and monitoring of neoadjuvant chemotherapy.

Role of PET in soft-tissue sarcoma

Imaging of local disease relies on MRI to define the extent of the soft-tissue tumor. However, soft-tissue sarcomas are heterogeneous tumors. Coregistration of MRI with FDG PET may be valuable in reducing sampling variation during the initial biopsy and then subsequently in planning the surgical approach. FDG PET can distinguish benign and low-grade malignancy from high-grade malignancy using delayed imaging. Lodge *et al.* (1999) demonstrated that the optimal time to scan the site of primary disease is at 4 hours after injection of FDG. FDG PET has also been used to identify malignant change in patients with neurofibromatosis type 1 with good separation of benign from malignant change seen using a cut-off SUV of 3.3 at 3 hours post injection (Ferner et al, 2000). Metastatic disease is found at presentation in about 10–25 percent of patients with soft-tissue sarcomas. FDG PET is less sensitive than CT in the detection of lung metastases. However, two thirds of metastases are seen outside the lungs and these may be visualized with FDG PET. In recurrence MRI is used to assess local disease, but FDG PET may be helpful if MR is equivocal, especially if patients have received radiotherapy. However, tissue almost always needs to be obtained for confirmation. FDG PET has been used to assess recurrent disease in limb stumps after amputation. Diffuse increased uptake is seen for up to 18 months after surgery, but focal uptake can be seen with tumor recurrence. Focal uptake also occurs in association with local infection/inflammation but this is usually easy to identify clinically in pressure points with local areas of skin breakdown. Focal uptake in the stump should always prompt examination to exclude local recurrence of tumor. Therefore, in initial staging, re-staging, and surveillance, a combination of MRI for local disease, CT for chest disease, and whole-body PET may be required to manage these rare and difficult tumors.

FDG PET can detect active disease in lytic lesions in multiple myeloma, with a higher sensitivity than plain radiography. It may have a role in staging in patients with apparently solitary plasmacytoma and in the detection of occult disease in patients with nonsecretory myeloma, where the lack of paraprotein makes it difficult to assess disease status and monitor treatment.

EXAMPLES TO ILLUSTRATE KEY ISSUES

| CASE 14.1 | Diagnosis: Sarcoma – directing biopsy |

Clinical history:

This patient was referred with a probable soft-tissue tumor in the right calf. PET/CT was requested to help direct biopsy of the tumor with MR registration.

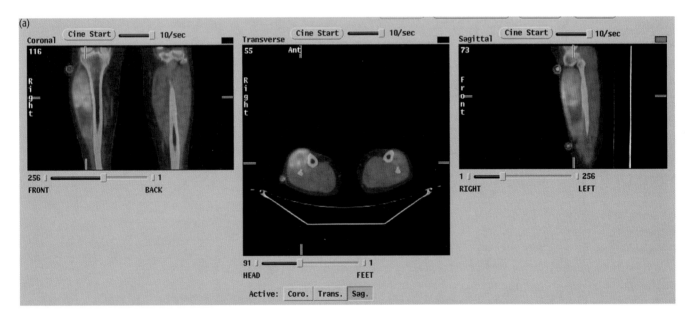

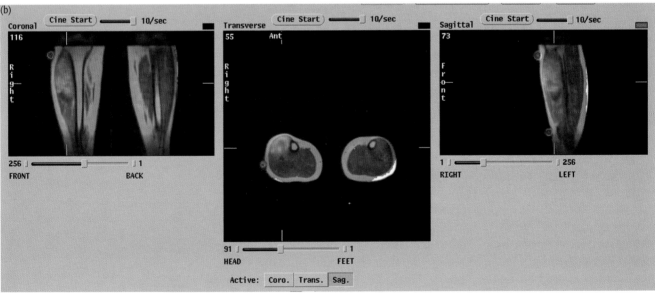

PET/CT findings:

There was intense uptake associated with a lesion in the right calf, the maximum SUV of the tumor was 4.9 at 4 hours after injection suggesting a malignant etiology. Orthogonal images are shown of the PET/CT scan with skin markers (a), which was then registered to the MR scan giving fused PET/MR images (b). These were then used to guide preoperative sampling. The biopsy and final surgical specimen revealed high-grade round cell liposarcoma. (A small lung nodule was seen in the right upper lobe of the lung, which was not FDG avid and was followed up by CT scan. The nodule did not alter on CT over time and is presumed to be benign.)

Key points:

1 PET can be used to help direct biopsy with MR registration.
2 There is clearer differentiation between high-grade and low-grade or benign lesions if scanning is delayed until 4 hours after injection (Lodge *et al.*, 1999).

CASE 14.2	Diagnosis: Sarcoma

Clinical history:

This patient was referred with a tumor in the right hamstrings. PET/CT was requested to direct biopsy.

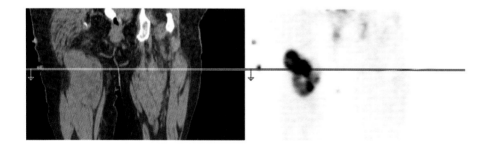

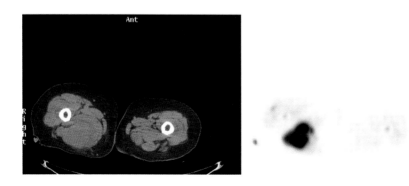
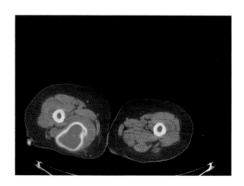

PET/CT findings:

There was avid uptake in the lesion in the right biceps femoris suggestive of a high-grade tumor. The maximum SUV was 18. Note the markers used for registration with the MRI for preoperative sampling. Abnormal uptake was not seen elsewhere. Biopsy of the most intense area of uptake revealed high-grade pleomorphic sarcoma.

Key point:

Obtaining a representative sample is especially important in these tumors as they can be heterogeneous. This can be important in planning the subsequent surgical approach for tumor resection.

CASE 14.3	Diagnosis: Sarcoma and neurofibromatosis

Clinical history:

This patient with neurofibromatosis type 1 had a malignant peripheral nerve sheath tumor removed from the left thigh 2 years earlier. Surveillance CT scanning had shown a soft-tissue mass adjacent to the liver, which was enlarging in size. The PET/CT was requested to determine whether this represented an enlarging neurofibroma or metastasis and if there were other sites of disease.

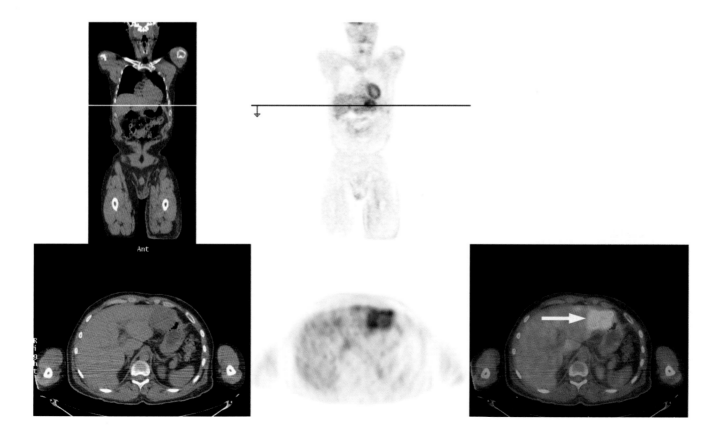

PET/CT findings:

There was intense FDG uptake in a large mass adjacent to the left lobe of the liver. The uptake increased on delayed imaging with a maximum SUV in the lesion of 9.0 at 4 hours after injection, consistent with a metastasis from soft-tissue sarcoma. The mass was removed at surgery. Multiple small intra-abdominal nodules were also present in the abdomen, which had not been identified on PET or CT. Histologic examination of the mass and three nodules removed from the surface of the falciform ligament revealed rhabdomyosarcoma.

Key points:

1 PET/CT can help to characterize lesions as 'malignant' or 'benign' in neurofibromatosis.
2 Delayed imaging at 4 hours allows clearer differentiation of benign from malignant disease.
3 Small-volume disease can be missed on PET and CT.

CASE 14.4	Diagnosis: Sarcoma

Clinical history:

This patient had a synovial sarcoma removed from the anterior abdominal wall 12 years previously. The patient re-presented with a probable recurrence in the left thigh and metastasis in the right lung on CT scanning. PET/CT was requested to exclude extrapulmonary disease.

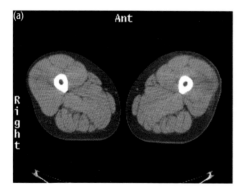

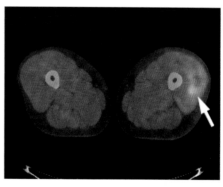
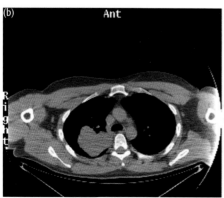
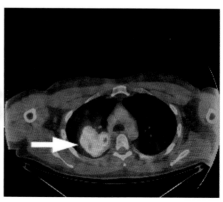

PET/CT findings:

Avid uptake was associated with a lesion in the vastus lateralis muscle of the left thigh (a) and within the right lung (b). The patient underwent local excision of the lesion in the thigh and right upper lobectomy. Histologic examination confirmed the presence of recurrence of synovial sarcoma in the thigh and metastatic disease in the lung.

Key point:

It is usually necessary to use several modalities in the assessment of these rare and 'difficult to manage' tumors; MRI is used for the assessment of local recurrence, CT for the assessment of pulmonary disease, and PET to exclude extrapulmonary disease.

CASE 14.5	Diagnosis: Sarcoma – restaging

Clinical history:

This patient had a leiomyosarcoma excised from the right chest wall followed by wedge resection of a lung metastasis in the left lower lobe. After surgery, a CT scan showed a new 1 cm nodule adjacent to the surgical sutures, the nature of which was uncertain. PET/CT was requested to determine whether the nodule reflected surgical changes or represented a new metastasis, and if there was metastatic disease outside the lung.

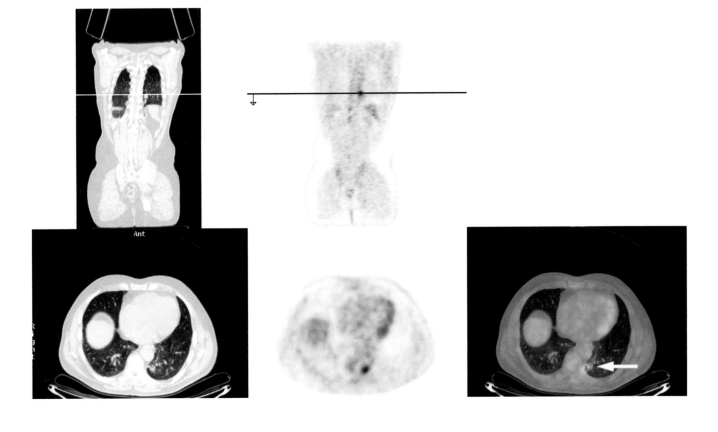

PET/CT findings:

Increased uptake was seen within the lung nodule in the left lower lobe consistent with a metastasis, but there was no evidence of extrapulmonary disease. A lung segmentectomy was performed and the lesion completely excised. Histologic examination indicated metastatic leiomyosarcoma.

Key point:

PET/CT can be used to restage disease in patients with isolated metastasis to determine if surgery is appropriate. However, CT is often more sensitive for the assessment of lung metastasis in soft-tissue sarcoma.

CASE 14.6	Diagnosis: Plasmacytoma

Clinical history:

This patient was diagnosed as having a plasmacytoma of the sixth left rib. PET/CT was requested to determine if there were additional sites of disease.

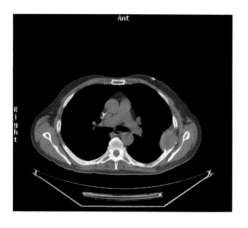

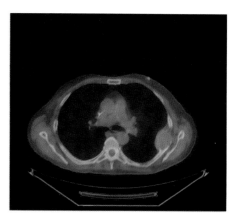

PET/CT findings:

Low-grade uptake was seen in a soft-tissue mass eroding the left sixth rib consistent with the known plasmacytoma. No other sites of disease were identified.

Key points:

1 Low or high grade uptake of FDG can be seen in plasmacytoma and in multiple myeloma. PET/CT is particularly useful in cases of 'nonsecretory' disease when there is no clinical marker.
2 PET/CT can differentiate between solitary and multiple sites of disease.

CONCLUSIONS

CURRENT INDICATIONS

Bone and Soft-tissue sarcoma

1 To direct initial biopsy
2 Staging at diagnosis
3 Restaging at relapse
4 Monitoring treatment response
5 Detection of disease in patients with apparently solitary plasmacytoma
6 Detection of relapse in patients with nonsecretory multiple myeloma

---

REFERENCES AND FURTHER READING

Aoki J, Watanabe H, Shinozaki T *et al.* (2001) FDG PET of primary benign and malignant bone tumors: standardized uptake value in 52 lesions. *Radiology* **219**, 774–7.

Ferner RE, Lucas JD, O'Doherty MJ *et al.* (2000) Evaluation of fluorodeoxyglucose positron emission tomography (FDG PET) in the detection of malignant peripheral nerve sheath tumours arising from within plexiform neurofibromas in neurofibromatosis 1. *J Neurol Neurosurg Psychiatry* **68**, 353–7.

Franzius C, Sciuk J, Daldrup-Link HE, Jurgens H, Schober O (2000) FDG-PET for detection of osseous metastases from malignant primary bone tumours: comparison with bone scintigraphy. *Eur J Nucl Med* **27**, 1305–11.

Franzius C, Bielack S, Flege S *et al.* (2002) Prognostic significance of F-FDG and (99m)Tc-methylene diphosphonate uptake in primary osteosarcoma [see comment]. *J Nucl Med* **43**, 1012–17.

Franzius C, Daldrup-Link HE, Wagner-Bohn A *et al.* (2002) FDG-PET for detection of recurrences from malignant primary bone tumors: comparison with conventional imaging. *Ann Oncol* **13**, 157–60.

Hain SF, O'Doherty MJ, Lucas JD, Smith MA (1999) Fluorodeoxyglucose PET in the evaluation of amputations for soft tissue sarcoma. *Nucl Med Comm* **20**, 845–8.

Hawkins DS, Rajendran JG, Conrad EU, Bruckner JD, Eary JF (2002) Evaluation of chemotherapy response in pediatric bone sarcomas by [F-18]-fluorodeoxy-D-glucose positron emission tomography. *Cancer* **94**, 3277–84 [erratum appears in *Cancer* **97**, 3130].

Jadvar H, Gamie S, Ramanna L, Conti PS (2004) Musculoskeletal system. *Semin Nucl Med* **34**, 254–61.

Lodge MA, Lucas JD, Marsden PK *et al.* (1999) A PET study of 18FDG uptake in soft tissue masses. *Eur J Nucl Med* **26**, 22–30.

Lucas JD, O'Doherty MJ, Wong JC *et al.* (1998) Evaluation of fluorodeoxyglucose positron emission tomography in the management of soft-tissue sarcomas. *J Bone Jt Surg [Br]* **80**, 441–7.

Lucas JD, O'Doherty MJ, Cronin BF *et al.* (1999) Prospective evaluation of soft tissue masses and sarcomas using fluorodeoxyglucose positron emission tomography. *Br J Surg* **86**, 550–6.

Orchard K, Barrington S, Buscombe J *et al.* (2002) Fluoro-deoxyglucose positron emission tomography imaging for the detection of occult disease in multiple myeloma. *Br J Haematol* **117**, 133–5.

Ries LAG, Eisner MP, Kosary CL *et al.*, eds (2004) *SEER Cancer Statistics Review, 1975–2001*. National Cancer Institute, Bethesda, MD, 2004. http://seer.cancer.gov/csr/1975_2001/

Schirrmeister H, Bommer M, Buck AK *et al.* (2002) Initial results in the assessment of multiple myeloma using 18F-FDG PET. *Eur J Nucl Med Mol Imaging* **29**, 361–6.

Schulte M, Brecht-Krauss D, Werner M *et al.* (1999) Evaluation of neoadjuvant therapy response of osteogenic sarcoma using FDG PET. *J Nucl Med* **40**, 1637–43.

Smith MA, O'Doherty MJ (2000) Positron emission tomography and the orthopaedic surgeon. *J Bone Jt Surg [Br]* **82**, 324–5.

CHAPTER 15
BRAIN TUMORS

INTRODUCTION AND BACKGROUND

Primary brain tumors have an incidence of approximately 12–15 per 100 000 of the population, and overall metastatic brain disease is more common. Usually, when a space-occupying lesion is the presenting clinical feature, a primary brain tumor rather than a metastasis is the cause – however, metastasis vs. primary tumor remains a key differential diagnostic point with histologic confirmation important when possible. In some studies, approximately 50 percent of the patients have presented with some form of epilepsy, although headaches, weakness, and altered mental state can be among the many possible presentations. Primary brain tumors are the most prevalent solid tumors in childhood and the spectrum is quite different from those in adults, with posterior fossa involvement more common in children. In many instances, biopsy of lesions carries significant risks. New treatments are being introduced, with little overall improvement in overall outcome yet seen. A wide range of therapeutic options are under study, including stereotactic biopsy and sterotactic surgery (which is frequently image guided), conformal radiotherapy, chemotherapy (more recently using agents which enhance the passage of the agents across the blood–brain barrier), and radioactive seed implantation, as well as newer biologic therapies, including vascular targeting agents and toxin conjugates. Nevertheless, the outlook remains poor, with survival less than 1 year for high-grade tumors. Imaging is increasingly required to detect disease, particularly recurrent disease, and in planning and guiding therapy and biopsy. Probably the biggest imaging difficulty at present is the failure of anatomic imaging methods to clearly differentiate recurrent tumor from scar and post-radiation effects.

Glioblastoma multiforme is the most malignant of the astrocytomas. Astrocytomas are divided into grades I–IV of malignancy with worsening prognosis. Spinal cord tumors are 10 times less frequent than brain tumors.

It is important to appreciate the changes in tumor distribution with age.

PATHOLOGY	PERCENT
Children /young adults	
Astrocytoma	60 (10 glioblastoma multiforme)
Medulloblastoma	20
Ependymoma	10
Others	10
Age >45 years	
Astrocytoma	85 (50 glioblastoma multiforme)

EPIDEMIOLOGY	
Incidence	
Men	8.9 new cases per 100 000/ 2535 cases UK
	6.7 new cases per 100 000/ 10 620 cases USA
Women	6.4 new cases per 100 000/ 1926 cases UK
	5.2 new cases per 100 000/ 7880 cases USA
Proportion of all cancers	1–2%
Age	
0–4 years	3 per 100 000
>65 years	20 per 100 000

> *Primary brain tumors generally have a poor prognosis and the higher grades, e.g. glioblastoma multiforme are essentially incurable.*

PROGNOSIS

Overall 5-year survival		
Adults	11–16%	
Children	64%	
Astrocytoma		
Low-grade	5-year survival	50–75%
Grades III and IV	Median survival	9–10 months

KEY MANAGEMENT ISSUES

KEY MANAGEMENT ISSUES

Initial management issues
- Diagnosis and grading of malignancy
- Extent for treatment planning
- Directing biopsy
- Functional assessment of perilesional cortex
- Prognosis

Post-treatment management
- Differential diagnosis of recurrence vs. radiation necrosis
- Directing biopsy
- Extent of tumor for treatment planning
- Monitoring therapy response (surgery/radiotherapy/chemotherapy)

Role of PET in primary brain tumors

Brain tumors are infrequent, but have been well studied by positron emission tomography (PET) over the past 25 years. Di Chiro and colleagues (1982) first recognized the potential of $[^{18}F]$2-fluoro-2-deoxy-D-glucose (FDG) for imaging brain tumors and reported on this approach. Based on this experience, several settings exist for the use of PET in the management of brain tumors. FDG is the most commonly used tracer, despite the limitation of its high uptake into normal brain tissue (which means background activity levels are high).

Recently it has been suggested that delayed imaging times beyond the typical 30–60 minutes may enhance the quality of FDG PET imaging of brain tumors. This is because delayed imaging times allow additional differentiation of the gray matter from the tumor due to faster dephosphorylation in the normal gray matter. It may be a reasonable strategy but has not been extensively explored.

Since the initial report from the National Institutes of Health group (Di Chiro *et al.*, 1982), many subsequent studies have examined the ability of FDG and PET to distinguish between histologically aggressive (high FDG uptake) and less aggressive (low FDG uptake) brain tumors, as well as viable tumor (persistent FDG uptake) from scar or necrosis post treatment (low or absent FDG uptake). One study did not show a separation between high- and low-grade gliomas, but, on average, the general trend of high FDG uptake substantially associated with more aggressive tumors seems true, although a great deal of overlap exists. Elevated FDG uptake in a brain tumor is generally associated with a poorer prognosis compared with brain tumors with lower levels of FDG uptake (Alavi *et al.*, 1988). Delbeke and colleagues (1995) investigated which FDG PET criteria should be used to separate high-grade from low-grade brain tumors before the patients received any treatment. They observed the best separating index to be a tumor/white matter uptake ratio of 1.5. At this cut-off level, the sensitivity and specificity of FDG-PET for high-grade tumors was 94 percent and 77 percent, respectively. Additional studies have generally shown a reasonably good correlation between the level of FDG uptake and the grade of the tumor in patients with brain tumors. These data have recently been validated in children (Borgwardt *et al.*, 2005), as well, but it should be realized that several types of pediatric brain tumor, such as pilocytic astrocytomas, can have intense FDG uptake similar to that of a high-grade tumor but be biologically relatively less aggressive (Fig. 15.1).

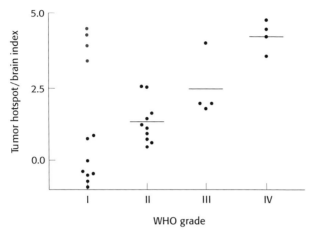

Figure 15.1 *FDG uptake in pediatric tumors correlates with the grade of malignancy, with the exception of the 'benign hypermetabolic' tumors. From Borgwardt L et al. (2005) Increased fluorine-18 2-fluoro-2-deoxy-D-glucose (FDG) uptake in childhood CNS tumors is correlated with malignancy grade: a study with FDG positron emission tomography/magnetic resonance imaging coregistration and image fusion.* J Clin Oncol **23**, 3030–3037. *Reprinted with permission from the American Society of Clinical Oncology*

There are several situations in which PET can be useful in brain tumor imaging. In actual practice, the post-treatment monitoring of brain tumors is the most common application in many medical centers. FDG allows detection of high-grade tumors, despite the fact that it has high uptake into normal brain tissue. After the completion of radiation therapy, contrast enhancement on computed tomography (CT) or magnetic resonance imaging (MRI) in the area of previous tumor mass may represent viable tumor or radiation necrosis, as both can demonstrate mass effect and both can have contrast enhancement. FDG uptake into such contrast-enhancing lesions strongly suggests the presence of viable tumor, whereas absence of FDG uptake suggests that necrosis is present (particularly if the tumor is of a higher grade and was visible on PET before the treatment). This emphasizes the importance of having a baseline FDG PET study, especially for lower-grade brain tumors, to be sure they are positive before treatment (i.e. have higher FDG uptake than white matter). Alternatively, as is shown in the case examples in this chapter, [11C]L-methionine can be very helpful in delineating the location of lower-grade brain tumors not well seen on PET with FDG. Indeed, [11C]L-methionine, although probably providing less robust prognostic data than FDG, has in most studies been shown to be superior to FDG for detection of recurrent brain tumors. To date, qualitative visual analysis, in which FDG uptake is compared with normal white or gray matter, is generally used for analysis in preference to quantitative analysis. This approach generally means that any focus of activity which has more intense tracer uptake than normal brain white matter is considered to represent viable tumor. The reason FDG uptake appears to correlate with survival and tumor grade is not yet fully clear. It may be related to the increased cellular density seen in high-grade tumors or may be related to increased FDG uptake in the more rapidly proliferating tumor cells. These correlations are often relatively modest but usually statistically relevant.

Representative studies comparing FDG PET and histology/outcome after brain tumor therapy include that of Di Chiro *et al.* (1987), who reported that PET with FDG appropriately diagnosed necrosis present in all 10 of the 10 patients with necrosis from a group of 95 suspected of having necrosis following brain tumor therapy. Valk *et al.* (1988) reported a rate of 84 percent accuracy of PET in determining if necrosis was present or absent following interstitial brachytherapy for brain tumors. They pointed out that PET scan results were more reliable predictors of outcome than histological results, which often showed some 'viable' cells after treatment but of questionable 'viability' clinically.

Some low-grade tumors have low FDG uptake, yet in other cases high uptake of FDG can be seen in tumors which have evidence of contrast enhancement on CT but are associated with a good prognosis – as in juvenile pilocytic astrocytomas (Fulham *et al.*, 1993). In the situation of low-grade gliomas, other tracers, such as [^{11}C]L-methionine, [^{11}C]thymidine, or [^{11}C]putrescine, may potentially represent reasonable choices for PET tumor imaging in the brain, in contrast with FDG only (Bergstrom *et al.*, 1987). These latter tracers have only a low level of uptake into normal brain and thus often allow for higher tumor/background uptake ratios than FDG. [^{11}C]L-Methionine has been shown not to accumulate in focal radiation necrosis in the relatively small numbers of patients studied to date and to accumulate in many low-grade gliomas. Bergstrom *et al.* (1987) reported that 7/11 low-grade gliomas had increased uptake of [^{11}C]L-methionine compared with normal brain. Roelcke and colleagues (1996) showed that [^{11}C]L-methionine uptake is correlated with ^{82}Rb uptake across a wide range of histologies. This is not the case with FDG. This observation suggests that a significant component of [^{11}C]L-methionine uptake into higher grade tumors may be due to blood–brain barrier alteration, as opposed to incorporation into tumor protein. This, coupled with Ogawa *et al.*'s (1995) report stating that there is some [^{11}C]L-methionine uptake into intracerebral hematomas not caused by tumors, indicates that some caution must still be exercised when attempting to determine if a focus of residual contrast enhancement after brain tumor therapy is due to necrosis or viable tumor, at least when using [^{11}C]L-methionine. Thus, FDG remains better established in this specific clinical setting.

Untreated central nervous system (CNS) lymphomas are well imaged by FDG PET, with FDG uptake into the lymphomas similar to that seen in high-grade gliomas. The uptake is higher in CNS lymphoma than in CNS infections – a situation which may be useful for diagnosis in the human immunodeficiency virus (HIV)-positive patient.

Although FDG is clearly valuable in imaging primary brain tumors, especially high-grade tumors, data on imaging intra-axial metastases to brain are much more limited. Griffeth *et al.* (1993) reported that FDG uptake into untreated metastases from a variety of cancers was inadequate for satisfactory visualization of metastases (up to a third of patients in their study). This is particularly the case when small lesions are located in close proximity to gray matter folds in the brain. This has also been reported by one of our centers (Larcos and Maisey, 1996), where several instances of failure to detect metastatic lung cancer to brain were reported.

Meningiomas can also be imaged with PET. In a series of 17 patients, Di Chiro *et al.* (1987) reported that those tumors with the highest FDG uptake appeared to have the most aggressive histologic appearance, whereas those with low FDG uptake appeared to have a less aggressive histology. Patients with tumors with low FDG uptake were found to have the greatest likelihood for long-term survival. It is uncertain if low FDG uptake in a meningioma would suggest that surgery could be delayed, but such metabolic information may be a useful adjunct in challenging cases.

Two other clinical issues in brain tumor management are well addressed by PET:

- localization of active tumor for biopsy is more accurate with PET than CT in some cases
- [^{15}O]water activation PET can also define areas of the cerebral cortex that are activated during motor or visual stimulation by undertaking [^{15}O]water blood flow studies at rest and during a task that activates the cerebral cortex.

These data on the exact location of functional cortical areas can then be superimposed on MRI structural data to assist planning of surgical procedures, the goal being to excise all the tumor but spare normal tissue as much as possible. In many centers, MRI has replaced PET for this role as [^{15}O]water studies are not widely available.

Brain tumor treatment is quite commonly monitored with PET if there is a difficult diagnostic question after treatment. A decline in FDG uptake in a tumor at several weeks to months after the conclusion of therapy suggests a good response of the tumor to treatment. In contrast, an increase in FDG uptake compared with the basal level, or persistent FDG uptake, would strongly suggest residual tumor being present despite treatment. Responses of glucose metabolism immediately after treatment are less clear, however, so assessing response is not currently justified if done only a few days after a treatment is given. Indeed, the optimal time to assess treatment is still unclear, but it would seem to be safest if done well after the treatment course is completed. Given the resolution of current PET devices, they are not expected to detect microscopic foci of tumor, so a negative scan does not completely exclude the possibility of residual tumor being present. The greatest difficulties in assessing treatment response with PET seem to be in patients with low-grade tumors. In this setting, [^{11}C]L-methionine may be useful if available.

EXAMPLES TO ILLUSTRATE KEY ISSUES

CASE 15.1	Diagnosis: Low-grade glioma

Clinical history:

This patient was referred with a left frontoparietal lesion present on MR scanning. PET was requested to characterize the lesion.

(a)

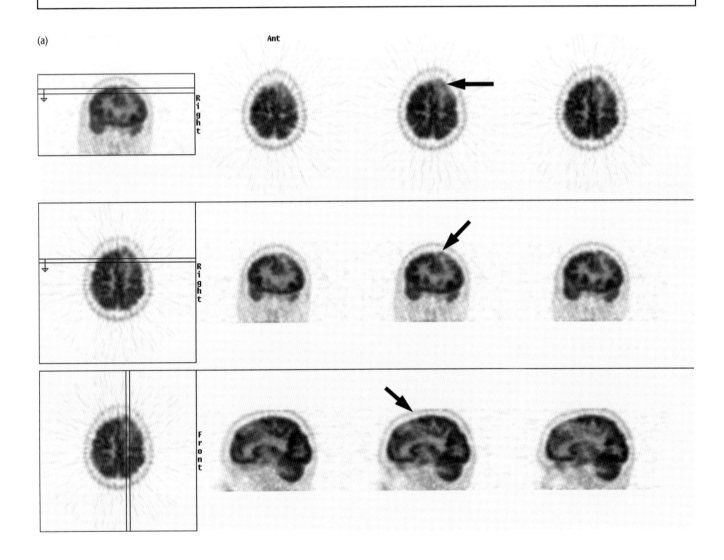

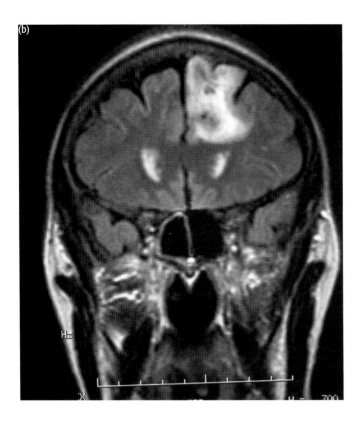

(b)

PET findings:

Only low-grade uptake was seen at the site of the lesion (a) seen on MRI (b) compatible with low-grade tumor.

Key point:

Low-grade tumors have uptake lower or equal to normal cortex on FDG scanning.

CASE 15.2 | **Diagnosis: Brain tumor – characterization of lesion**

Clinical history:

This patient was referred with focal seizures and a tumor in the right parietal lobe. The patient was not keen to have a biopsy. PET was requested to characterize the lesion.

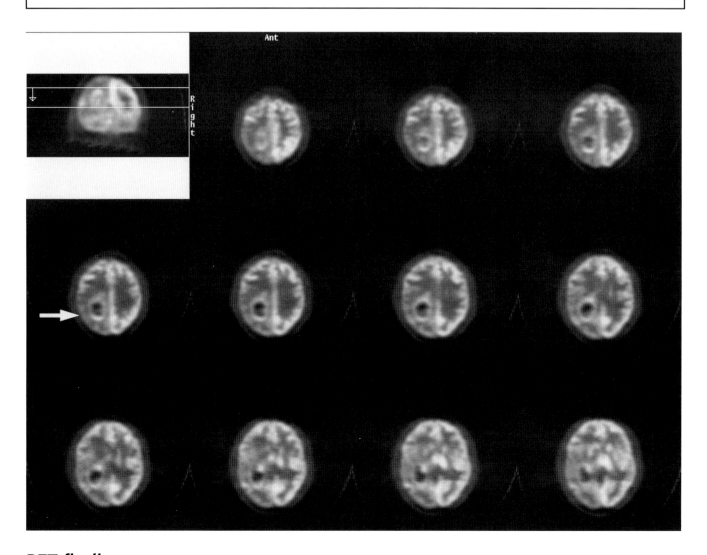

PET findings:

A rim of high FDG uptake was present around a photopenic centre indicative of a high-grade tumor with central necrosis. The patient was referred for radiotherapy.

Key points:

1 PET can characterize primary brain tumors as high- or low-grade and give useful prognostic information when planning treatment.
2 PET can direct biopsy of tumor when there is central necrosis.
3 Since metastases can also present as solitary brain masses, whole-body PET may also be considered reasonable if the tumor histology is not known.

CASE 15.3 | Diagnosis: Brain metastases from lung cancer

Clinical history:

This elderly patient presented with confusion, dysphasia and dysarthria, and right-sided weakness. CT scan of the brain showed metastases. Chest radiograph and CT scan of the chest did not show an obvious primary. PET was requested to locate a primary tumor.

(a)

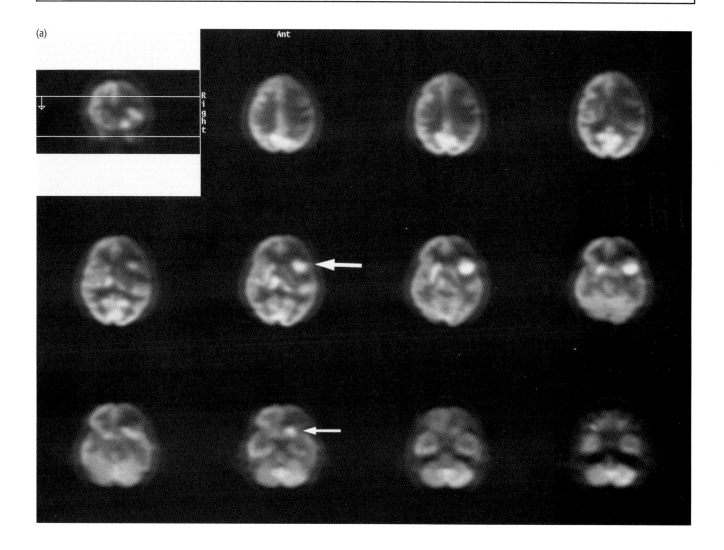

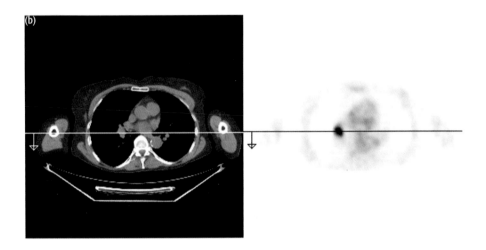

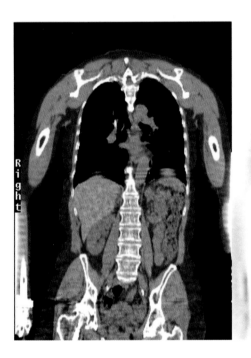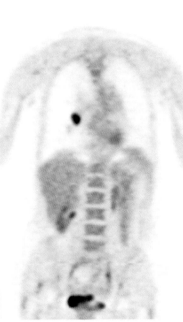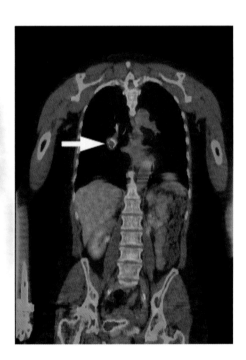

PET findings:

Uptake was increased in a large focus in the left parietal lobe and a smaller focus in the left frontotemporal region (a). There was also ipsilateral hypometabolism in the peritumoral region and basal ganglia and thalamus on the left. In addition there was reduced right cerebellar metabolism consistent with crossed cerebellar diaschisis. Increased uptake was also seen at the right lung hilum (b) suggesting a lung primary tumor. Bronchoscopy was performed, and malignant squamous cells obtained from bronchoalveolar lavage.

Key points:

1 Uptake in brain metastases can be variable and some metastases from lung cancer may have uptake similar to normal cortex. PET may miss metastatic brain disease. MRI or CT are usually better for detection of brain secondaries.
2 PET can be used to detect the primary site where there are known secondaries.

| CASE 15.4 | Diagnosis: Benign tumor – hamartoma |

Clinical history:

This 3-year-old child was investigated for complex partial seizures. She was found to have a lesion on MRI (a,b) in the right frontal lobe. PET was requested to characterize the lesion.

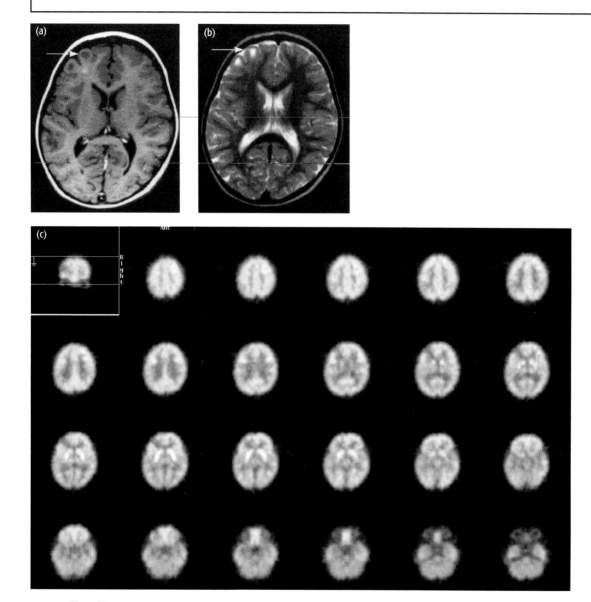

PET findings:

There was only low-grade uptake at the site of the lesion suggestive of a benign or low-grade tumor (c). At surgery the lesion proved to be a hamartoma.

Key point:

PET can characterize brain lesions and determine appropriate management; in this case surgery was undertaken not because of suspected malignancy but to control the epilepsy.

CASE 15.5	Functional assessment of perilesional cortex

History:

PET was requested to establish the proximity of tumor to important functional brain areas to determine the feasibility of surgery.

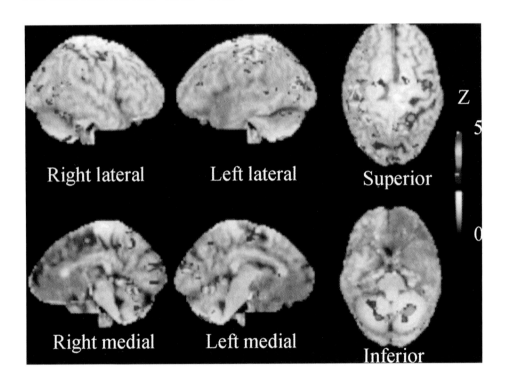

PET study:

An activation study was undertaken while the patient was tapping his finger. Note that due to the mass lesions normal brain might be significantly displaced.

Key point:

The color bar (Z score) refers to the number of standard deviations by which the uptake differs from normal data.

CASE 15.6	Diagnosis: Recurrent high-grade tumor

Clinical history:

This patient was referred with a history of glioblastoma multiforme treated with surgery, chemotherapy, and radiotherapy 4 years earlier. MRI showed a 5 cm mass with edema suggestive of recurrent tumor (a).

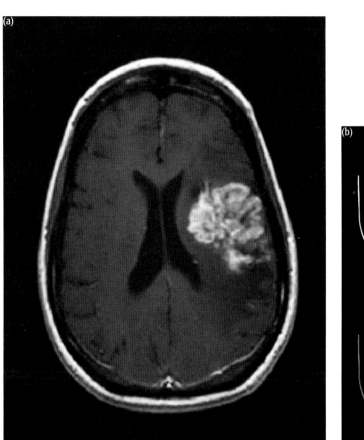

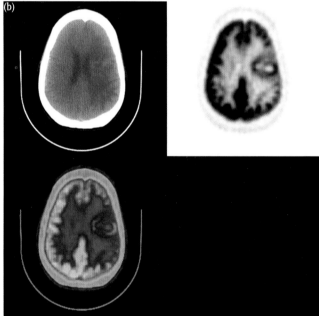

PET findings:

Increased metabolic activity was associated with the mass in the inferoposterior aspect of the left frontal lobe compatible with recurrence (b). Note also the diffuse decreased activity in the left frontal region, consistent with post-radiation changes (b).

Key point:

PET can identify metabolic changes associated with recurrent tumor.

CASE 15.7	Diagnosis: High-grade recurrence

Clinical history:

This 46-year-old man had been previously treated with radiotherapy and chemotherapy for high-grade glioma. He presented with symptoms suggestive of recurrence. PET was requested to determine if there was recurrence and the extent of disease.

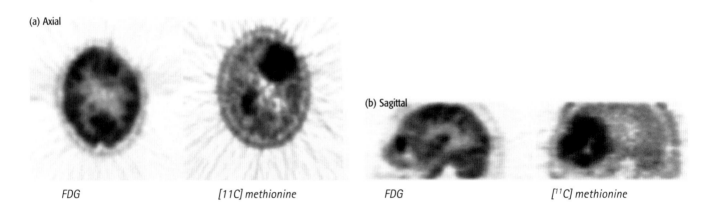

(a) Axial

FDG 　　　　　　　[11C] methionine 　　　　　　　(b) Sagittal

FDG 　　　　　　　[¹¹C] methionine

PET findings:

There was high-grade uptake of FDG in the left frontal lobe and of [¹¹C]methionine in the left frontal and the right parietal lobes, indicating recurrence at these sites.

Key points:

1 FDG and methionine are complementary tracers in scanning brain tumors.
2 Note that FDG confirmed recurrence but the uptake of methionine was greater relative to FDG, such that the extent of recurrent tumor, especially in the right parietal lobe, can only be appreciated with methionine.
3 Methionine often shows uptake in both low- and high-grade tumors so does not give the same prognostic information as FDG but the higher contrast between methionine and normal brain can be an advantage when scanning low-grade tumors.
4 False-positive uptake can occur with methionine where there is disruption of the blood–brain barrier by processes other than tumor, including intracerebral hematoma.

CASE 15.8	Diagnosis: Post-treatment fibrosis

Clinical history:

This young child had undergone multiple surgery, chemotherapy, and radiotherapy for an anaplastic ependymoma. Although she was neurologically stable with a left hemiplegia, she complained of new headaches. MRI showed an enhancing region in the right parietal lobe suggestive of recurrent disease. PET was requested to determine if this represented post-treatment change or recurrent tumor.

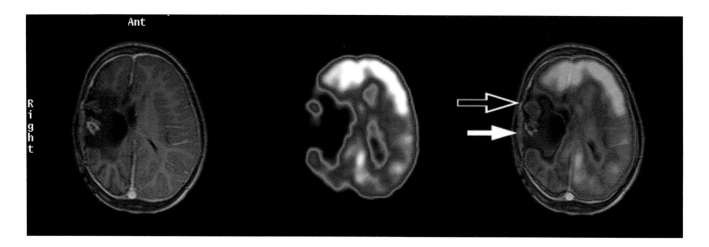

PET findings:

The PET was registered to the MR scan. The area of enhancing tissue seen on MRI did not take up FDG (solid arrow) indicating this was likely to be scar or inflammatory tissue. The small focus of FDG uptake (broken arrow) also present in the right parietal region corresponded to an island of normal cortex on MRI. There was no evidence of disease recurrence. The child remained well on follow-up.

Key points:

1 PET can differentiate active malignancy from post-treatment change.
2 PET findings should be interpreted in context with anatomic imaging.

CASE 15.9	Diagnosis: Medulloblastoma – treatment response

Clinical history:

This child had an incomplete resection of a medulloblastoma. PET was requested to assess the extent of residual tumor and to monitor the effects of chemotherapy treatment.

(a)

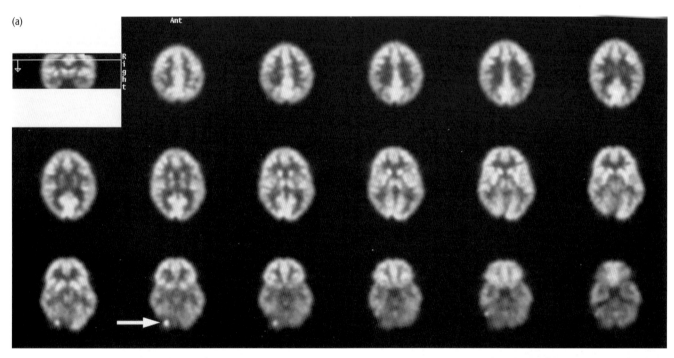

(b)

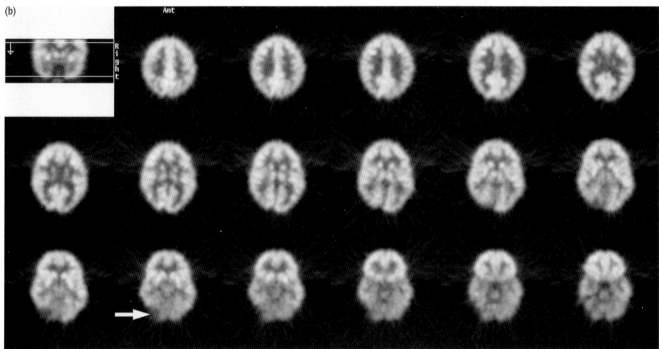

PET findings:

There was high uptake in the tumor in the right cerebellar hemisphere prior to chemotherapy (a) which completely resolved following treatment (b). She remains disease free several years later.

Key points:

PET can provide helpful information in monitoring treatment with chemotherapy in selected cases.

CASE 15.10	Diagnosis: Lymphoma and HIV encephalopathy

Clinical history:

This patient with HIV disease was referred with a lesion on MRI in the right parietal lobe, the nature of which was uncertain.

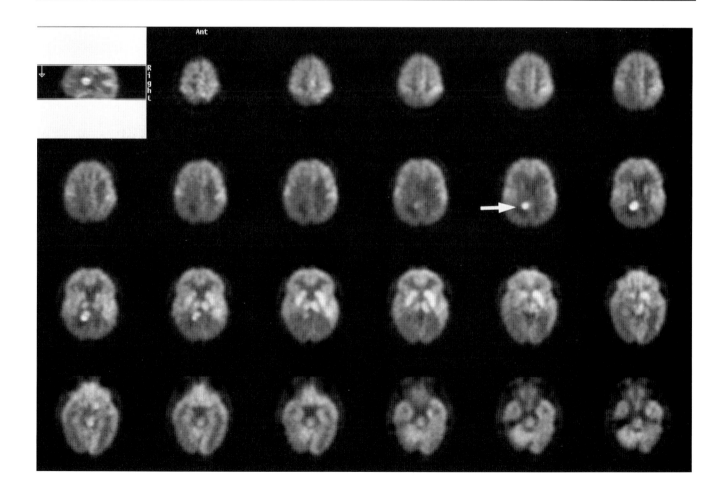

PET/CT findings:

There was a focus of intense uptake in the right parietal lobe posterior to the thalamus. Biopsy of the lesion revealed lymphoma. Note also global reduction of uptake in the cerebral cortex with preservation of uptake in the basal ganglia and thalamus – typical features of HIV encephalopathy.

Key points:

PET can help to differentiate between intracerebral infection (commonly toxoplasmosis) which has no or low-grade FDG uptake and intracerebral malignancy (commonly lymphoma) in patients with HIV disease presenting with neurological illness. Contrast this with Case 15.11.

CASE 15.11	Diagnosis: Cerebral toxoplasmosis

Clinical history:

This patient with newly diagnosed HIV presented with a 6-week history of headache and increasing confusion associated with fever. MRI showed a lesion centered on the right lentiform nucleus with surrounding edema and mass effect, consistent with toxoplasmosis or lymphoma (a). PET was requested to characterize the lesion.

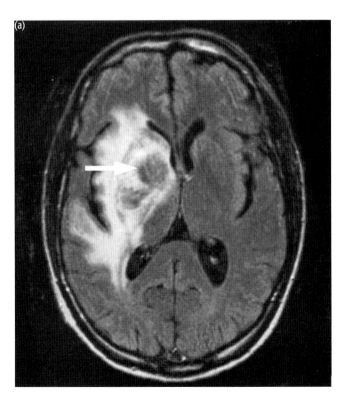

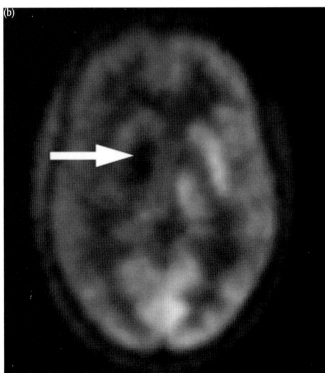

PET findings:

There was a photopenic defect corresponding to the lesion on MRI consistent with toxoplasmosis and not lymphoma (b). Note also diffuse reduction in the right frontoparietal region. The patient was treated with antitoxoplasmosis therapy and showed good clinical response.

Key point:

Contrast with Case 15.10 which showed high uptake of FDG in cerebral lymphoma.

CONCLUSIONS

CURRENT CLINICAL INDICATIONS

1 Diagnosis of recurrence when differentiation of scar/necrosis unclear on MRI/CT
2 Diagnosis when there is contraindication to biopsy or failed biopsy
3 Direction of biopsy where the site of tumor is unclear on MRI
4 Planning treatment when the extent of tumor is unclear on MRI
5 Monitoring response to chemotherapy/radiotherapy
6 Helping assess grade of tumor
7 Suspected high-grade transformation of low-grade tumor
8 Differentiation of intracerebral malignancy from infection in HIV disease

POSSIBLE INDICATIONS

1 Prediction of chemotherapy response
2 Conformal or brachytherapy planning
3 Activation studies to locate normal functional cortical regions preoperatively

REFERENCES AND FURTHER READING

Alavi JB, Alavi A, Chawluk J *et al.* (1988) Positron emission tomography in patients with glioma. *Cancer* **62**, 1074–8.

Barker FG 2nd, Chang SM, Valk PE, Pounds TR, Prados MD (1997) 18-Fluorodeoxyglucose uptake and survival of patients with suspected recurrent malignant glioma. *Cancer* **79**, 115–26.

Bergstrom M, Lundqvist H, Ericson K *et al.* (1987) Comparison of the accumulation kinetics of L-(methyl-11C)-methionine and D-(methyl-11C)-methionine in brain tumors studied with positron emission tomography. *Acta Radiol* **28**, 225–9.

Borgwardt L, Hojgaard L, Carstensen H *et al.* (2005) Increased fluorine-18 2-fluoro-2-deoxy-D-glucose (FDG) uptake in childhood CNS tumors is correlated with malignancy grade: a study with FDG positron emission tomography/magnetic resonance imaging coregistration and image fusion. *J Clin Oncol* **23**, 3030–7.

Delbeke D, Meyerowitz C, Lapidus R *et al.* (1995) Optimal cutoff levels of 18F fluorodeoxyglucose uptake in the differentiation of low-grade from high-grade brain tumors with PET. *Radiology* **195**, 47–52.

Di Chiro G, DeLaPaz RL, Brooks RA *et al.* (1982) Glucose utilization of cerebral gliomas measured by [^{18}F] fluorodeoxyglucose and positron emission tomography. *Neurology* **32**, 1323–9.

Di Chiro G, Hatazawa J, Katz DA *et al.* (1987) Glucose utilization by intracranial meningiomas as an index of tumor aggressivity and probability of recurrence: a PET study. *Radiology* **164**, 521–6.

Francavilla TL, Miletich RS, Di Chiro G. (1989) Positron emission tomography in the detection of malignant degeneration of low-grade gliomas. *Neurosurgery* **24**, 1–5.

Fulham MJ, Melisi JW, Nishimiya J *et al.* (1993) Neuroimaging of juvenile pilocytic astrocytomas: an enigma. *Radiology* **189**, 221–5.

Giammarile F, Cinotti LE, Jouvet A *et al.* (2004) High and low grade oligodendrogliomas (ODG): correlation of amino-acid and glucose uptakes using PET and histological classifications. *J Neurooncol* **68**, 263–74.

Griffeth LK, Rich KM, Dehdashti F *et al.* (1993) Brain metastases from non-central nervous system tumors: evaluation with PET. *Radiology* **186**, 37–44

Hoffman JM, Waskin HA, Schifter T *et al.* (1993) FDG-PET in differentiating lymphoma from nonmalignant central nervous system lesions in patients with AIDS. *J Nucl Med* **34**, 567–75.

Hustinx R, Pourdehnad M, Kaschten B, Alavi A. (2005) PET imaging for differentiating recurrent brain tumor from radiation necrosis. *Radiol Clin North Am* **43**, 35–47.

Ito M, Lammertsma AA, Wise RJ *et al.* (1982) Measurement of regional cerebral blood flow and oxygen utilisation in patients with cerebral tumours using ^{15}O and positron emission tomography: analytical techniques and preliminary results. *Neuroradiology* **23**, 63–74.

Larcos G, Maisey MN (1996) FDG-PET screening for cerebral metastases in patients with suspected malignancy. *Nucl Med Commun* **17**, 197–8.

O'Doherty MJ, Barrington SF, Campbell M, Lowe J, Bradbeer CS (1997) PET scanning and the HIV positive patient. *J Nucl Med* **38**, 1575–83.

Ogawa T, Shisodo F, Kanno I *et al.* (1993) Cerebral glioma: evaluation with Methionine PET. *Radiology* **186**, 45–53.

Ogawa T, Hatazawa J, Inugami A *et al.* (1995) Carbon-11-methionine PET evaluation of intracerebral hematoma: distinguishing neoplastic from non-neoplastic hematoma. *J Nucl Med* **36**, 2175–9.

Patronas NJ, Di Chiro G, Brooks RA *et al.* (1982) Work in progress: [18F] fluorodeoxyglucose and positron emission tomography in the evaluation of radiation necrosis of the brain. *Radiology* **144**, 885–9.

Pirotte B, Goldman S, Bidaut LM *et al.* (1995) Use of positron emission tomography (PET) in stereotactic conditions for brain biopsy. *Acta Neurochir* **134**, 79–82.

Pirotte B, Goldman S, Massager N *et al.* (2004) Combined use of 18F-fluorodeoxyglucose and 11C-methionine in 45 positron emission tomography-guided stereotactic brain biopsies. *J Neurosurg* **101**, 476–83.

Roelcke U, Radu E, Ametamey S *et al.* (1996) Association of [82]rubidium and ^{11}C-methionine uptake in brain tumors measured by positron emission tomography. *J Neuro Oncol* **27**, 163–72.

Spence AM, Mankoff DA, Muzi M (2003) Positron emission tomography imaging of brain tumors. *Neuroimaging Clin North Am* **13**, 717–39.

Spence AM, Muzi M, Mankoff DA *et al.* (2004) 18F-FDG PET of gliomas at delayed intervals: improved distinction between tumor and normal gray matter. *J Nucl Med* **45**, 1653–9.

Tsuyuguchi N, Takami T, Sunada I *et al.* (2004) Methionine positron emission tomography for differentiation of recurrent brain tumor and radiation necrosis after stereotactic radiosurgery – in malignant glioma. *Ann Nucl Med* **18**, 291–6.

Utriainen M, Metsahonkala L, Salmi TT *et al.* (2002) Metabolic characterization of childhood brain tumors: comparison of 18F-fluorodeoxyglucose and 11C-methionine positron emission tomography. *Cancer* **95**, 1376–86.

Valk P, Budinger T, Levin V *et al.* (1988) PET of malignant cerebral tumors after interstitial brachytherapy. *J Neurosurg* **69**, 830–8.

Van Laere K, Ceyssens S, Van Calenbergh F *et al.* (2005) Direct comparison of 18F-FDG and 11C-methionine PET in suspected recurrence of glioma: sensitivity, inter-observer variability and prognostic value. *Eur J Nucl Med Mol Imaging* **32**, 39–51.

CHAPTER 16

PEDIATRIC ONCOLOGY

EVA A WEGNER

INTRODUCTION

The role of positron emission tomography (PET) in adult oncology has been well documented (Gambhir *et al.*, 2001). There are fewer evidence-based guidelines available for scanning in pediatric oncology. The extensive knowledge of PET scanning in adults is often extrapolated to children, notwithstanding the differences in tumor types and disease behavior, normal variants, and scan procedures and protocols. However, the role of PET in pediatric oncology is slowly emerging, as PET and PET/CT scanning in children becomes more widespread.

CLINICAL APPLICATIONS

PET scanning can be used for accurate initial staging of cancer, early prediction of response to treatment, evaluation of residual masses, in biopsy planning, in radiotherapy planning, and to establish suspected disease recurrence (Table 16.1). In a review of our 10-year experience at Guy's and St Thomas' Clinical PET Centre, PET altered the management of 24 percent of children with cancer (Wegner *et al.*, 2005). This is comparable with management changes due to a PET scan seen in adults with cancer (30 percent) (Gambhir *et al.*, 2001). The referring clinicians considered PET to be helpful in 75 percent of the pediatric cases scanned, even if the results did not lead to management change. In these cases PET was considered 'helpful' because it confirmed clinical suspicion, clarified equivocal results of other studies, confirmed the need for further treatment or guided biopsy (Wegner *et al.*, 2005). Krasin *et al.* (2004) argue that the PET scan can be used to modify the radiation dose and the volume of radiotherapy field in children with cancer.

In pediatric oncology, the most common diagnoses for which PET scanning has been used are Hodgkin disease (HD) and non-Hodgkin lymphoma (NHL), central

Table 16.1 Indications (percent) for scanning in pediatric oncology at Guy's and St Thomas' Clinical PET Centre over 10 years (Wegner *et al.*, 2005)

Reason for referral for a PET scan	Diagnosis				
	Lymphoma *n*=63	CNS tumors *n*=62	Sarcoma *n*=30	Neurofibroma *n*=16	Other *n*=18
Help with diagnosis	5	23	}30	–	17
Staging	8	5		–	11
Monitoring disease	5	19	50	–	}33
Therapy response	17	}26	7	–	
Residual mass	49		–	–	–
Suspected recurrence	16	27	13	–	39
Suspected malignant transformation	–	–	–	100	–

nervous system (CNS) tumors, and bone and soft-tissue sarcoma. PET has also been used for imaging neuroblastoma, malignant peripheral nerve sheath tumors, Wilms tumors, and occasionally for other malignancies such as testicular or thyroid cancer (Shulkin, 1997; Wegner *et al.*, 2005).

Childhood lymphoma represents 10–15 percent of pediatric malignancies. It differs from adult HD and NHL in terms of histopathology and therapeutic strategies, and therefore the results of studies in adults should not be extrapolated to children. With cure rates of up to 90 percent, the therapeutic strategies aim to minimize treatment and the long-term sequelae. Nonetheless, aggressive, early treatment is required for high-grade, extensive forms of the disease. The role of PET in adult patients with lymphoma has been extensively documented. Many of such studies included patients under the age of 18 years. Relatively few studies concentrate on the role of PET in pediatric lymphoma. These data are, however, slowly emerging. A PET scan takes a relatively short time to acquire, results can be obtained on the same day and it has a significantly lower radiation dose than [^{67}Ga]citrate, which, until recently, has been the standard imaging modality used in lymphoma (Stabin and Gelfand, 1998). Montravers *et al.* (2002) reported that PET had 100 percent sensitivity in staging and restaging childhood lymphoma. PET detected more sites than conventional imaging and upstaged the disease in 24–50 percent of cases. Management was changed in 10–32 percent of cases (Montravers *et al.*, 2002; Depas *et al.*, 2005; Hermann *et al.*, 2005; Wegner *et al.*, 2005). The negative predictive value of PET following treatment was 89–93 percent (Depas *et al.*, 2005; Hermann *et al.*, 2005).

Imaging of CNS tumors was one of the first clinical applications of PET scanning. Much work has been done in adult neuro-oncology, however these data cannot be extrapolated to children, considering the differences in histologic tumor types and different tumor behavior in children. It has been shown that the intensity of [^{18}F]2-fluoro-2-deoxy-D-glucose (FDG) uptake correlates with the grade of brain tumours, while [^{11}C]methionine can delineate the extent of the disease. PET therefore has a role in assessing the tumor grade and thus indirectly assessing the prognosis, localizing the best site for biopsy, assessing the response to treatment, differentiating radiation necrosis from tumor recurrence in the presence of equivocal anatomic imaging, and excluding high-grade transformation (Robinson *et al.*, 1999). In one study PET altered management of CNS tumors in 16 percent of cases, most commonly by changing from active treatment to observation (Wegner *et al.*, 2005).

COMMON PITFALLS

Accuracy of PET findings can vary depending on tumor type, location, and scan timing in relation to treatment. The possible sources of error have been described previously (Cook *et al.*, 1999, 2004). Normal scan appearances in children may be different than in adults. FDG uptake in brown fat or skeletal muscles is common in young patients and may mimic malignancy. This is particularly true in children with lymphoma, as the brown fat is located in the areas commonly involved in disease such as the neck, the mediastinum, the axillae, the supraclavicular fossae, and the paraspinal regions (Hany *et al.*, 2002; Yeung *et al.*, 2003). Keeping the patient in a warm environment and administration of oral diazepam may reduce the tracer uptake in the brown fat and the muscle (Barrington and Maisey, 1996).

FDG uptake in thymic tissue is a further unique problem frequently encountered in children. This phenomenon is observed equally in children before or after chemotherapy (73 percent vs. 75 percent, respectively). It is thought to be due to increased metabolic activity in the normal thymus before puberty and/or due to reactive thymic hyperplasia, for example following treatment, acute infection, or stress (Brink et al., 2001). FDG-avid thymic tissue has also been demonstrated in 34 percent of healthy young adults on screening PET scans (Nakahara et al., 2001). Familiarity with normal appearances is essential to distinguish between physiologic thymic uptake and active disease in the mediastinum. This is particularly important in children with potentially curable diseases such as lymphoma, as they often have residual tissue in the mediastinum following treatment. The normal thymic appearances can be described as homogeneous λ-shaped uptake in the anterior mediastinum. In contrast, abnormal uptake may be focal or markedly increased in a disproportionally enlarged thymus or within the mediastinal mass. Presence or absence of active disease determines further chemotherapy and/or radiotherapy, which carry the risks of short-term and long-term complications, such as secondary malignancies and cardiovascular disease (Valagussa et al., 1992; Boivin et al., 1995).

It is important to recognize the normal developmental changes in cerebral glucose metabolism. In newborns, the most metabolically active areas are the sensorimotor cortex, thalamus, brain stem, and the cerebellar vermis. The uptake in the parietal, temporal, and primary visual cortex is similar to that of an adult brain by 2–3 months, followed by the frontal cortex at 6–12 months. At 2–3 years the FDG uptake has the same distribution as in an adult brain, however, it is more intense. This gradually decreases to the level seen in adult brains by early teenage years (Chugani et al., 1986).

PRACTICAL ASPECTS

Patient cooperation is a significant issue in imaging children. PET scanning usually requires the patient to remain still for a prolonged period of time. Fortunately, due to advances in technology allowing shorter scanning times and larger fields of view, the length of time required for PET imaging has reduced substantially. Most children with cancer have had previous imaging (computed tomography (CT) or magnetic resonance imaging (MRI)) and can cooperate with a PET study. Successful imaging can be facilitated by providing a relaxed, child-oriented environment, and staff experienced in pediatric venipuncture and dealing with children. With adequate preparation and communication with both the parents and the child it is possible to obtain good quality diagnostic images (Pintelon et al., 1992; Borgwardt et al., 2003; Roberts and Shulkin, 2004). The parents usually know if the child had any problems cooperating with imaging previously and if sedation or general anesthetic will be required. If so, guidelines are available for sedation of children (Pintelon et al., 1992; Weiss, 1993).

DOSIMETRY

As with all imaging using ionizing radiation, dosimetry requires special consideration in children undergoing PET scanning. The administered activity can be calculated as: the patient's weight (kg) multiplied by the adult activity (MBq) and divided by 70 kg. An alternative method involves calculating the dose based on the body surface area (Paediatric Task Group of the European Association of Nuclear Medicine, 1990). The effective dose (ED) following an FDG PET study was calculated (from animal and human data) by Stabin et al. (1998), based on administered activity of 2.59 MBq/kg. The ED for a newborn child was 1.9 mSv, for a

1-year-old 2.5 mSv, for a 5-year-old 2.8 mSv, for a 10-year-old 3.2 m Sv, and for 15-year-old 4.3 mSv. In comparison, adult ED was calculated to be 4.4 mSv. Ruotsalainen *et al.* (1996) calculated that following an FDG PET study in a newborn child, the bladder wall received 1.03 ± 2.10 mGy/MBq and the heart received 0.89 ± 0.26 mGy/MBq. This appears to be lower than the radiation doses received in many other nuclear medicine studies and significantly lower than the ED following [^{67}Ga]-citrate study (Ruotsalainen *et al.*, 1996; Stabin *et al.*, 1998). It needs to be stressed that in both these studies the calculated radiation doses from FDG were based on administered activity which is lower than usually given in clinical practice.

With the continuing improvement in technology and the development of a new generation of scanners with higher sensitivity (such as PET/CT), there is potential for further reduction in administered activity. The dosimetry related to the CT component of the PET/CT will depend on a variety of factors. Recently high-resolution CT scans of the chest in children were evaluated using 34 mAs, 50 mAs, and 180 mAs (Lucaya *et al.*, 2000). Good quality images were obtained using the 34 mAs settings in cooperative children and 50 mAs in non-cooperative children. The results suggested that more work needs to be done on optimizing CT acquisition protocols in the combined PET/CT scanners to further reduce radiation doses to children.

EXAMPLES TO ILLUSTRATE KEY ISSUES

CASE 16.1	Diagnosis: Hodgkin disease – treatment response

Clinical history:

This teenager presented with cough and wheeze, which did not respond to antibiotic treatment and steroids. A chest radiograph revealed a mediastinal mass. Biopsy of the mass showed T lymphoblastic lymphoma. PET/CT was requested to stage the disease at diagnosis and to monitor treatment.

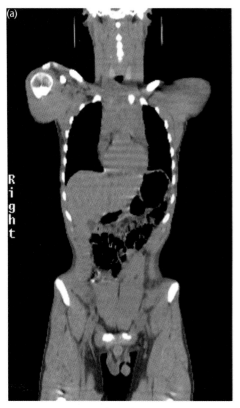
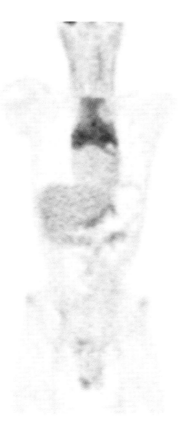
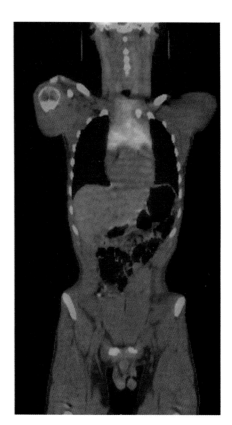

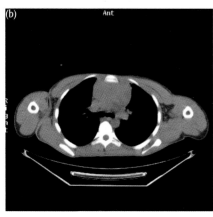
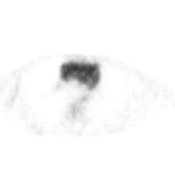
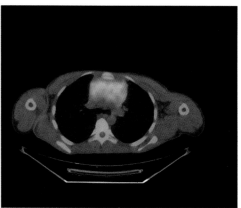

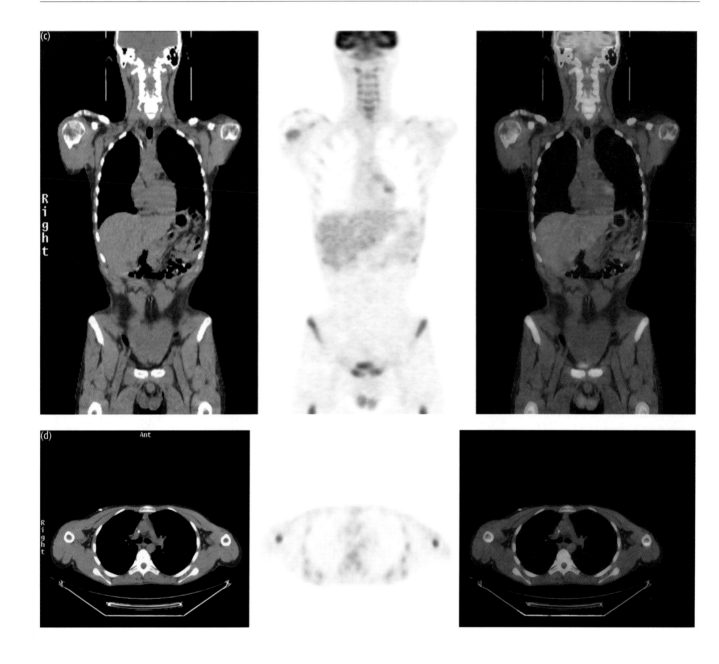

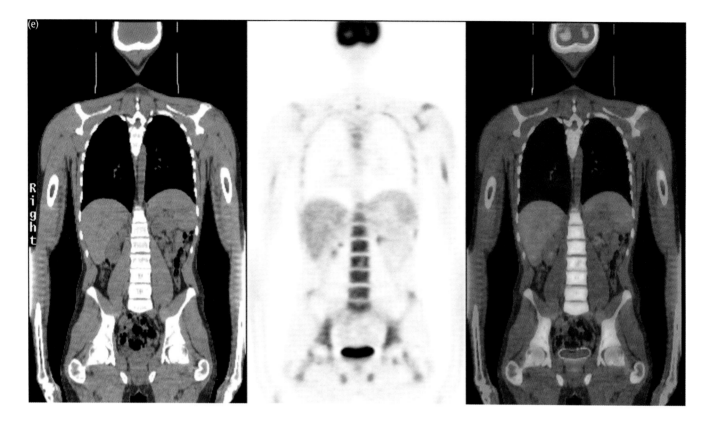

PET/CT findings:

There was high uptake of FDG in the mediastinal mass at staging (a, b) which resolved completely at the end of chemotherapy (c, d) Note the diffusely increased uptake in the bone marrow secondary to treatment (e).

Key points:

1 PET/CT is used to stage pediatric and adult lymphoma as it is more sensitive than CT.
2 The staging scan is helpful as a baseline to assess treatment response.
3 PET/CT influences management in pediatric oncology practice in a similar way to adult oncology practice.

CASE 16.2	Diagnosis: Hodgkin disease – treatment response

Clinical history:

Scan 1, (a): This 12-year-old child had residual right paratracheal lymphadenopathy and an anterior mediastinal mass at the end of six cycles of chemotherapy. PET was requested to determine disease activity in the residual lymphadenopathy.

Scan 2, (b): The child was treated with further high-dose chemotherapy. PET/CT was requested to evaluate treatment response.

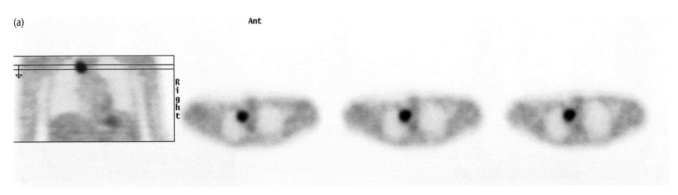

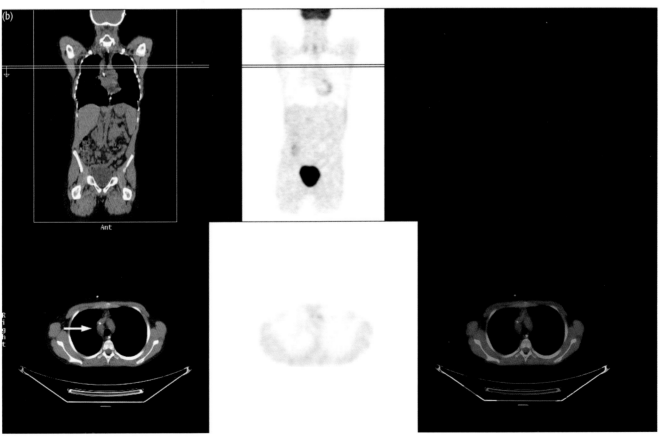

PET/CT findings:

Scan 1, (a) (PET scan): High uptake in the right paratracheal region was indicative of residual active lymphoma at this site.

Scan 2, (b) (PET/CT scan): Following further treatment there was complete resolution of uptake in the residual right paratracheal lymphadenopathy (see arrow).

Key points:

1 PET/CT is used to assess disease response in refractory lymphoma, as in adult practice.
2 The CT scan in this child was acquired using a lower dose of 30 mA than is used in adults, with satisfactory image quality for localization purposes.

CASE 16.3	Diagnosis: Neurofibromatosis – malignant change?

Clinical history:

This 12-year-old child was diagnosed as having an enlarging paraspinal thoracic neurofibroma. PET/CT was requested to characterize the lesion and to determine if there was likely to be malignant change.

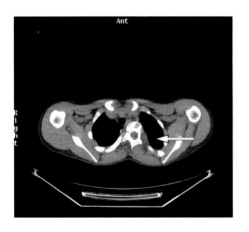 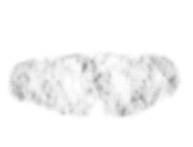 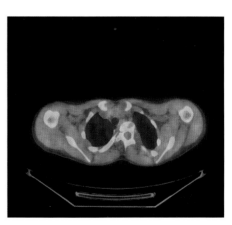

PET/CT findings:

There was no uptake in the neurofibroma (see arrow) and no evidence of malignant transformation. The lesion continued to enlarge and was excised 6 months later. It was a benign plexiform neurofibroma.

Key point:

Plexiform neurofibromata can undergo malignant change. The metabolic activity within a neurofibroma can help to differentiate benign from malignant disease and guide management.

CASE 16.4	Diagnosis: Recurrent brain tumor

Clinical history:

This 11-year-old boy had a history of mixed astrocytoma/oligodendroglioma which was resected 6 years earlier. He had received radiotherapy for recurrence 5 months earlier. He developed some new symptoms and had an MR scan which showed an enhancing lesion in the right parietal lobe, which was consistent with either inflammation and fibrosis due to radiotherapy or residual/recurrent disease. PET/CT was requested to characterize the lesion.

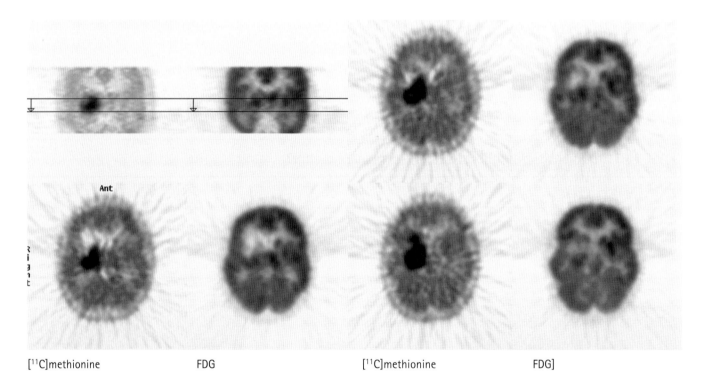

[¹¹C]methionine   FDG   [¹¹C]methionine   FDG]

PET/CT findings:

Sequential axial slices are shown of the brain after injection of [¹¹C]methionine and FDG, which demonstrated recurrent tumor with high- and low-grade components.

Key points:

1 FDG assesses tumor grade and methionine delineates tumor extent.
2 PET can differentiate between radiation necrosis and tumor recurrence where anatomic imaging is inconclusive.

REFERENCES AND FURTHER READING

Barrington SF, Maisey MN (1996) Skeletal muscle uptake of fluorine-18-FDG: effect of oral diazepam. *J Nucl Med* 37, 1127–9.

Boivin JF, Hutchinson GB, Zauber AG *et al.* (1995) Incidence of second cancers in patients treated for Hodgkin's disease. *J Natl Cancer Inst* 87, 732–4.

Borgwardt L, Larsen HJ, Pedersen K, Hojgaard L (2003) Practical use and implementation of PET in children in a hospital PET centre. *Eur J Nucl Med Mol Imaging* 30, 1389–97.

Brink I, Reinhardt MJ, Hoegerle S *et al.* (2001) Increased metabolic activity in the thymus gland studied with 18-FDG PET: Age dependency and frequency after chemotherapy. *J Nucl Med* 42, 591–5.

Chugani HT, Phelps ME (1986) Maturation changes in cerebral function in infants determined by 18FDG positron emission tomography. *Science* 231, 840–3.

Cook GJR, Maisey MN, Fogelman I (1999) Normal variants, artefacts and interpretative pitfalls in PET imaging with 18-fluoro-2-deoxyglucose and carbon-11-methionine. *Eur J Nucl Med* 26, 1363–78.

Cook GJR, Wegner EA, Fogelman I (2004) Pitfalls and artefacts in 18FDG PET and PET/CT oncologic imaging. *Semin Nucl Med* 34, 122–33.

Depas G, De Barsy C, Jerusalem G *et al.* (2005) 18F-FDG PET in children with lymphomas. *Eur J Nucl Med Mol Imaging* 32, 31–8.

Gambhir SS, Czernin J, Schwimmer J *et al.* (2001) A tabulated summary of the FDG PET literature. *J Nucl Med* 42, 1S–93S.

Hany TF, Garehpapagh E, Kamel EM *et al.* (2002) Brown adipose tissue: a factor to consider in symmetrical tracer uptake in the neck and upper chest region. *Eur J Nucl Med Mol Imaging* 29, 1393–8.

Hermann S, Wormanns D, Pixberg M *et al.* (2005) Staging in childhood lymphoma. *Nuklearmedizin* 44, 1–7.

Krasin MJ, Hudson MM, Kaste SC (2004) Positron emission tomography in pediatric radiation oncology: integration in the treatment-planning process. *Pediatr Radiol* 34, 214–21.

Lucaya J, Piqueras J, Garcia-Pena P *et al.* (2000) Low-dose high-resolution CT of the chest in children and young adults: dose, cooperation, artifact incidence, and image quality. *Am J Roentgenol* 175, 985–92.

Montravers F, McNamara D, Landman-Parker J *et al.* (2002) [(18)F]FDG in childhood lymphoma: clinical utility and impact on management. *Eur J Nucl Med Mol Imaging* 29, 1155–65.

Nakahara T, Fujii H, Ide M *et al.* (2001) FDG uptake in the morphologically normal thymus: comparison of FDG positron emission tomography and CT. *Br J Radiol* 74, 821–4.

Paediatric Task Group of the European Association of Nuclear Medicine: Piepsz A, Hahn K, Roca I *et al.* (1990) A radiopharmaceutical schedule for imaging in paediatrics. *Eur J Nucl Med* 17, 127–9.

Pintelon H, Dejonckheere M, Piepsz A (1997) Pediatric nuclear medicine: a practical approach. *Q J Nucl Med* 41, 263–8.

Roberts EG, Shulkin BL (2004) Technical issues in performing PET studies in paediatric patients. *J Nucl Med Technol* 32, 5–9.

Robinson RO, Ferrie CD, Capra M, Maisey MN (1999) Positron emission tomography in the central nervous system. *Arch Dis Child* 81, 263–70.

Ruotsalainen U, Suhonen-Polvi H, Eronen E *et al.* (1996) Estimated radiation dose to the newborn in FDG-PET studies. *J Nucl Med* 37, 387–93.

Shulkin BL (1997) PET applications in pediatrics. *Q J Nucl Med* 41, 281–91.

Stabin MG, Gelfand MJ (1998) Dosimetry of pediatric nuclear medicine procedures. *Q J Nucl Med* 42, 93–112.

Valagussa P, Santoro A, Bonadonna G (1992) Thyroid, pulmonary and cardiac sequelae after treatment for Hodgkin's disease. *Ann Oncol* 3, 111–15.

Wegner EA, Barrington SF, Kingston JE *et al.* (2005) The impact of PET scanning on management of paediatric oncology patients. *Eur J Nucl Med Mol Imaging* 32, 23–30.

Weiss S (1993) Sedation of paediatric patients for nuclear medicine procedures. *Semin Nucl Med* 3, 190–8.

Yeung HWD, Grewal RK, Gonen M, Schoder H, Larson SM (2003) Patterns of 18F-FDG uptake in adipose tissue and muscle: a potential source of false-positives for PET. *J Nucl Med* 44, 1789–96.

PART III
Other applications of PET

CHAPTER 17
NEUROLOGY AND PSYCHIATRY

INTRODUCTION AND BACKGROUND

Early research and clinical applications of positron emission tomography (PET) were almost exclusively devoted to the brain. These early studies used single-slice, small-volume PET scanners and provided immense amounts of data that have driven forward our understanding of brain function, in particular, a better understanding of changes in cerebral circulation including:

- relations between blood flow, blood volume, and oxygen extraction using [^{15}O]water, [^{15}O]carbon monoxide and [^{15}O]oxygen gas tracers and variations that occur during and after stroke
- developmental changes in regional glucose metabolism and the patterns of changes in dementias
- sites of cerebral sensorimotor control by [^{15}O]water perfusion activation studies
- a huge amount of information about the distribution of brain receptors (benzodiazepine, opioid, monoamineoxidase-B, and histamine receptors and others) in normal and various psychiatric states.

In spite of these advances in our understanding of basic physiology and pathophysiology that have arisen from PET studies, there are still relatively few clinical applications.

[^{18}F]2-Fluoro-2-deoxy-D-glucose (FDG) is the most important tracer, because glucose is the major energy substrate for brain and much is known about the relation between glucose metabolism and FDG uptake. Flow studies with [^{15}O]water have been used in the assessment of cerebrovascular disease to measure transient ischemia but usually [^{15}O]water shows a distribution similar to FDG. However, [^{15}O]water flow studies do have a role in activation studies where the short half-life of the tracer enables repeated testing under different experimental conditions. [^{11}C]L-Methionine is important in brain tumors and [^{11}C]flumazenil is sometimes used in the assessment of partial epilepsies.

CLINICAL APPLICATIONS OF PET IN NEUROLOGY AND PSYCHIATRY
Dementia
Brain tumors
Epilepsy
Human immunodeficiency virus (HIV) disease

NORMAL APPEARANCES

An example of a normal FDG brain scan is shown on the following pages. Axial slices are shown of the FDG PET images from vertex to cerebellum (a). Representative slices from the PET, CT and fused datasets are also shown in axial (b), coronal (c), and sagittal (d) planes. Note the artifact on the CT images from surface electroencephalography (EEG) electrodes as this was a study performed in a patient for investigation of partial epilepsy who turned out to have a normal scan.

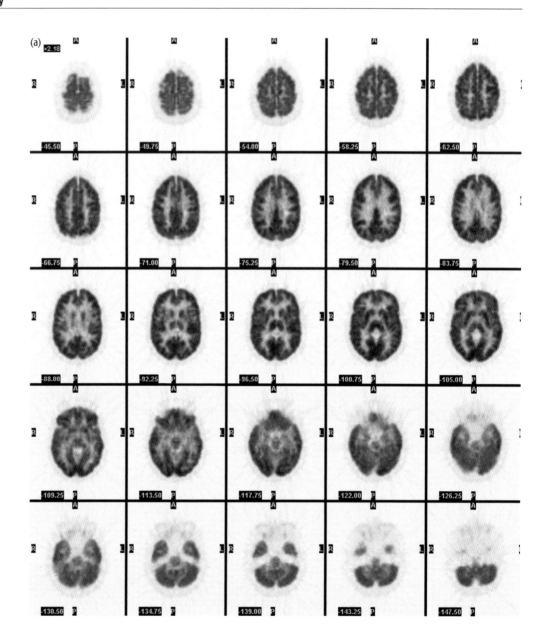

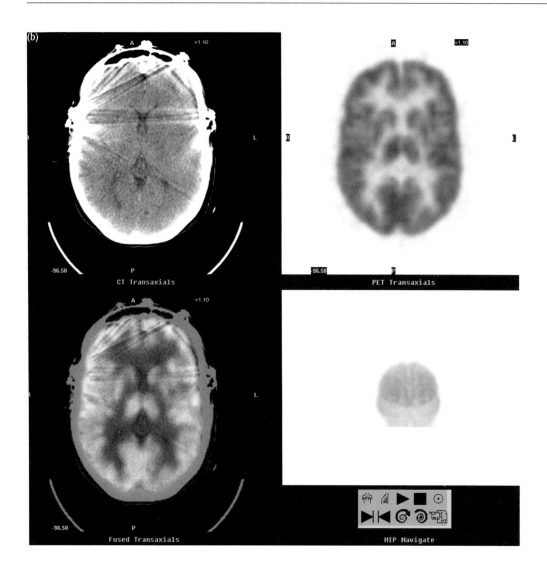

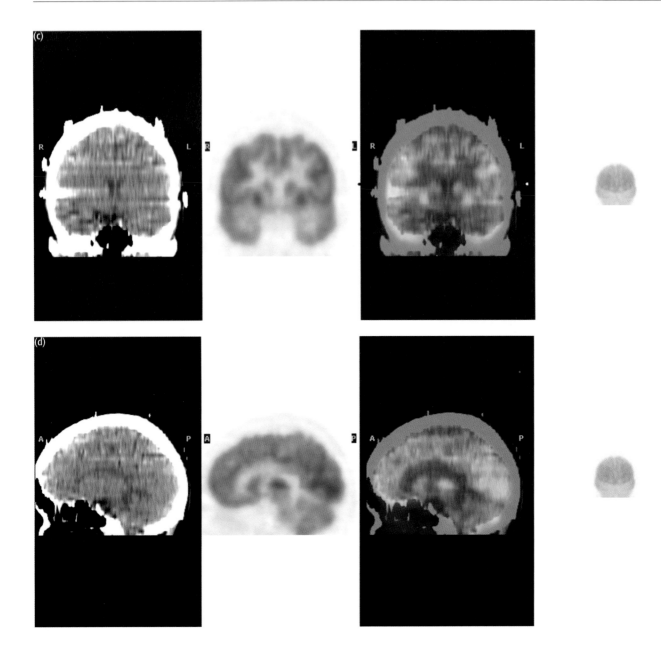

1 Dementia

Dementia is defined as loss of memory and at least one other area of complex behavior sufficient to interfere with daily life. It is an increasing problem for society and usually a personal and family tragedy. It will get worse, as it has been estimated that up to 5 percent of people over 65 and up to 25 percent of those over 80 will have some form of dementia.

CAUSES OF DEMENTIA

Degenerative
Alzheimer disease
Frontal lobe degeneration
Pick disease
Olivopontocerebellar degeneration
Lewy body disease
Huntington disease
Parkinson disease

Vascular
Multiple infarct dementia
Small vessel (Binswanger disease)

Trauma
Multiple
Subdural/extradural

Infective
HIV disease
Creutzfeldt–Jacob disease

Other causes
Hydrocephalus
Metabolic causes
Pseudodementia

Investigation in the first instance is directed toward detection of treatable disease, e.g. brain tumor, hypothyroidism, hydrocephalus. Alzheimer disease and vascular dementia are responsible for up to 50 percent of all cases of dementia. Lewy body dementia, which is associated with parkinsonism and increased risk of autonomic failure, is responsible for up to 20 percent of cases.

Investigation is directed at excluding treatable causes and defining the likely progress of the disorder. There are typical findings with FDG PET in Alzheimer disease and other types of dementia. As would be expected, metabolic changes occur before structural changes and FDG PET abnormalities may precede structural changes by as much as 12–18 months. Early detection is becoming increasingly important because treatments for Alzheimer disease which enhance cholinergic activity work only on intact synapses and are designed to slow the process. Such treatments may delay the median time to functional decline and the necessity for institutional care. FDG PET scanning has been used in combination with genetic testing to identify individuals at high risk. There is particular interest in the preclinical detection of disease, with regard to the testing of new drugs in the research setting.

IMAGING FINDINGS IN THE DEMENTIAS

MR imaging	FDG PET imaging
Alzheimer disease	
Early: normal or hippocampal atrophy	Temporoparietal and cingulate hypometabolism
Advanced: frontal, parietotemporal atrophy	Temporoparietal hypometabolism with sparing of subcortical structures, primary visual and sensorimotor cortex; later also frontal hypometabolism, cortical atrophy, and thalamic separation
Multiple infarct dementia	
White matter signals and cortical and subcortical infarcts	Focal asymmetric cortical and deep hypometabolic areas
Pseudodementia	
Normal	Normal or frontal hypometabolism
Frontal dementias	
Early: normal	Frontal: frontal lobe hypometabolism
Late: frontal atrophy	Pick: frontal + temporal hypometabolism
Trauma	
Mild: normal	Focal hypometabolism
Severe: atrophy	Focal hypometabolism
HIV	
Normal	Diffuse cortical hypometabolism with sparing of deep structures
Huntingdon disease	
Early: normal	Hypometabolism of caudate nucleus
Late: caudate atrophy	
Lewy body disease	
Early: nil	Alzheimer disease-like picture but with reduced visual cortex metabolism
Late: atrophy	

KEY MANAGEMENT ISSUES

KEY MANAGEMENT ISSUES

Early diagnosis of Alzheimer disease vs. benign memory loss
Differential diagnosis of dementia
Differentiation from pseudodementia/depression

EXAMPLES TO ILLUSTRATE KEY ISSUES

CASE 17.1	Diagnosis: Alzheimer dementia

Clinical history:

This patient presented with word-finding difficulties and memory impairment. Cognitive testing revealed a global pattern of impairment but with the left hemisphere more severely affected – possibly Alzheimer disease. PET was requested to determine the etiology of dementia.

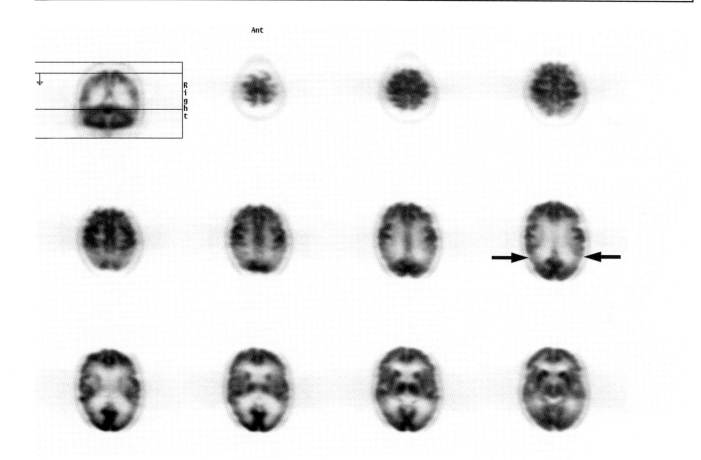

PET findings:

There was bitemporal, posterior parietal, and temporal hypometabolism consistent with Alzheimer disease.

Key point:
Preservation of cortical uptake in the posterior cingulate cortex weighs against Lewy body dementia.

CASE 17.2	Diagnosis: Alzheimer-type dementia

Clinical history:

This patient was referred with cognitive impairment, in particular with problems with expression of language. Clinical features were suggestive of frontotemporal dementia or Pick disease or Alzheimer disease. PET was requested to characterize the type of dementia.

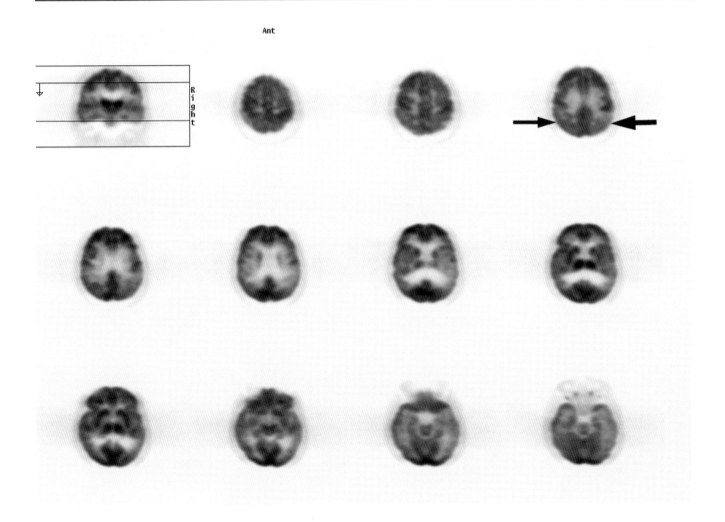

PET findings:

The scan showed reduced uptake in the temporoparietal lobes bilaterally, more marked on the left than the right suggestive of early Alzheimer disease.

Key points:

1 The features of early Alzheimer disease are those of bilateral temporoparietal hypometabolism, frequently asymmetric, which later extends to involve the frontal lobes.
2 Pick disease and frontotemporal dementia have reduced uptake frontally.

CASE 17.3	Diagnosis: Advanced Alzheimer disease

Clinical history:

This patient had advanced Alzheimer disease.

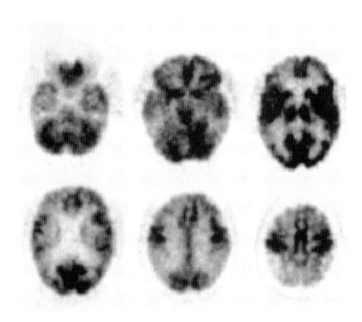

PET findings:

Metabolism was reduced bilaterally in the parietal, temporal and frontal cortices. Activity was relatively preserved in the motor cortices, anterior cingulate cortex (top left midline), basal ganglia, thalamus, and the structures of the posterior fossa.

Key point:

Late in Alzheimer disease, changes extend into the frontal lobes.

| CASE 17.4 | Diagnosis: Alzheimer disease |

Clinical history:

This patient had advanced Alzheimer disease.

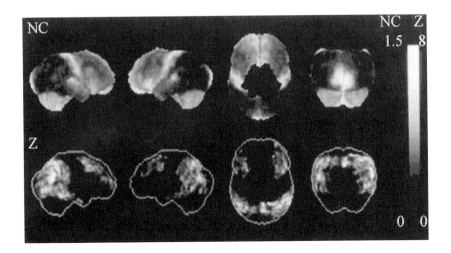

PET findings:

This statistical stereotactic surface projection image shows reduced glucose metabolism compared with normal data. The Z score refers the number of standard deviations by which the FDG uptake in this patient differed from the normal data.

Key point:

Comparison of patient data with 'normal' databases is increasingly being used in clinical practice.

CASE 17.5	Diagnosis: Pick disease

Clinical history:

This patient presented with clinical features suggestive of frontal lobe dementia. PET was requested to determine the type of dementia.

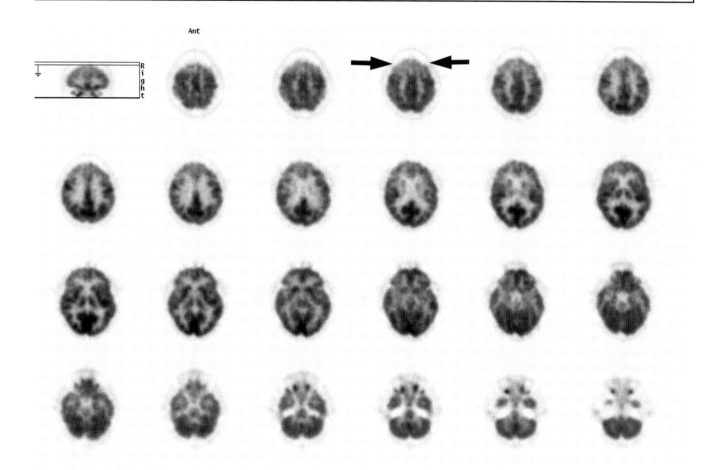

PET findings:

There was bilateral reduction in uptake in the frontal lobes, consistent with a diagnosis of Pick disease.

Key point:

The features of Pick disease on FDG scanning are of bilateral frontal and sometimes temporal hypometabolism.

| CASE 17.6 | Diagnosis: Huntington disease |

Clinical history:

This patient was asymptomatic but at risk for Huntington disease.

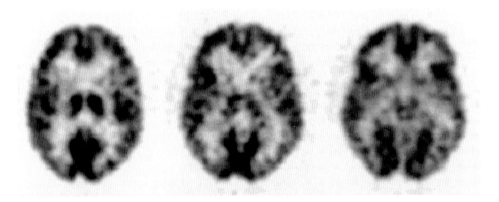

PET findings:

Metabolism in the caudate nuclei was reduced in advance of atrophy.

Key point:

In some instances of Huntington disease, metabolic features on PET may be visualized in advance of the clinical signs or symptoms.

CASE 17.7	Diagnosis: Lewy body dementia

Clinical history:

This elderly patient presented with decreasing cognitive function. PET was requested to characterize the dementia.

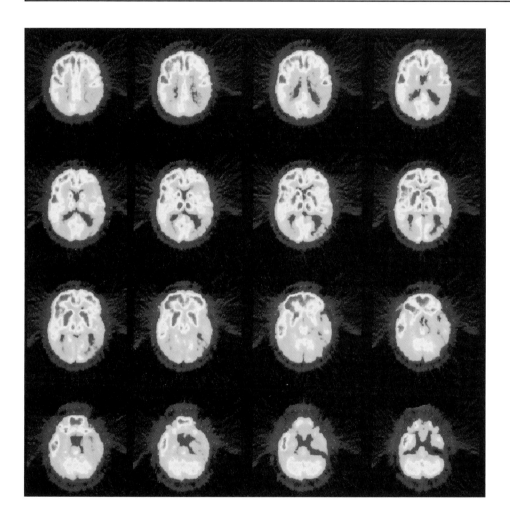

PET findings:

Metabolism was reduced in the parietotemporal association cortices and frontal association cortex. There was asymmetric (more severe on the left) but bilateral involvement of the cerebral hemispheres.

Key points:

1 The pattern of reduction in metabolism in the association cortices in Lewy body dementia is similar to that seen in Alzheimer disease. Moreover, in both dementias metabolic activity in the primary sensorimotor cortex and subcortical structures (thalamus, striatum, and cerebellum) is relatively preserved.
2 Cerebral hemispheres are involved bilaterally but the involvement may be asymmetric.
3 In addition, metabolic reduction is often seen in the occipital cortex – a finding that could be a diagnostic discriminator for Lewy body dementia.

CONCLUSIONS

CURRENT CLINICAL INDICATIONS
1 Early symptoms when MRI normal
2 Parkinson disease with dementia
3 HIV with dementia or neurological symptoms ± fever
4 Differential diagnosis when MRI is equivocal
5 Differentiating severe depression with dementia features

2 Epilepsy

Epilepsy is a common condition; approximately 1 in 40 of the population will have a fit sometime in their lifetime, and there is about 1:200 prevalence in the population. Over the past 20 years imaging studies have generated a mass of important data increasing our understanding of the causes, pathophysiology, and the treatment of this condition. MRI forms the mainstay of imaging for epilepsy, and increasingly functional MRI and magnetic resonance spectroscopy are playing a role. It is in the area of potentially surgically treatable partial epilepsy that PET studies have an important role. MRI is used as the primary imaging investigation to exclude treatable mass lesions and the common causes of partial epilepsy: hippocampal sclerosis and malformation of cortical development, and vascular malformations and acquired cortical damage. There remains a group of patients (10–40 percent, depending on the sophistication of the MRI techniques) in whom the imaging is normal, equivocal, or discrepant with electroencephalography (EEG). It is these patients who will benefit from PET studies. The results of surgery for temporal lobe epilepsy (TLE) are better than for extratemporal epilepsy and the majority of surgical procedures carried out are to cure TLE.

An epileptogenic focus studied in the interictal period is an area of decreased flow and decreased metabolism. Such an area will usually be larger than the pathologic abnormality, probably due to deafferentation of the surrounding tissue which may include the ipsilateral thalamus and frontal lobes. Patients with TLE in whom there is clear lateralization of the focus with FDG PET, and the findings are concordant with scalp EEG and video telemetry, may be able to proceed to surgery without the need for prior invasive EEG.

Ictal scans result in increased metabolism and flow. Ictal PET scans are unusual and tend to occur 'by accident', as PET imaging is not suited to ictal studies. The uptake period for FDG in the brain is typically between 30 and 60 minutes. A seizure usually lasts less than a few minutes and the peri-ictal 'increased' metabolism is usually masked by the interictal 'reduced' metabolism that is present during the rest of the uptake period. This contrasts with single photon emission computed tomography (SPECT) where there is high first-pass extraction of perfusion tracers such as 99m-technetium hexamethylpropyleneamine-oxime (HMPAO) and 99m-technetium-ethyl cysteinate dimer. The complexity of ictal imaging, however, is a drawback of the technique and injection ideally needs to take place within 2 minutes of the onset of the seizure for accurate assessment of the focus. A series by Won *et al.* (1999) comparing interictal PET with ictal SPECT suggested PET was more sensitive than SPECT but that both techniques had high accuracy and either could be used.

There is considerable overlap between the rate of FDG uptake in normal brain and sites of epileptic foci. Therefore absolute quantitation is not applied clinically. Typically asymmetry of greater than 10–15 percent is taken as representing significant hypometabolism. Use of asymmetry indices of 10–15 percent or more have been shown to be statistically significantly associated with a successful outcome to surgery. Bilateral hypometabolism on PET may be associated with a poorer surgical outcome.

Accuracy of FDG PET in extratemporal epilepsy is variable and that of other imaging techniques is less good than for TLE. However, focal abnormalities on PET may help to decide that the patient should proceed to invasive EEG testing and can help to choose the sites to place intracranial electrodes.

Reduction in tracer uptake with $[^{11}C]$flumazenil, which binds to benzodiazepine receptors within the benzodiazepine-GABA$_A$ complex, has been reported in both temporal and extratemporal epilepsy. Initial reports suggested that the reduction in benzodiazepine binding imaged using $[^{11}C]$flumazenil appeared to be better circumscribed than change in flow or metabolism and to be closely correlated with the ictal onset zone. However, in a larger study by Ryvlin *et al.* (1998) involving 100 patients undergoing evaluation for surgery who had video telemetry, EEG, MRI, FDG, and $[^{11}C]$flumazenil PET, $[^{11}C]$flumazenil did not provide data that was superior to FDG PET overall in TLE. Flumazenil was slightly more sensitive than FDG but was falsely lateralizing in some patients in whom the FDG was normal. Others have reported increases in binding outside the affected hippocampus in temporal lobe white matter and in the frontal and parietal cortex. In the study by Ryvlin *et al.* flumazenil was more sensitive than FDG in the detection of the focus in patients with cryptogenic frontal lobe epilepsy but neither tracer was able to localize the lesion accurately enough to replace the need for invasive EEG. In a small number of patients with bitemporal abnormalities in the study $[^{11}C]$flumazenil helped to confirm bilateral involvement. Hence $[^{11}C]$flumazenil shows promise for lateralization in extratemporal epilepsy and in the detection of bitemporal epilepsies but its role requires further evaluation in larger series of patients.

KEY MANAGEMENT ISSUES

KEY MANAGEMENT ISSUES
Lateralization of partial epilepsy (when MRI is normal or conflicts with EEG findings) to avoid invasive EEG
Direction of placement of electrodes when invasive EEG is required
Prediction of surgical outcome
Assistance in management of pediatric 'malignant' epilepsies

Role of PET in epilepsy

TEMPORAL AND FRONTAL LOBE EPILEPSY	
Temporal lobe epilepsy	Extratemporal epilepsy
Hypometabolic foci in 75–90%	Hypometabolic foci in 30–80%
Hypometabolic focus larger than pathologic lesion	Hypometabolic focus larger than pathologic lesion
No extra information when MRI definite	90% with hypometabolism have MRI abnormality
Extent and severity of hypometabolism correlates with a good surgical outcome	Poorer surgical outcome; ~50% of patients have significant reduction in seizure frequency compared with up to 90% of those with TLE and clear evidence of a focus

There are many forms of complex pediatric seizure syndromes; often they are resistant to medical therapy and patients may be considered for surgery. PET findings may assist surgical assessment, including the assessment of functional integrity of brain outside the epileptic focus. These syndromes often have normal MRI findings, and may have single or multiple hypometabolic foci.

PEDIATRIC SYNDROMES
West syndrome
Lennox–Gastaut syndrome
Infantile spasms
Landau–Kleffner syndrome
Rasmussen syndrome

EXAMPLES TO ILLUSTRATE KEY ISSUES

CASE 17.8	Diagnosis: Temporal lobe epilepsy

Clinical history:

This patient with history of complex partial seizures was referred for assessment prior to epilepsy surgery. PET was requested to locate the site of a focus for epilepsy.

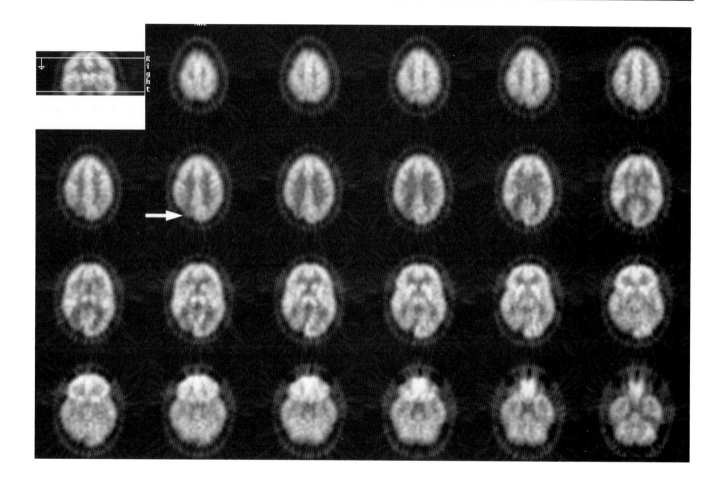

PET findings:

There was right temporal hypometabolism on this interictal scan suggestive of a right temporal focus for epilepsy.

Key points:

1 Decreased FDG uptake on PET is the typical finding on interictal scans surrounding the epileptogenic region.
2 PET can help to identify the origin of an epileptic focus but changes on PET are frequently larger and more diffuse than the focus.

| CASE 17.9 | Diagnosis: Temporal lobe epilepsy |

Clinical history:

This patient was referred with a history of focal seizures. Clinical features and video telemetry suggested a right temporal lobe focus. MRI showed right mesial temporal sclerosis but suggested there were might also be left hippocampal atrophy. PET was requested to determine the site of an epileptic focus with a view to surgery.

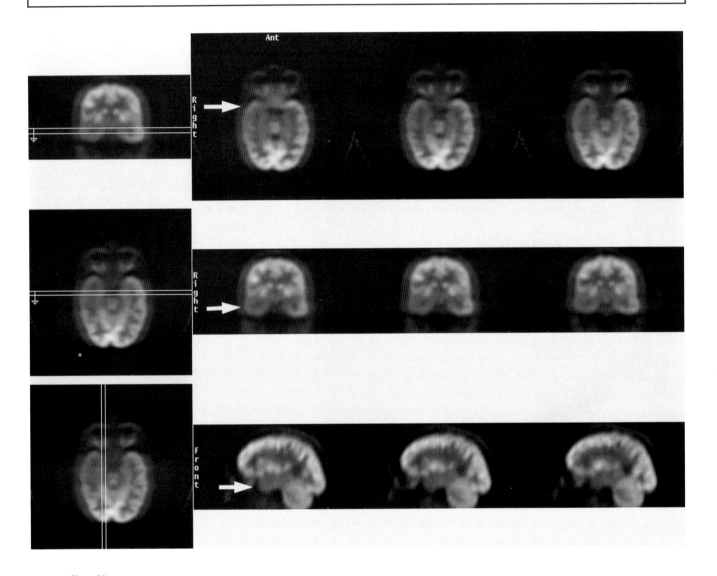

PET findings:

There was hypometabolism in the right temporal lobe suggestive of a right temporal lobe focus.

Key point:

PET has little to add if there are concordant features on clinical assessment, EEG, and MRI. However, when there are discordant features, PET can be helpful in identifying a focus.

CASE 17.10	Diagnosis: Epilepsy – occipital focus

Clinical history:

This patient had a long history of complex partial seizures resistant to medical treatment. MR showed right occipital microgyria. However, foramen ovale telemetry and scalp EEG monitoring showed bilateral synchronous onset of seizure activity. PET was requested to determine whether there were unilateral or bilateral changes in metabolism.

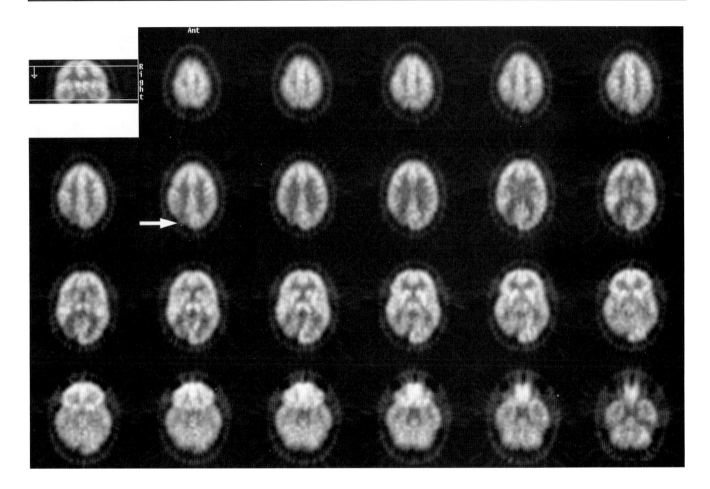

PET findings:

There was hypometabolism in the right occipital lobe. The site of seizure onset was subsequently confirmed as the right occipital lobe with subdural telemetry. The patient underwent surgery with significant improvement in seizure frequency.

Key point:

PET added weight to the MR findings and provided the impetus for further investigation with subdural telemetry.

CASE 17.11	Diagnosis: Rasmussen syndrome

Clinical history:

This child had progressive right hemiparesis with diffuse changes on MRI in the left hemisphere suggestive of Rasmussen syndrome.

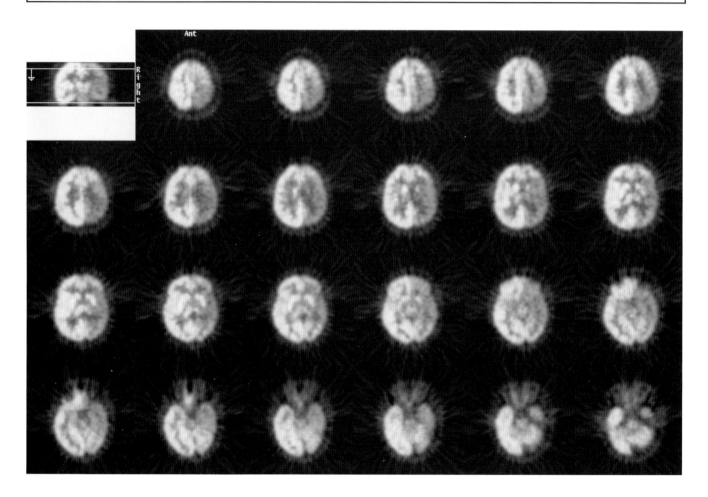

PET findings:

There was diffuse hypometabolism throughout the left hemisphere. The diagnosis of Rasmussen disease was confirmed at surgery when hemispherectomy was performed.

Key point:

The typical appearances of Rasmussen syndrome are of diffuse change in the affected hemisphere.

CONCLUSIONS

CURRENT CLINICAL INDICATIONS
1 Selection for TLE surgery where MRI normal or conflicts with EEG
2 To direct placement of electrodes for invasive EEG (especially extratemporal epilepsy)
3 To assist in the management of selected pediatric 'malignant' epilepsies

POSSIBLE INDICATIONS
1 Detection of bilateral temporal abnormalities which might preclude surgery
2 Functional assessment prior to surgery in children

REFERENCES AND FURTHER READING

Antonini A, Kazumata K, Feigin A *et al.* (1998) Differential diagnosis of parkinsonism with [18F]fluorodeoxyglucose and PET. *Mov Disord* **13**, 268–74.

Barrington S, Koutroumanidis M, Agathonikou A *et al.* (1998) Clinical value of 'ictal' FDG-PET and the routine use of simultaneous scalp EEG studies in patients with intractable partial epilepsies. *Epilepsia* **39**, 753–66.

Burdette JH, Minoshima S, Vander Borght T, Tran DD, Kuhl DE (1996) Alzheimer disease: improved visual interpretation of PET images by using three-dimensional stereotaxic surface projections. *Radiology* **198**, 837–43.

Duncan JS (1999) Positron emission tomography receptor studies. *Adv Neurol* **79**, 893–9.

Ferrie CD, Marsden PK, Maisey MN, Robinson RO. Cortical and subcortical glucose metabolism in childhood epileptic encephalopathies. *J Neurol Neurosurg Psychiatry* **63**, 181–7.

Grady CL, Haxby JV, Horwitz B *et al.* (1988) Longitudinal study of the early neuropsychological and cerebral metabolic changes in dementia of the Alzheimer type. *J Clin Exp Neuropsychol* **10**, 576–96.

Hammers A, Koepp MJ, Hurlemann R *et al.* (2002) Abnormalities of grey and white matter [11C]flumazenil binding in temporal lobe epilepsy with normal MRI. *Brain* **125**, 2257–71.

Henry TR, Van Heertum R (2003) Positron emission tomography and single photon emission computed tomography in epilepsy care. *Semin Nucl Med* **33**, 88–104.

Hwang SI, Kim JH, Park SW *et al.* (2001) Comparative analysis of MR imaging, positron emission tomography, and ictal single-photon emission CT in patients with neocortical epilepsy. *AJNR Am J Neuroradiol* **22**, 937–46.

Imamura T, Ishii K, Sasaki M *et al.* (1997) Regional cerebral glucose metabolism in dementia with Lewy bodies and Alzheimer's disease: a comparative study using positron emission tomography. *Neurosci Lett* **235**, 49–52.

Juhasz C, Chugani DC, Muzik O *et al.* (2001) Relationship of flumazenil and glucose PET abnormalities to neocortical epilepsy surgery outcome. *Neurology* **56**, 1650–8.

Koutroumanidis, M, Barrington, S, Agathonikou A *et al.* (1998) Interictal regional slow activity in temporal lobe epilepsy correlates with lateral temporal hypometabolism as imaged with FDG-PET. Neurophysiologic and metabolic implications. *J Neurol Neurosurg Psychiatry* **65**, 170–6.

Koutroumanidis M, Binnie C, Panayiotopoulos C (1998) Positron emission tomography in partial epilepsies: the clinical point of view. *Nucl Med Commun* **19**, 1123–6.

Koutroumanidis M, Hennessy MJ, Seed PT *et al.* (2000) Significance of interictal bilateral temporal hypometabolism in temporal lobe epilepsy. *Neurology* **54**, 1811–21.

Lamusuo S, Pitkanen A, Jutila L *et al.* (2000) [11C]Flumazenil binding in the medial temporal lobe in patients with temporal lobe epilepsy: correlation with hippocampal MR volumetry, T2 relaxometry, and neuropathology. *Neurology* **54**, 2252–60.

Manno EM, Sperling MR, Ding X *et al.* (1994) Predictors of outcome after anterior temporal lobectomy: positron emission tomography. *Neurology* **44**, 2331–6.

Mielke R, Kessler J, Szelies B *et al.* (1996) Vascular dementia: perfusional and metabolic disturbances and effects of therapy. *J Neural Transm Suppl* **47**, 183–91.

Neuroimaging Subcommision of the International League Against Epilepsy (2000) Commission on Diagnostic Strategies: recommendations for functional neuroimaging of persons with epilepsy. *Epilepsia* **41**, 1350–6.

Reiman EM, Caselli RJ, Yun LS *et al.* (1996) Preclinical evidence of Alzheimer's disease in persons homozygous for the epsilon 4 allele for apolipoprotein E. *N Engl J Med* **334**, 752–8.

Robinson RO, Ferrie CD, Capra M, Maisey MN (1999) Positron emission tomography and the central nervous system. *Arch Dis Child* **81**, 263–70.

Rossor MN, Kennedy AM, Frackowiak RS (1996) Clinical and neuroimaging features of familial Alzheimer's disease. *Ann N Y Acad Sci* **777**, 49–56.

Ryvlin P, Bouvard S, Le Bars D *et al.* (1998) Clinical utility of flumazenil-PET versus [18F]fluorodeoxyglucose-PET and MRI in refractory partial epilepsy. A prospective study in 100 patients. *Brain* **121**, 2067–81.

Savic I, Thorell JO, Roland P (1995) [11C]flumazenil positron emission tomography visualizes frontal epileptogenic regions. *Epilepsia* **36**, 1225–32.

Savic I, Persson A, Roland P *et al.* (1998) In-vivo demonstration of reduced benzodiazepine receptor binding in human epileptic foci. *Lancet* **2**, 863–6.

Small GW, Leiter F (1998) Neuroimaging for diagnosis of dementia. *J Clin Psychiatry* **59**(Suppl 11), 4–7.

Spencer SS (2002) When should temporal-lobe surgery be treated surgically? *Lancet Neurol* **1**, 1375–82.

Theodore WH (2002) When is positron emission tomography really necessary in epilepsy diagnosis? *Curr Opin Neurol* **15**, 191–5.

Van Heertum RL, Greenstein EA, Tikofsky RS (2004) 2-Deoxy-fluoroglucose-positron emission tomography imaging of the brain: current clinical applications with emphasis on the dementias. *Semin Nucl Med* **34**, 300–12.

Wiebe S, Blume WT, Girvin JP, Eliasziw M, Effectiveness and Efficiency of Surgery for Temporal Lobe Epilepsy Study Group (2001) A randomized, controlled trial of surgery for temporal-lobe epilepsy. *N Engl J Med* **345**, 311–18.

Won HJ, Chang KH, Cheon JE *et al.* (1999) Comparison of MR imaging with PET and ictal SPECT in 118 patients with intractable epilepsy. *AJNR Am J Neuroradiol* **20**, 593–9.

CHAPTER 18
CARDIOLOGY

INTRODUCTION AND BACKGROUND

The frequency of coronary artery disease in the developed world is high although cancer has now replaced coronary artery disease as the major cause of death in North America.

Within the overall spectrum of coronary artery disease, patients with left ventricular dysfunction pose particular problems and consume an increasingly large proportion of healthcare costs devoted to cardiac disease. Such patients are at increased risk from surgical procedures and percutaneous coronary intervention. However, some of these patients may benefit significantly in terms of symptom improvement, enhanced quality of life, and improved survival if they undergo successful revascularization. The major determinant of whether revascularization results in functional improvement is the extent of hibernating myocardium present.

Rahimtoola (1985) first used the term 'hibernating myocardium' to describe the 'smart heart' that could adapt to low flow by downgrading function and be restored to full function with revascularization. The original description implied that resting flow in areas of cardiac dysfunction was always impaired although it is now recognized that coronary flow reserve may be reduced while there is normal flow at rest. The term 'repetitive stunning' is sometimes used to refer to the situation where there is chronic impairment of function secondary to intermittent but frequent and repeated episodes of ischemia yet the resting blood flow remains normal.

> *No matter what nomenclature is used, chronic cardiac dysfunction secondary to resting ischemia or intermittent ischemia can be improved if the muscle is revascularized. It is this broader meaning that is usually nowadays meant by 'hibernating myocardium'.*

DEFINITIONS	
Viable myocardium	Myocardium that has or retains the ability to contract
Hibernating myocardium	Chronic reversible ischemic dysfunction
Stunned myocardium	Acute reversible ischemic dysfunction
Infarction/scar	Irreversible myocardial damage unable to contract

The challenge for imaging is to identify and distinguish those patients with chronic left ventricular dysfunction who have sufficiently extensive areas of hibernating myocardium and who should be revascularized from those who have large areas of infarcted myocardium even with some small areas of hibernating myocardium in whom the risks and financial costs associated with revascularization are not justified.

In a recent meta-analysis which included results from 24 studies involving 3088 patients, the annual mortality among patients with 'viability' was 16 percent with medical treatment compared with 3.2 percent among those who underwent revascularization (p<0.0001). Most data suggest that revascularization does not confer any survival benefit on patients with 'nonviable' dysfunctional myocardium. Only one study has suggested that patients with severe coronary artery disease (three-vessel disease and/or left main stem stenosis) did better with revascularization than medical treatment even without evidence of viability, although the reduction in relative risk was much higher for those patients with viability.

KEY MANAGEMENT ISSUES

> **KEY MANAGEMENT ISSUES**
> Selection of patients with left ventricular dysfunction for revascularization
> Evaluation before cardiac transplantation

Role of PET in hibernating myocardium

PET flow/metabolism studies are generally regarded as the gold standard for imaging hibernation. Other techniques, such as stress echocardiography, have higher specificity but are less sensitive in patients who have severe impairment of function and large areas of akinesis. Glucose metabolism is preserved or increased in hibernating myocardium because of increased expression of glucose transporters and glycolysis, possibly in response to increased glycogen synthesis secondary to other mechanisms such as translocation of glyceraldehyde-3-phosphate dehydrogenase (GADPH).

> *With increasing ischemia, glucose – first aerobic then anaerobic glycolysis – is increasingly the critical substrate. This is the basis for FDG as a PET metabolic tracer.*

> **SUBSTRATE METABOLISM**
> Fatty acid oxidation supplies >50% of myocardial fuel in the fasting state
> Postprandially, glucose and insulin increase Glut 4 transport at the myocardial surface and glucose oxidation to >50% of myocardial fuel
> During severe exercise lactate oxidation increases and may supply >50% of myocardial fuel
> Prolonged fasting may result in ketones providing significant fuel

The presence of $[^{18}F]$2-fluoro-2-deoxy-D-glucose (FDG) uptake in sites of normal or impaired flow can be used to distinguish viable from infarcted myocardium where both flow and glucose metabolism are impaired. The sensitivity of FDG PET for the detection of hibernating myocardium is approximately 85–90 percent with a specificity of 70–75 percent.

The use of PET in the selection of candidates for surgery can reduce perioperative mortality and complication rates. The 30-day mortality among patients selected for surgery using PET has been reported to be less than 1 percent compared with between 11 percent and 20 percent for those who were revascularized without undergoing PET viability assessment preoperatively. The use of inotropes, ventilatory and mechanical support, and incidence of cardiac arrest was also significantly lower among patients who had preoperative PET. The use of PET to select patients for surgery is also cost effective. A low perioperative mortality of 2.2 percent was maintained in patients diverted to revascularization from cardiac transplantation, which is an increasing use for PET with the shortage of donor hearts.

Perhaps because of the development of PET centers remote from a cyclotron, the use of single photon emission computed tomography (SPECT) tracers to investigate flow has increased, with FDG PET reserved for the assessment of metabolism only. This is more practical for facilities without a cyclotron on site, as PET perfusion tracers such as water or ammonia have ultrashort half-lives and rubidium, which is produced in a generator, is more costly than technetium flow tracers. PET perfusion tracers can reliably be used for the detection and assessment of ischemia in coronary artery disease, but the cost associated with PET compared with SPECT means that PET imaging is almost exclusively directed to the imaging of hibernation. Imaging for the assessment of ischemia is reserved for selected cases only. PET can occasionally be helpful in the differentiation of ischemic from nonischemic cardiomyopathy.

PET TRACERS FOR CLINICAL CARDIOLOGY

[^{13}N]Ammonia	
[^{15}O]Water	Flow
^{81}Rb	
FDG	
[^{11}C]Acetate	Metabolism

Perfusion imaging is usually performed in PET only alongside imaging of metabolism for viability assessment. Where a cyclotron is available, [^{13}N]ammonia is the tracer of choice. ^{82}Rb which is generator produced is an alternative if there is no cyclotron. FDG is the most commonly used tracer. [^{11}C]acetate has been used to assess fatty acid metabolism but is not widely applied.

Effort is being concentrated in the gating of cardiac imaging so that simultaneous assessment of function and metabolism can be performed. In the future PET/CT may be used for simultaneous assessment of coronary anatomy using CT angiography, cardiac function, perfusion and metabolism.

PATIENT PREPARATION

Glucose loading
Glucose and variable insulin doses
Euglycemic insulin clamp (only selected cases)
Fatty acid lowering regimens

Patients usually undergo scanning after an oral glucose load because uptake in the fasting state may be variable in the myocardium resulting in poor quality images. Extra insulin may be given to enhance uptake in the myocardium, especially in diabetic patients. The use of a hyperinsulinemic euglycemic clamp gives better image quality than more simple approaches but does not alter the ratio of uptake in normal vs. hibernating vs. infarcted myocardium and is generally used in clinical studies only where more simple approaches have failed.

EXAMPLES TO ILLUSTRATE KEY ISSUES

CASE 18.1	Diagnosis: Coronary artery disease – viability?

Clinical history:

This patient had three-vessel coronary artery disease with impaired left ventricular function (ejection fraction 25 percent). He had symptoms of heart failure without angina. PET/CT was requested to determine whether there was significant hibernating myocardium.

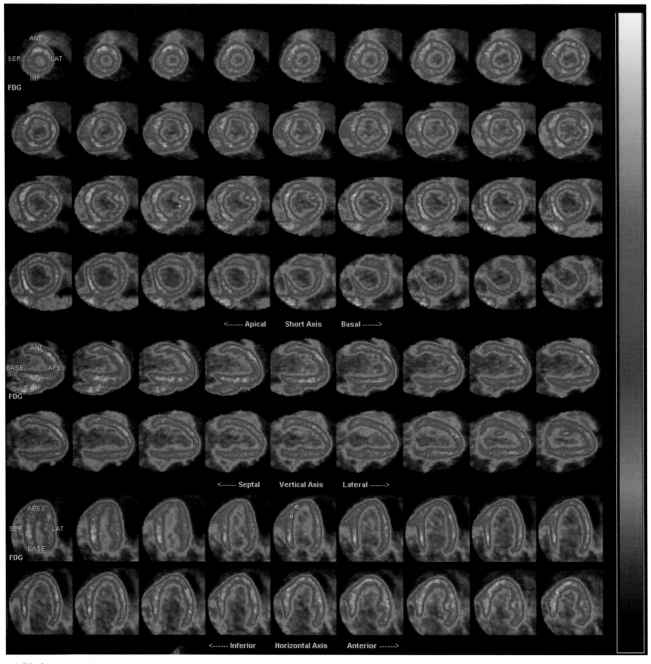

(a) [¹³N]Ammonia (perfusion).

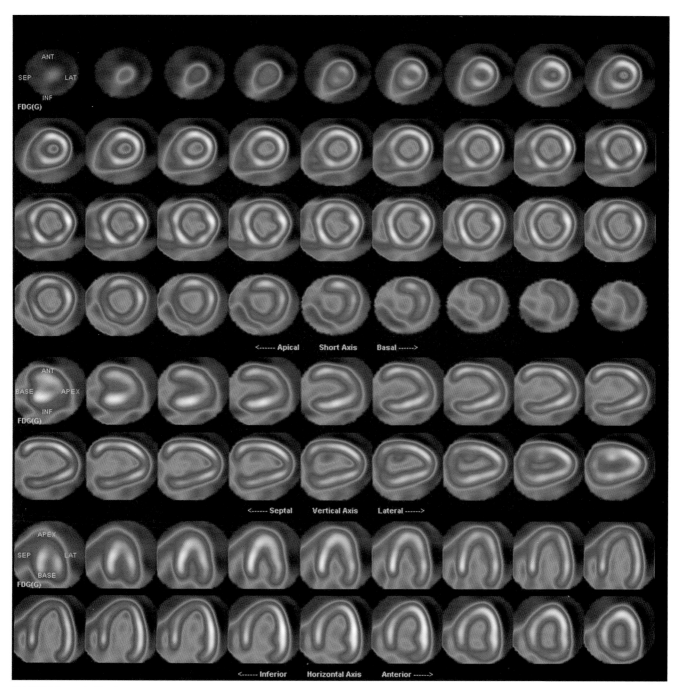

(b) ¹⁸FDG (metabolism).

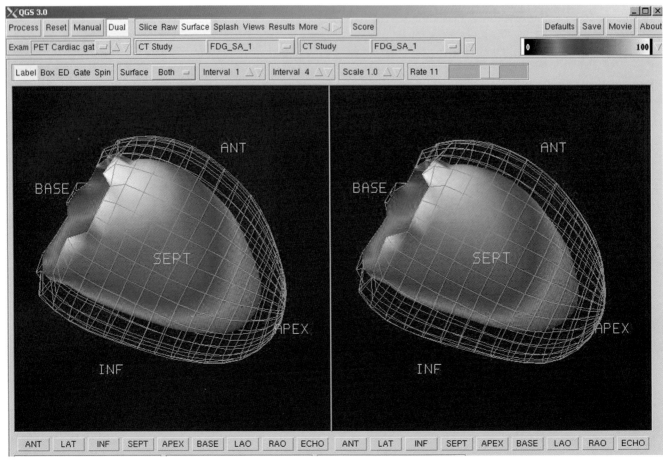

(c) Surface views: end diastole and end systole. Endocardial (inner) and epicardial (outer) surfaces are shown. INF, inferior; ANT, anterior; SEPT, septum

PET/CT findings:

There was reduction of perfusion (ammonia) in the proximal anterolateral wall and proximal inferior wall (a) with good metabolism (FDG) throughout the left ventricle (b) despite global impairment in contractility predictive of extensive hibernation (c).

Key points:

1 Dysfunctional myocardium with normal or impaired resting perfusion and preserved FDG metabolism is predictive of hibernating myocardium.
2 The resting ejection fraction and the extent of the area of hibernation influences the degree of functional recovery and symptomatic improvement.

CASE 18.2 | Diagnosis: Coronary artery disease – viability?

Clinical history:

This patient had two previous coronary artery bypass surgery operations and a history of ventricular tachycardia. He had severe breathlessness due to impaired left ventricular function (ejection fraction ~20 percent). PET/CT was requested to determine if there was viable myocardium amenable to revascularization.

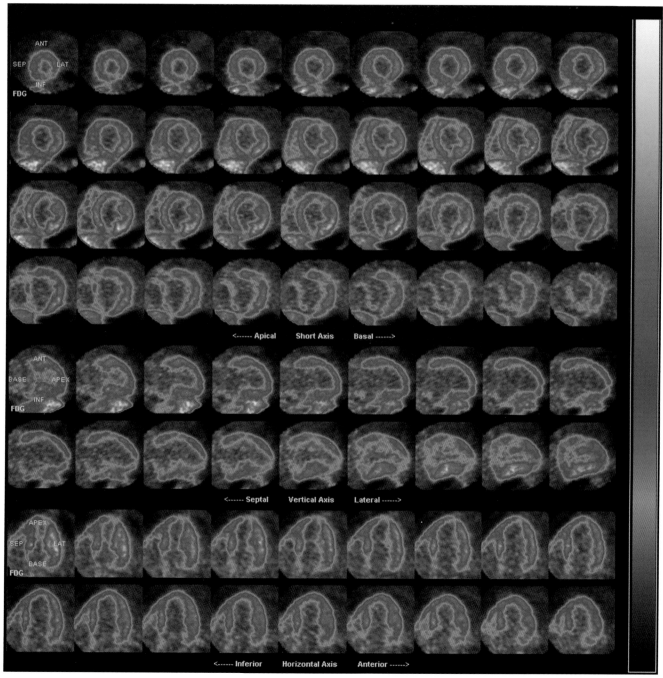

(a) [^{13}N]Ammonia (perfusion).

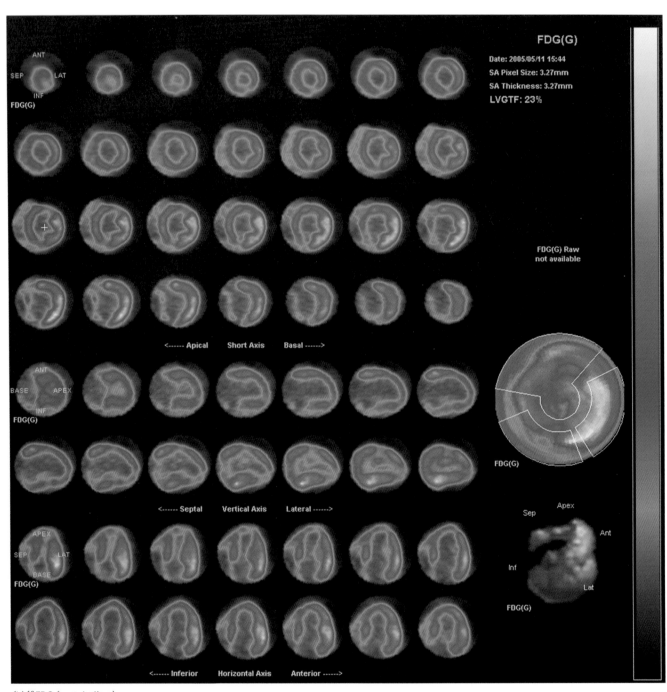

(b) ¹⁸FDG (metabolism).

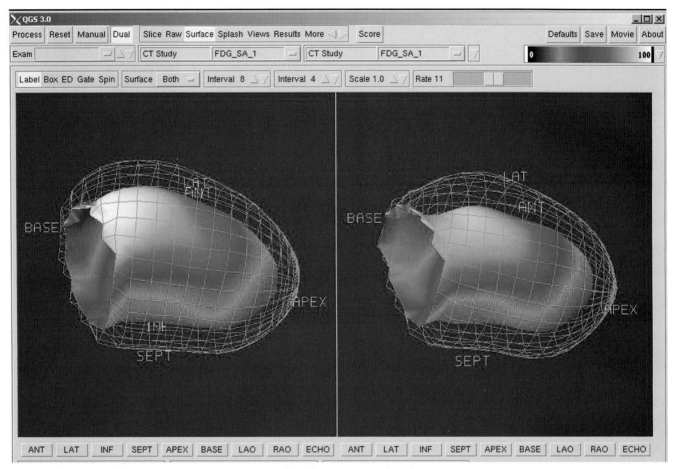

(c) Surface views: end diastole and end systole. Endocardial (inner) and epicardial (outer) surfaces are shown. LAT, lateral; ANT, anterior; INF, inferior; SEPT, septum

PET/CT findings:

There was matched reduction of perfusion (ammonia) (a); and metabolism (FDG) (b) in the septum, the mid and distal anterior wall, and most of the inferior wall indicating nonviable myocardium. These areas showed impaired contractility (c). (Note marked liver uptake in the prefusion images). The remainder of the left ventricle showed normal perfusion, metabolism, and wall motion.

Key point:

Matched reduction of perfusion and metabolism indicates nonviable myocardium, and it is unlikely that revascularization of these areas would improve function.

CASE 18.3	Diagnosis: Coronary artery disease – viability?

Clinical history:

This patient had previous coronary artery bypass surgery. He had symptoms of heart failure with impaired left ventricular function (ejection fraction ~20 percent). Coronary angiography showed a patent left internal mammary artery graft to the left anterior descending artery, a large occluded first obtuse marginal branch of the left circumflex artery and an ostial stenosis of the right coronary artery (RCA), which was stented. Initially there was some symptomatic relief but symptoms recurred within a few months of stenting. PET/CT was requested to determine if there was viable myocardium in the territories of the circumflex and/or the RCA, which would influence the surgical approach.

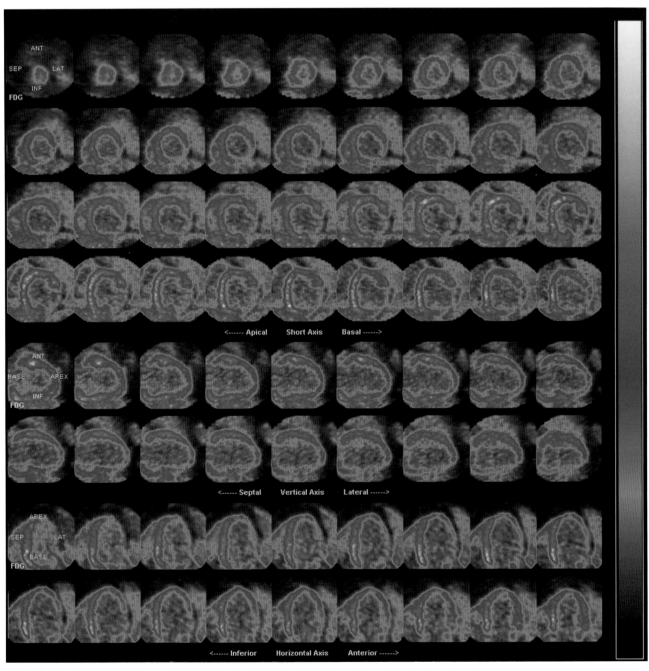

(a) [^{13}N]Ammonia (perfusion).

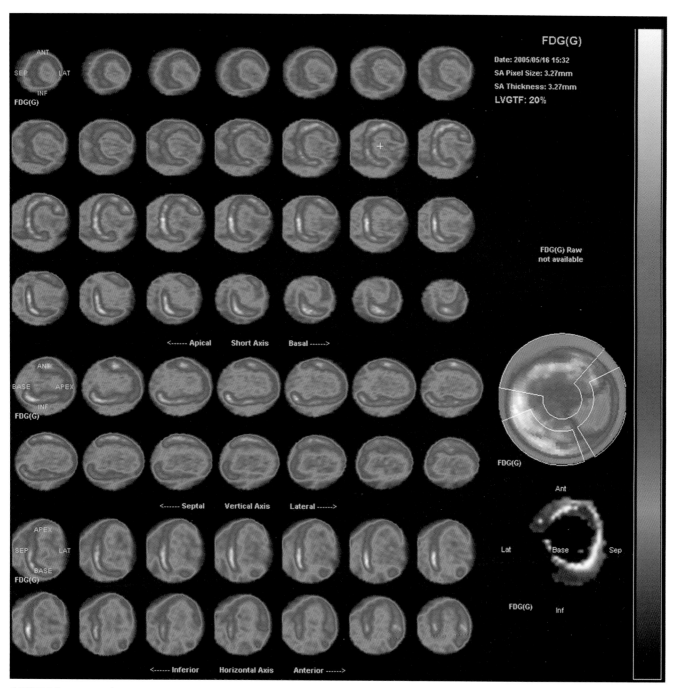

(b) ^{18}FDG (metabolism).

PET/CT findings:

There was matched reduction of perfusion (ammonia) (a) and metabolism (FDG) (b) at the apex in the lateral wall extending into the inferior wall at the base of the heart and in the basal anterior wall. In addition there was reduction in metabolism in the basal anteroseptal wall (b). These walls also showed impaired contractility representing nonviable myocardium. The remainder of the myocardium had good FDG uptake and contractility. Correlation with angiography indicated the majority of the area of nonviable myocardium was supplied by the first obtuse marginal branch and that the RCA stent was working well.

Key point:

Matched reduction of perfusion and metabolism indicates nonviable myocardium.

CASE 18.4	Diagnosis: Coronary artery disease – viability?

Clinical history:

This patient was referred for assessment of viability of the inferior wall to determine if it should be revascularized.

(a)

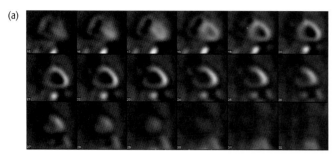

(b)

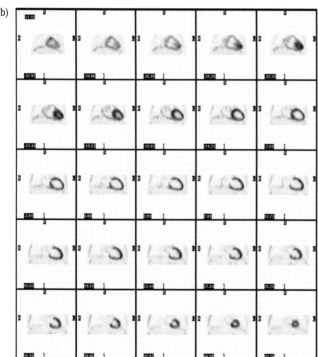

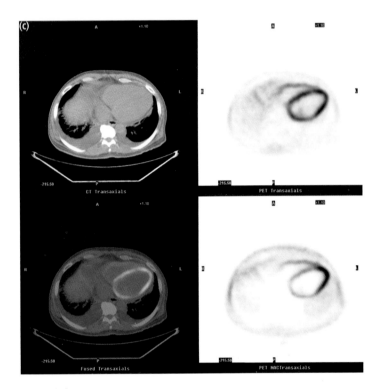

PET/CT findings:

Coronal perfusion images are shown with [99mTc] sestamibi (a). There was significant reduction in resting perfusion in the inferior wall suggesting this area might be nonviable or that uptake was reduced due to attenuation. Corresponding images are shown with FDG (b) indicating that the inferior wall had good uptake of FDG and that this wall was viable. Note that on the nonattenuation-corrected transaxial images (bottom right in image c) with FDG there is reduced uptake in the inferior wall yet normal uptake in the attenuation-corrected images (top right in image c).

Key point:

Problems with attenuation in the inferior wall (often in men) and in the anterior wall (in women) can be overcome using attenuation-corrected PET.

CASE 18.5 | Diagnosis: Coronary artery disease – viability?

Clinical history:

This patient with poor left ventricular function was referred for assessment of myocardial viability.

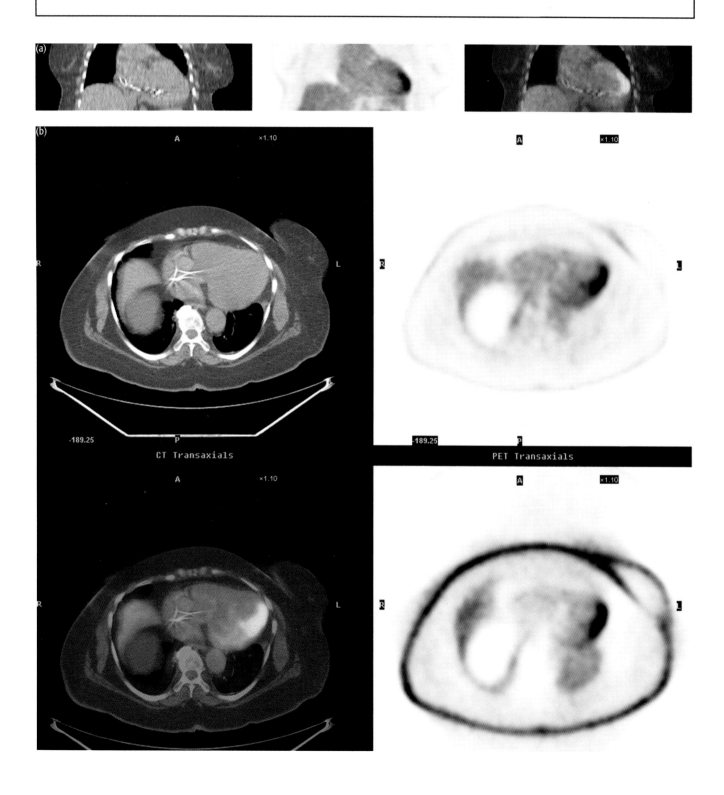

PET/CT findings:

There was poor uptake of FDG in the inferior wall and basal anterior wall (a), and the septum and the posterolateral wall (b) indicating that much of the left ventricular muscle was nonviable.

Key point:

Patients with large regions of 'nonviable' myocardium on PET are at increased operative risk compared with patients with viable myocardium.

CONCLUSIONS

REFERENCES AND FURTHER READING

Afridi I, Grayburn P, Panza JA *et al.* (1998) Myocardial viability during dobutamine echocardiography predicts survival in patients with coronary artery disease and severe left ventricular systolic dysfunction. *J Am Coll Cardiol* **32**, 921–6.

Allman KC, Shaw L, Hachamovitch R, Udelson JE (2002) Myocardial viability testing and impact of revascularization on prognosis in patients with coronary artery disease and left ventricular dysfunction: a meta-analysis. *J Am Coll Cardiol* **39**, 1151–8.

Barrington S, Chambers J, Hallett W *et al.* (2004) Comparison of sestamibi, thallium, echocardiography and PET for the detection of hibernating myocardium. *Eur J Nucl Med* **31**, 355–61.

Bax JJ, Wijns W, Cornel JH *et al.* (1997) Accuracy of currently available techniques for prediction of functional recovery after revascularization in patients with left ventricular dysfunction due to chronic coronary artery disease: comparison of pooled data. *J Am Coll Cardiol* **30**, 1451–60.

Chaudhry F, Tauke J, Alessandrini R *et al.* (1999) Prognostic implications of myocardial contractile reserve in patients with coronary artery disease and left ventricular dysfunction. *J Am Coll Cardiol* **34**, 738.

Depre C, Vanoverschelde JL, Melin JA *et al.* (1995) Structural and metabolic correlates of the reversibility of chronic left ventricular ischemic dysfunction in humans. *Am J Physiol* **268**, H1265–H1275.

Di Carli MF, Maddahi J, Rokhsar S *et al.* (1998) Long-term survival of patients with coronary artery disease and left ventricular dysfunction: implications for the role of myocardial viability assessment in management decisions. *J Thorac Cardiovasc Surg* **116**, 997–1004.

Dreyfus GD, Duboc D, Blasco A *et al.* (1994) Myocardial viability assessment in ischemic cardiomyopathy: benefits of coronary revascularization. *Ann Thorac Surg* **57**, 1402–7.

Elsasser A, Schlepper M, Klovekorn W *et al.* (1997) Hibernating myocardium: an incomplete adaptation to ischaemia. *Circulation* **96**, 2920–31.

Fath-Ordoubadi F, Pagano D, Marinho NV, Keogh BE, Bonser RS, Camici PG (1998). Coronary revascularization in the treatment of moderate and severe postischemic left ventricular dysfunction. *Am J Cardiol* **82**, 26–31.

Flameng WJ, Shivalkar B, Spiessens B *et al.* (1997) PET scan predicts recovery of left ventricular function after coronary artery bypass operation. *Ann Thorac Surg* **64**, 1694–701.

Haas F, Haehnel CJ, Picker W *et al.* (1997) Preoperative positron emission tomographic viability assessment and perioperative and postoperative risk in patients with advanced ischemic heart disease. *J Am Coll Cardiol* **30**, 1693–700.

Jacklin PB, Barrington SF, Roxburgh JC *et al.* (2002) The cost-effectiveness of pre-operative positron emission tomography in ischaemic heart disease. *Ann Thorac Surg* **73**, 1403–9.

Knuuti MJ, Nuutila P, Ruotsalainen U *et al.* (1992) Euglycemic hyperinsulinemic clamp and oral glucose load in stimulating myocardial glucose utilization during positron emission tomography. *J Nucl Med* **33**, 1255–62.

Landoni C, Lucignani G, Paolini G *et al.* (1999) Assessment of CABG-related risk in patients with CAD and LVD. Contribution of PET with [18F]FDG to the assessment of myocardial viability. *J Cardiovasc Surg* **40**, 363–72.

Lewis P, Nunan T, Dynes A, Maisey M (1996) The use of low-dose intravenous insulin in clinical myocardial F-18 FDG PET scanning. *Clin Nucl Med* **21**, 15–18.

Pagano D, Townend JN, Littler WA *et al.* (1998) Coronary artery bypass surgery as treatment for ischemic heart failure: the predictive value of viability assessment with quantitative positron emission tomography for symptomatic and functional outcome. *J Thorac Cardiovasc Surg* **115**, 791–9.

Pasquet, A, Robert, A, D'Hondt AM *et al.* (1999) Prognostic value of myocardial ischaemia and viability in patients with chronic left ventricular ischaemic dysfunction. *Circulation* **100**, 141–8.

Pitt M, Lewis M, Bonser RS (2001) Coronary artery surgery for ischemic heart failure: risks, benefits, and the importance of assessment of myocardial viability. *Prog Cardiovasc Dis* **43**, 373–86.

Rahimtoola SH. A perspective on the three large multicenter randomized clinical trials of coronary bypass surgery for chronic stable angina. *Circulation* **72**, V123–V135.

Vanoverschelde JL, Wijns W, Depre C *et al.* (1993) Mechanisms of chronic regional postischemic dysfunction in humans. New insights from the study of noninfarcted collateral-dependent myocardium. *Circulation* **87**, 1513–23.

CHAPTER 19
INFECTION AND INFLAMMATION

INTRODUCTION AND BACKGROUND

[^{18}F]2-Fluoro-2-deoxy-D-glucose (FDG) was developed as an agent for brain imaging but was soon found to have broad applicability in tumor imaging. It was initially thought that FDG had low uptake in inflammation, but experimental studies of inflammation and infection using relevant models showed that increased glucose utilization was typical of both human inflammatory and infectious diseases. In the past several years FDG PET has been used increasingly widely to detect infections, to determine if infection, tumor, or inflammation is responsible for a fever of unknown origin (FUO), to assess patients with sarcoidosis, to assess the activity of vasculitis, and to determine if inflammatory bowel disease is active, among other indications. These applications are not as mature as those in cancer imaging but are expected to grow substantially in the coming years.

KEY MANAGEMENT ISSUES

KEY MANAGEMENT ISSUES
Determination of the source of FUO
Detection of infection
Assessment of infection vs. loosening in painful prostheses
Detection and assessment of activity of inflammatory processes, e.g. vasculitis, sarcoidosis, arthritides

Role of PET in infection and inflammation

Early case reports of brain abscesses demonstrated that FDG can accumulate in infections. Follow-up studies in animal models and in humans showed high uptake of FDG into infectious processes, and an early report showed that 10/11 infections were detected in humans. Much larger studies have now been performed and have generally shown 80–100 percent sensitivity for detection of infection. Challenges can include tracer uptake in inflamed joints, especially when used in the setting of prosthesis imaging for determining loosening vs. infection, which can lower the specificity of the technique. Certainly, patients with diabetes are not as effectively imaged as patients with normal blood sugar levels, although this has been studied only to a limited extent.

Although FDG can be used to label leukocytes, there is not convincing evidence that this approach is superior to simply injecting FDG intravenously. Challenges in infection detection, in addition to uptake near joints and around normal painless and noninfected prostheses include uptake into surgical scars, which can be intense. In general, infections are somewhat more diffuse in distribution than surgical margins and can be distinguished based on the shape and knowledge of the timing of the surgery.

FUO can have a variety of causes which include infection, tumor, and immunologic diseases. FDG PET is a reasonable tool in the work-up of such patients, because it can detect abnormalities associated with all three processes.

Inflammatory cells and bacteria in infection use glucose. This can be exploited with FDG PET imaging. If a patient has poor glucose control, this method may not work as well due to competition between glucose and FDG uptake.

Infected joints can have increased uptake but many noninfected joints have moderate to intense tracer uptake. This can decrease the specificity of the imaging test. Thus it is not generally recommended that FDG replace leukocyte imaging for detection of infected joints and prostheses. Results in the literature are mixed, but caution must be used before diagnosing such an infectious process.

FDG PET can be a useful tool in the management of patients with FUO to direct biopsy and make the diagnosis in a timely fashion.

PGL in HIV can be associated with low, moderate, or high uptake, and this should not be confused with lymphoma.

Increased FDG uptake in inflamed blood vessels is commonly seen. Takayasu arteritis is one such process in which PET can be useful.

Separation of blood pool from blood vessel wall uptake can be challenging in some instances and delayed imaging may be useful. Typically, FDG uptake is separate from calcifications and is seen in over half of patients over 50 years of age, at some level of intensity.

Sarcoidosis can have intense FDG uptake. Uptake rises with time from injection, thus dual timepoint (early and delayed) imaging does not consistently separate infection/inflammation from tumor.
*   Sarcoidosis can occur anywhere in the body. In the mediastinum, sarcoid often involves multiple lymph nodes and can be confused with NHL. In bone FDG-avid sarcoid can mimic bone metastases.*

In human immunodeficiency virus (HIV) infection, HIV can affect T lymphocytes and other tissues located throughout the body. It has been shown that FDG uptake can occur into reactive lymph nodes, and that diffuse FDG uptake in nodes can be seen. It has been suggested that varied nodal groups are involved at varying times of the disease, with a peripheral to central spread. It is important to recognize HIV adenopathy, also referred to as persistent generalized lymphadenopathy (PGL), and not to assume that nodal uptake represents disseminated lymphoma (although it is clear that patients with HIV are at increased risk of non-Hodgkin lymphoma (NHL) and other cancers). Biopsy may be required to differentiate between these conditions.

Vasculitis is sometimes challenging to diagnose clinically and can present somewhat insidiously. By definition, increased white cell accumulation (inflammation) occurs in vasculitis and this process is one which is suitable for imaging with FDG PET. It has been suggested that FDG PET is more sensitive than magnetic resonance imaging (MRI) for vasculitis and better able to assess treatment response. The use of PET has been described in Takayasu arteritis and other vasculitides.

Increased FDG accumulation in blood vessels has also been seen in patients who have atherosclerosis, and there is an age-associated increase in FDG uptake in blood vessels, likely due in part to an inflammatory component of vasculitis. PET/computed tomography (CT) studies have shown the vascular signal from FDG typically to be in a different site than calcifications in patients with atherosclerosis.

Sarcoidosis has been shown to have intense FDG uptake when active. This is true in lymph nodes, the pulmonary parenchymal tissue, and in systemic sarcoidosis. Although often viewed as an annoying source of false-positive PET images in patients with known or suspected cancer, the ability to noninvasively quantify the activity of sarcoidosis is likely to have increasing value over the coming years. However, the precise role of PET with FDG in sarcoidosis management remains in evolution. Anecdotally, we have seen growth in clinical referrals for possible sarcoidosis in our practices.

Inflammatory bowel disease is yet another process in which white cell infiltration is a very prominent feature of the illness. There have been small reports about increased FDG uptake in inflamed bowel. One of the major challenges in PET imaging is to distinguish normal bowel activity of FDG from that in actively inflamed bowel. The precise role of PET in this clinical setting is in evolution, and PET is not yet routinely applied in most centers as the evidence base is limited.

Inflammatory arthritides typically have increased glycolytic activity when they are active and proliferating. A common incidental finding on PET imaging is increased periarticular uptake of FDG. When this is in joints typically affected by inflammatory joint disease, it must not be confused with tumor or infection. PET has been used in the experimental setting to follow the efficacy of therapies for inflammatory arthritides.

Although some view FDG as a highly 'nonspecific' tracer, this nonspecificity for cancer makes it of broad utility for a wide variety of processes in the body using glucose. Infection and inflammation are two processes which use glucose avidly and whereas there are already many promising uses of FDG, it is probable that even more will develop in the coming years. Since inflammatory processes are common, it is suggested that the ability to recognize and not confuse inflammation with active tumor is a most critical aspect of the interpretation of PET images. In so doing, the presence and activity of inflammatory processes can be managed.

EXAMPLES TO ILLUSTRATE KEY ISSUES

CASE 19.1	**Diagnosis: Head and neck abscess**

Clinical history:

This patient with a history of T2 N2b squamous cell carcinoma of the right buccal retromolar trigone was treated with surgery, which included a transoral excision of a buccal and alveolar cancer with a marginal mandibulectomy on the right side followed by bilateral neck radiation. He was admitted a year after completion of radiotherapy with cellulitis of the right cheek, and a fistula to the right cheek with exposed bone.

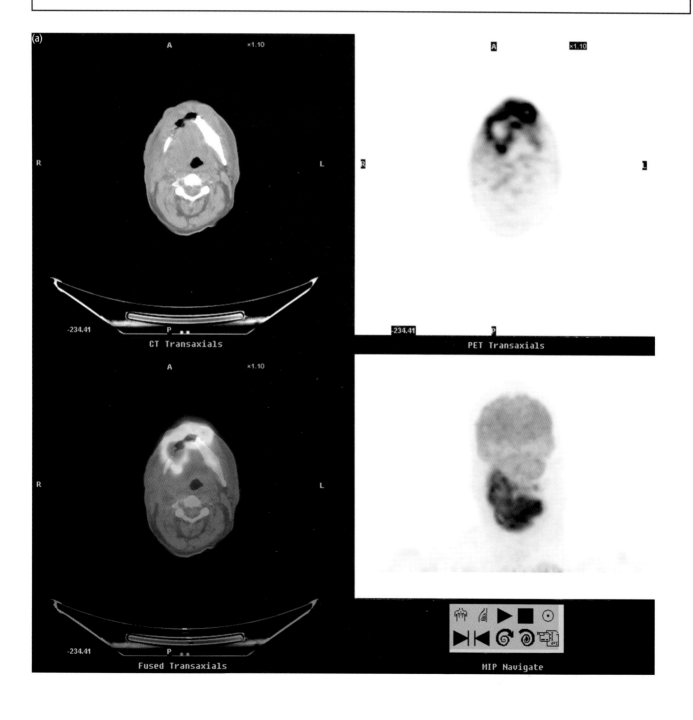

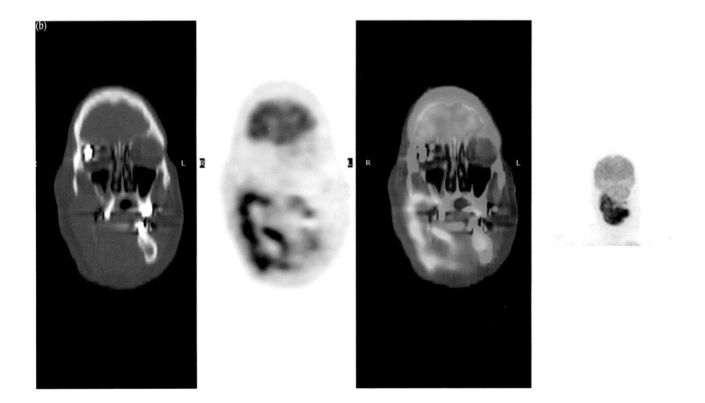

PET/CT findings:

There was massive abnormal focal uptake of FDG with a central photopenic area centred on the surgical defect on the right extending across the midline, anterior to the left mandible (a). The focus also extended medially and inferiorly to the right oropharynx and right base of the tongue (b).

The findings were most consistent with a large abscess and accompanying cellulitis. However, embedded malignancy was also possible. The lesion was subsequently biopsied and debrided and found to be due to infection with no evidence of cancer then or during clinical follow-up.

Key point:

High FDG uptake is seen in bacterial abscesses. Usually the history differentiates infectious uptake from recurrent cancer although, as in this case, recurrent malignancy can be difficult to exclude completely on PET/CT.

| CASE 19.2 | Diagnosis: Pneumonia |

Clinical history:

This patient had a 2-month history of cough. A mass was seen on CT in the right middle lobe of the lung with no improvement with antibiotic treatment. Percutaneous biopsy and bronchoscopy did not reveal evidence of malignancy, but the clinical likelihood of cancer was high. PET/CT was requested to characterize the lesion.

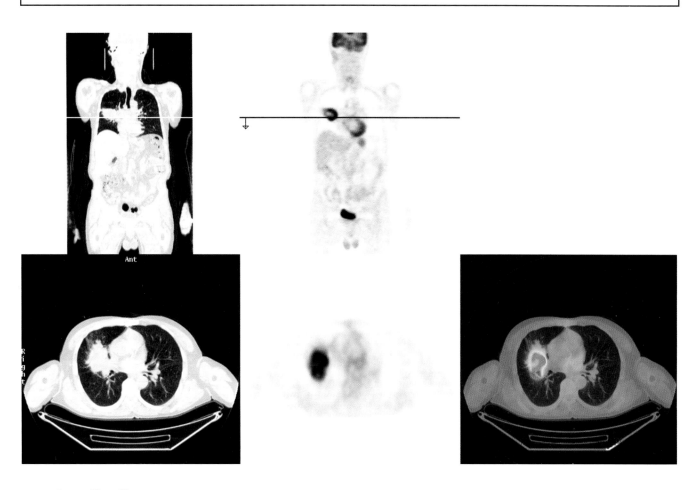

PET/CT findings:

There was high uptake within the mass in the right middle lobe, suggestive of primary lung malignancy. The mass was resected and showed features consistent with organizing pneumonia but no malignancy.

Key point:

FDG is not specific for cancer and shows high uptake within infection which can sometimes be indistinguishable from malignancy.

CASE 19.3	Diagnosis: J tube infection

Clinical history:

This patient had a purulent discharge associated with a J tube.

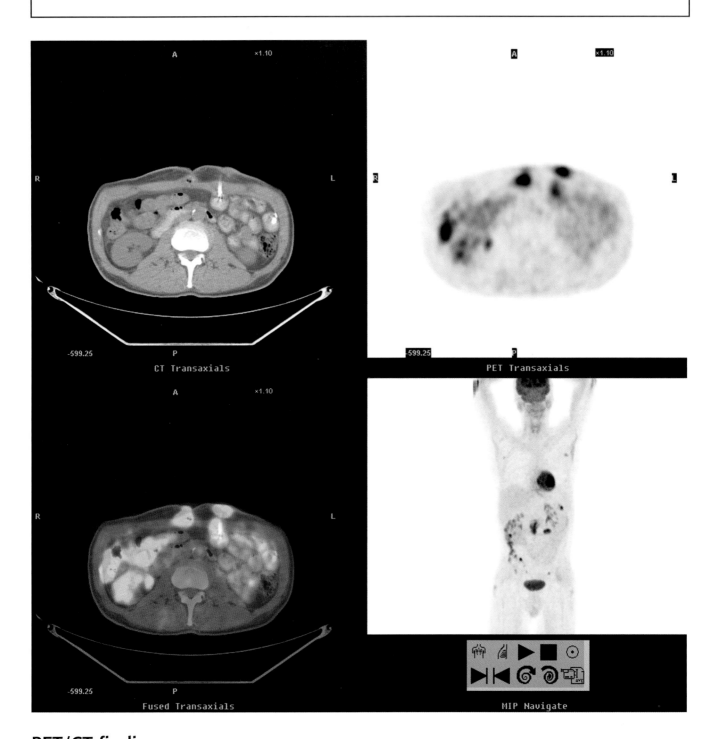

PET/CT findings:

High uptake of FDG was associated with the tube and gas in the anterior abdominal wall, which is typical of bacterial infection. Physiologic uptake is seen elsewhere in the bowel and in the right kidney.

CASE 19.4	Diagnosis: Osteomyelitis

Clinical history:

This patient presented with clinical symptoms suggestive of osteomyelitis around the left knee.

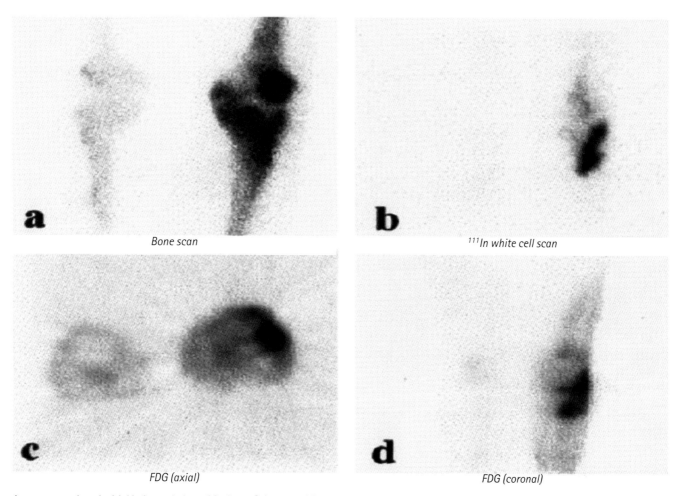

Bone scan

^{111}In white cell scan

FDG (axial)

FDG (coronal)

Images reproduced with kind permission of Springer Science and Business Media from Sugawara Y, Braun DK, Kison PV (1998) Rapid detection of human infections with fluorine-18 fluorodeoxyglucose and positron emission tomography: preliminary results. Eur J Nucl Med Mol Imaging **25**, 1238–43

PET findings:

There was high uptake of FDG in a focal distribution (c, d), similar to the distribution of abnormal white cell accumulation in an ^{111}In-labeled white cell scan (b), but less diffuse than the uptake on bone scanning (a) indicating that FDG was localizing to the infectious region in bone.

Case 19.5	Diagnosis: Cellulitis

Clinical history:

This elderly patient with chronic lymphoid leukemia presented with superficial ulcers on her left ankle.

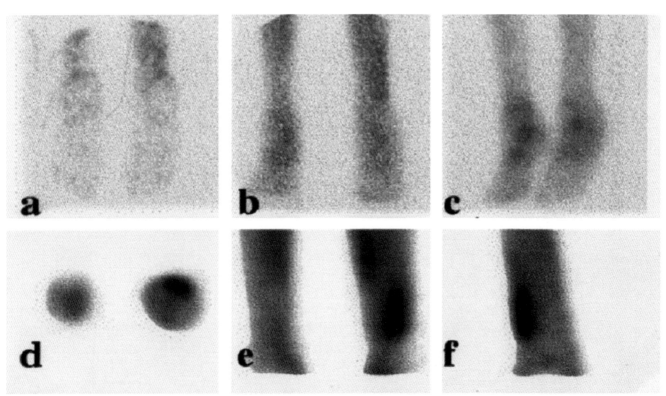

Images reproduced with kind permission of Springer Science and Business Media from Sugawara Y, Braun DK, Kison PV (1998) Rapid detection of human infections with fluorine-18 fluorodeoxyglucose and positron emission tomography: preliminary results. Eur J Nucl Med Mol Imaging 25, 1238–43

PET findings:

There was high uptake of FDG in a focal distribution (d–f) at the site of the ulcers consistent with cellulitis. On the bone scan faint uptake was seen in the arterial and blood pool phases of the triple phase scan (a, b) but none in the delayed images, consistent with cellulitis and no osteomyelitis.

| **CASE 19.6** | **Diagnosis: Inguinal abscess** |

Clinical history:

This patient with diabetes mellitus presented with a left inguinal abscess.

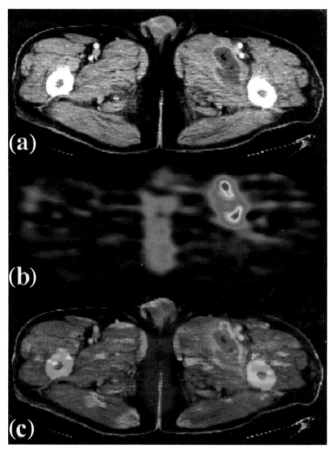

Images reproduced with kind permission of Springer Science and Business Media from Sugawara M, Braun DK, Kison PV (1998) Rapid detection of human infections with fluorine-18 fluorodeoxyglucose and positron emission tomography: preliminary results. Eur J Nucl Med Mol Imaging **25**, *1238–43*

PET/CT findings:

High uptake of FDG was seen on a PET scan (b) at the site of the abscess in the adductor compartment of the left thigh imaged on CT 24 hours before (a). Fused PET/CT images are shown (c).

Key point:

Patients with diabetes are at increased risk of developing bacterial infection. Usually the clinical history serves to differentiate high FDG uptake in infection from malignancy.

CASE 19.7 | **Diagnosis: Rheumatoid arthritis**

Clinical history:

This patient presented with rheumatoid arthritis.

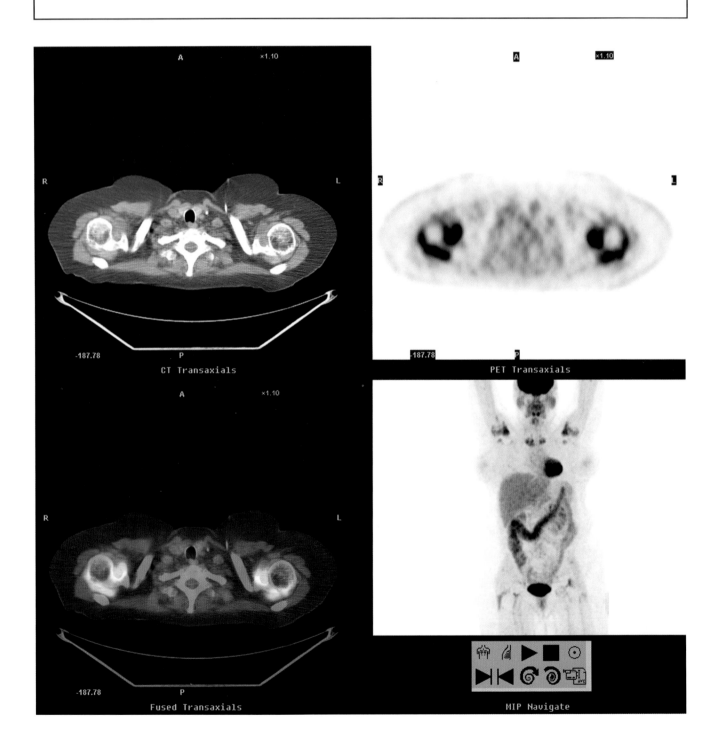

PET/CT findings:

There was high uptake associated with an active synovitis in the shoulder joints.

Key point:

Increased FDG uptake is seen in inflammatory joint disease and should not be confused with infection.

CASE 19.8	Diagnosis: PGL associated with HIV

History:

This patient had PGL associated with HIV.

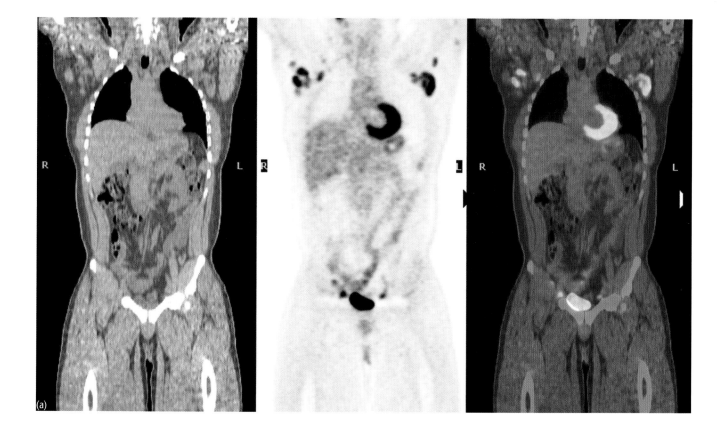

(a)

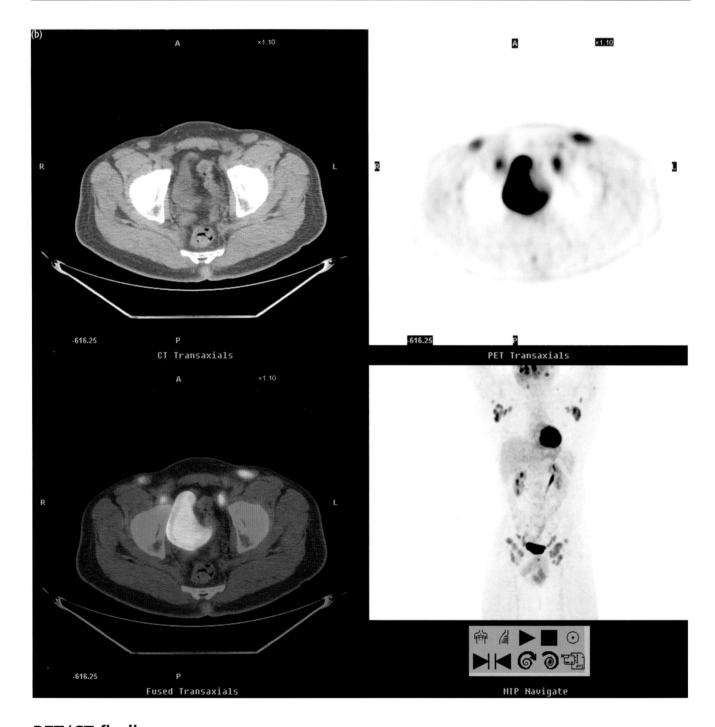

PET/CT findings:

High-grade uptake was associated with peripheral lymph nodes in this patient due to PGL. Note uptake in cervical (a, b), bilateral axillary (a, b) inguinal (a, b), and external iliac (b) nodes.

Key points:

1 In this patient the FDG nodal uptake was due to HIV adenopathy or PGL, however, appearances can be identical with lymphoma.
2 Biopsy may be required to differentiate between HIV adenopathy and infection, granulomatous disease, or malignancy.

CASE 19.9	Diagnosis: Vasculitis

Clinical history:

This patient presented with a 6-week history of FUO with raised inflammatory markers. CT scan of chest, abdomen, and pelvis was normal and blood cultures were negative. PET/CT was requested to determine a source for the FUO.

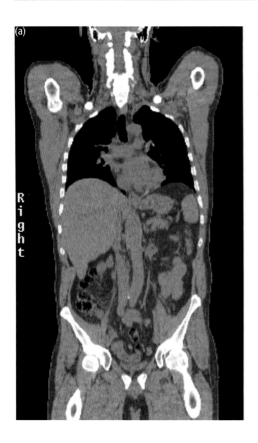
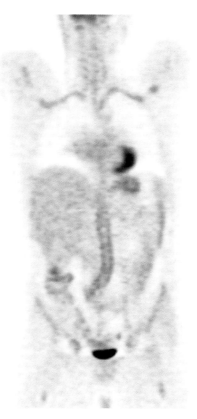
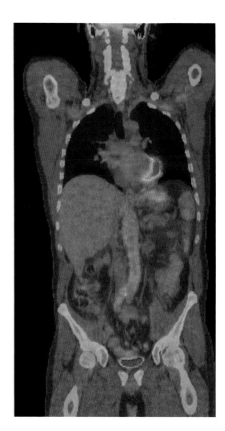

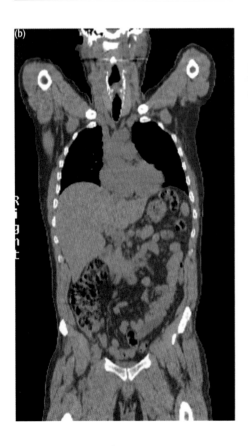
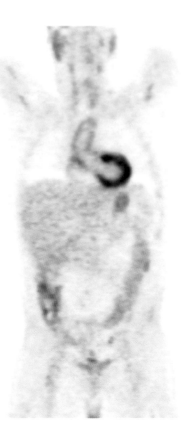
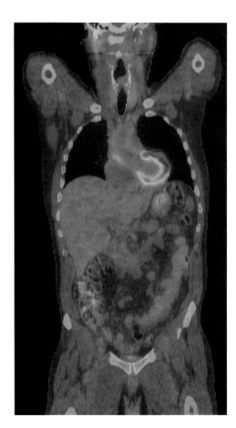

PET/CT findings:

There was high uptake in large vessels in the abdominal aorta and subclavian arteries, (a) and in the aortic arch and carotid vessels (b) most consistent with a large-vessel arteritis such as Takayasu arteritis.

Key points:

1 PET/CT can detect the source of FUO where other tests are negative.
2 PET/CT can be used to assess the activity of vasculitis.

| CASE 19.10 | Diagnosis: Sarcoidosis |

Clinical history:

This patient presented with a posterior uveitis. MRI showed no orbital abnormality but high signal in the cervical cord consistent with either sarcoidosis or demyelination. Clinically the diagnosis was thought most likely to be sarcoid.

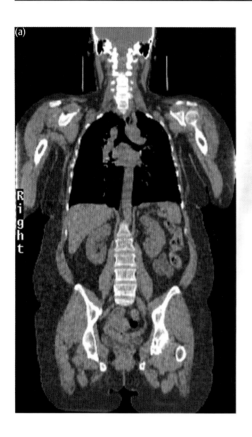
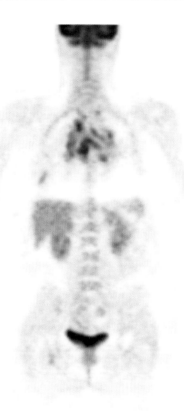
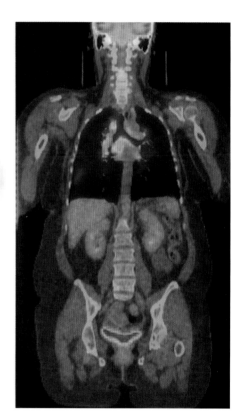

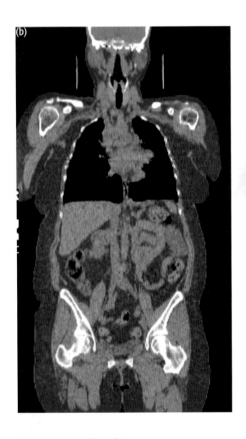
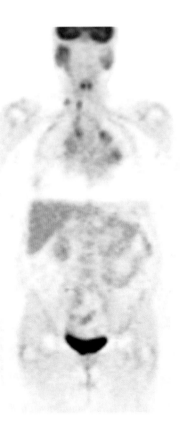
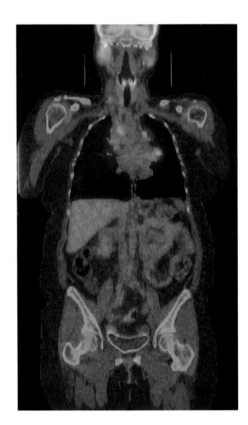

PET/CT findings:

There was high uptake in mediastinal and hilar glands (a), right cervical nodes (b), and both parotid glands, typical of sarcoidosis.

> **Key point:**
>
> In this case the history and pattern of distribution pointed to a diagnosis of sarcoidosis but the intensity and distribution of uptake can sometimes be similar with lymphoma and sarcoid.

CASE 19.11 | Diagnosis: Crohn disease

Clinical history:

This patient had active Crohn disease.

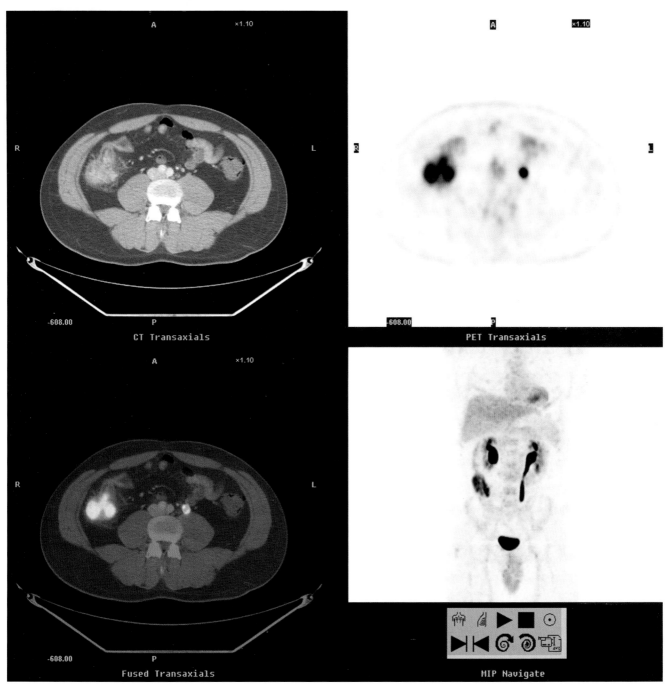

Images kindly supplied by Dr Phillip Ginsburg, Johns Hopkins Hospital

PET/CT findings:

High-grade uptake in the terminal ileum was associated with the active Crohn disease.

Key point:

High uptake is associated with inflammatory bowel disease when active but can also be seen in normal bowel. This may limit the usefulness of FDG PET to assess activity of disease.

CASE 19.12	Diagnosis: Crohn disease

Case history:

This patient with known active Crohn disease was referred for evaluation of a lung mass.

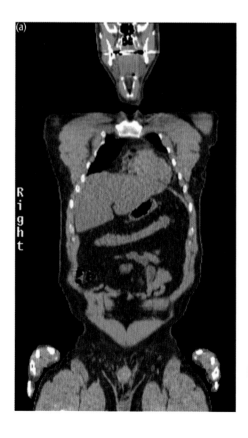 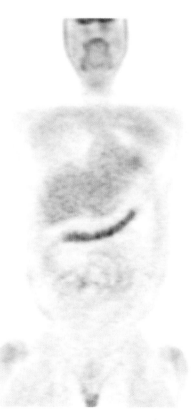 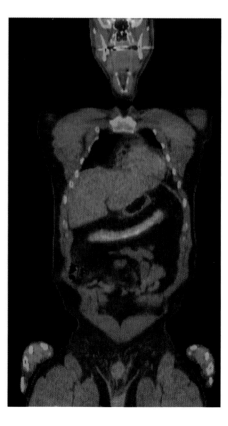

(b)

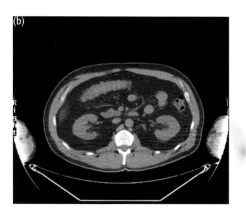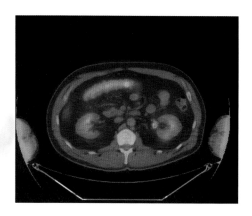

PET/CT findings:

The lung mass (not shown) did not take up FDG but there was diffuse increased uptake of tracer in the transverse colon associated with the typical cobblestone appearance on CT in known active Crohn disease.

Key point:

Increased FDG uptake occurs in association with active inflammatory bowel disease.

CONCLUSIONS

FURTHER READING

El-Haddad G, Zhuang H, Gupta N, Alavi A (2004) Evolving role of positron emission tomography in the management of patients with inflammatory and other benign diseases. *Semin Nucl Med* **34**, 313–29.

Guhlmann A, Brecht-Krauss D, Suger G *et al.* (1998) Chronic osteomyelitis: detection with FDG PET and correlation with histopathologic findings. *Radiology* **206**, 749–54.

Ichiya Y, Kuwabara Y, Sasaki M *et al.* (1996) FDG-PET in infectious lesions: The detection and assessment of lesion activity. *Ann Nucl Med* **10**, 185–91.

Keidar Z, Militianu D, Melamed E, Bar-Shalom R, Israel O (2005) The diabetic foot: initial experience with 18F-FDG PET/CT. *J Nucl Med* **46**, 444–9.

Love C, Marwin SE, Tomas MB (2004) Diagnosing infection in the failed joint replacement: a comparison of coincidence detection 18F-FDG and 111In-labeled leukocyte/99mTc-sulfur colloid marrow imaging. *J Nucl Med* **45**, 1864–71.

O'Doherty MJ, Barrington SF, Campbell M, Lowe J, Bradbeer CS (1997) PET scanning and the HIV positive patient. *J Nucl Med* **38**, 1575–83.

Reinartz P, Cremerius U, Schaefer WM *et al.* (2005) Radionuclide imaging of the painful hip arthroplasty. *J Bone Joint Surg [Br]* **87**, 465–70.

Stumpe KD, Notzli HP, Zanetti M *et al.* (2004) FDG PET for differentiation of infection and aseptic loosening in total hip replacements: comparison with conventional radiography and three-phase bone scintigraphy. *Radiology* **231**, 333–41. Epub 2004 Mar 24.

Sugawara Y, Braun DK, Kison PV *et al.* (1998) Rapid detection of human infections with fluorine-18 fluorodeoxyglucose and positron emission tomography: preliminary results. *Eur J Nucl Med* **25**, 1238–43.

Tahara T, Ichiya Y, Kuwabara Y *et al.* (1989) High [18F]-fluorodeoxyglucose uptake in abdominal abscesses: a PET study. *J Comput Assist Tomogr* **13**, 829–31.

Walter MA, Melzer RA, Schindler C *et al.* (2005) The value of [18F]FDG-PET in the diagnosis of large-vessel vasculitis and the assessment of activity and extent of disease. *Eur J Nucl Med Mol Imaging* **32**, 674–81.